A Brain Is Born

A Brain Is Born

Exploring The Birth And Development Of The Central Nervous System

John E. Upledger
D.O., O.M.M.

North Atlantic Books
Berkeley, California
and
UI Enterprises
Palm Beach Gardens, Florida

A Brain Is Born: Exploring the Birth and Development of the Central Nervous System

Throughout the book the term CranioSacral Therapy is used to denote Upleger CranioSacral Therapy®.

Published by

North Atlantic Books   The Upledger Institute, Inc.
P.O. Box 12327   and   11211 Prosperity Farms Road, D-325
Berkeley, California 94712   Palm Beach Gardens, Florida 33410-3487

Cover and design by Karin Hernandez and Paula Morrison
Illustrations by Älice Quaid

Printed in the United States of America

Library of Congress Cataloging-in-Publication Data

Upledger, John E., 1932–
     A brain is born : exploring the birth and development of
the central nervous system / John Upledger.
          p.   cm.
     "Sponsored by the Society for the Study of Native Arts and
Sciences"—T.p. verso.
     Includes bibliographical references and index.
     ISBN 1-55643-236-4
     1. Central nervous system—Growth.   2. Craniosacral
therapy.   I. Society for the Study of Native Arts and
Sciences.   II. Title.
     [DNLM: 1. Central Nervous System—embryology.
2. Central Nervous System—growth & development.
3. Infant, Newborn—physiology.   4. Abnormalities—
etiology.   5. Osteopathic Medicine—methods.   WL
300U67b   1996]
QP356.25.U65   1996
612.8—dc20
DNLM/DLC
for Library of Congress   96-29184
                                                   CIP

     3   4   5   6   7   8   9   /   03   02   01   00

To Nature and her genius.

Table of Contents

Section VI   The Newborn Evaluation   207

Foreword by James S. Gordon, M.D.

At its origins and in its heart, medicine is about balance. The work of medicine is the work of restoring wholeness, of helping to bring the malfunctioning part into the harmony of the whole. Its highest and best practice depends on maintaining balance between technique and art, between the outer knowing of science and the inner knowing of intuition. Great and gifted physicians have always understood this.

John Upledger knows and lives this truth. John began as a clinician working, as osteopaths do, with his hands and on the body's tissues. He became a researcher, and a professor of biomechanics at Michigan State University. He explores the physiology and anatomy of the craniosacral system, the movement of the cerebrospinal fluid, and the structure of the tissues which produce, confine and absorb it. His laboratory explorations led him back out to work with the living bodies of people who had been hurt by accident and illness. Soon, work with the body revealed to John the connections among physical, mental, emotional and spiritual experience. He developed CranioSacral Therapy and SomatoEmotional Release℠, ways to help his patients to recover and re-integrate memories and possibilities that had been locked in cramped muscles and constricted cranial rhythms; to help them to restore balance in and among body, mind and spirit.

A Brain is Born is part of John's work, his effort to help his patients, and to restore a balance between the knowledge of professionals and the uncertainty of those who come for help. He began this book as an instructional manual for parents whose children were suffering from central nervous system dysfunction. It is an effort to make embryology, and particularly the complex steps and intricate anatomy of brain development, available to all. It is a guide to help parents and therapists understand the ways that nature sometimes stumbles, and how and why certain children have been affected. It is a map of the terrain that the CranioSacral Therapist must navigate as he or she tries to coax disrupted nature back into balance.

This is not an easy book — the course that the brain takes in its development is complex — but John has made the path as clear as he can. The illustrations are well-done, and there is a lightness in the writing that helps us along this journey. John's authorial voice reassures us that we really can make sense of all this science. There is a sense of wonder, too, at Nature — who makes this growth and development possible, and a pleasure in all the paths it takes. As we read what John writes, we come to believe, as he does, that science can be put in the service of a healing art.

This is, as John intended, a book for physicians, therapists and lay persons, particularly parents. But it is also a text for those who are doing CranioSacral Therapy, and a rich and lively reminder for those of us who have forgotten the marvels of our own and our patients' growth and development.

James S. Gordon, M.D.

Foreword by Sharon Weiselfish, Ph.D., P.T.

John Upledger's philosophies of care, techniques, protocols, and literature for research bias are foundations for the field of Cranial Therapy. His contributions to healthcare have been integral to progress in Osteopathy, Physical Therapy, Occupational Therapy, Neurorehabilitation, Chiropractic and Dentistry. His books are used nationally and internationally for teaching and studying the craniosacral system, including CranioSacral Therapy, Cranial Osteopathy, Sacro-occipital Technique, and all other manual therapies that affect the central nervous system. His procedures are integrated into the practices of hospital-based therapists, private practitioners, school therapists, and every field, discipline and matrix that affects patient care today. CranioSacral Therapy for headache patients, low-back-pain patients, clients with sciatica, shoulder girdle pain, facial pain and temporomandibular joint involvement, is practiced with the understanding that Dr. Upledger's therapeutic intervention is beneficial, and necessary for total recovery.

A Brain is Born delves into the mysteries of brain development in John Upledger's typical informative, giving, factual manner, and provides the reader with translation, interpretation and application for recognizing the potential of the human brain to heal.

Can the brain heal? Is the plasticity, discussed in John's book, sufficient for recovery of the neurologic patient? Is it possible for the stroke victim, the brain-trauma client and the cerebral palsy child to normalize by facilitating healing with CranioSacral Therapy and other manual therapy techniques? Evidently so. Is this widely recognized? Leading neuroscientists in the field of neurologic research affirm: the brain can heal, neuronal regeneration is evidently possible throughout life, and all ages of patients can potentially make a transition towards better quality of life based on neural recovery, rather than compensation and coping.

Will we see a change in the fields of neurorehabilitation during the next decade? Absolutely! With John's gift of information, his vision, his clarity of description and his explanations, he is guiding us, the clinicians, into unknown territory: recovery for the neurologic patient. His contribution will become evident as we utilize his techniques, incorporate his philosophies, and discover the meaning of his words in this book and others.

In attempting to provide the reader with an understanding of the results of CranioSacral Therapy, I am constrained. I have yet to see a patient plateau, and therefore cannot give limitations and delimitations for easier acceptance. Possibly reading this book, *A Brain Is Born,* will provide you with a unique appreciation for the wonder of the human organism, specifically the unlimited potential of the body to adapt during embryologic development, and throughout the growth and development of the central nervous system. This infinite potential is evident in the process of a brain being born. There is an unlimited potential for your patients, your family members, your friends, as well as for you, the reader, the clinician, the researcher and the teacher.

May you enjoy the information in this book as I have. With the images presented, you can be transported to the 21st century of information, technology and outcome for your clients and others significant to you who are affected in any way by a neurologic dysfunction.

God grants us the ability to contribute during this lifetime. For all of us who have learned from and trained under John Upledger, I thank him for this added contribution to growth and development of healthcare, patient progress, and my own further enlightenment.

Sharon Weiselfish, Ph.D., P.T.

Foreword by
Douglas W. Wolff, D.O., Neurology

Telling the tale of the unfolding of the human being is a most prodigious task. From a drop of jelly we begin the formation of complex neuroanatomic circuitry, an awesome array of sophisticated neurochemical relays. The union of sperm and egg produces a genetic blueprint to direct the processes of cellular migration to birth and development.

By examining the process from an inside perspective, as if one were right there, Upledger elevates us to a new level of understanding (sublime in synchrony with the very essence of nature's design). The integration with the craniosacral perspective allows us to develop therapeutic strategies; tapping into nature's limitless utility, allowing us a gentler way to intercede with potential problems. For example, hydrocephalus, attention-deficit disorder and seizures.

Anyone who has observed complex clinical phenomena, such as behavioral alteration, motor dysfunction or neuroendocrine derangement, and has tried to understand the relationship of neuroanatomical, neurochemical, cytoarchtectic structure with something as evanescent as emotion and energy flow, knows that the infinite is approached and it humbles us. It also allows us to sense the purpose of structure/function relationships.

While tracing the embryological development, Upledger shows us the range of possibilities of pathological substrates that lead to the common maladies of today. *A Brain is Born* is a powerful integration of all the developmental processes of the human nervous system with CranioSacral Therapy. Implicit in its telling is that nature knows best.

It is a great honor and a privilege to participate in this seminal work.

Douglas W. Wolff, D.O., Neurology

Introduction

A Brain is Born was actually begun in the late 1970s, while I was conducting a clinic at Michigan State University for brain-dysfunctioning children. Early on in the clinic's lifetime, it became very clear that the parents of these young clinic patients suffered more agony than was perhaps necessary, simply because they had little, or perhaps no understanding of how or why these problems happened. In their lack of understanding frequently blossomed the guilt that so often flourishes when you are not quite sure whether or not you contributed to the cause of a problem, either through ignorance, negligence or intention. In order to help these caring parents understand what had happened to their children, we spent hours explaining the possibilities to them. Then came a 46-page booklet entitled "Your Child's Brain," written by one of my graduate students, Sister Anne Brooks (now an osteopathic physician and surgeon) and me.

After I left the university and returned to Florida to practice, our clinical work focused less specifically upon children, and more upon brain and spinal cord dysfunctioning patients of all ages. The need for more and deeper explanations about these dysfunctions, how and why they happened, and what could be done about them, grew. The sense of guilt carried by significant others, as well as parents, became more and more apparent. The treatment for this guilt became more and more apparent also. This treatment was the explanation and understanding of how things work and, in these patients, how things didn't work within their brains and spinal cords.

Ultimately, in 1993 it was decided that I should do a video that would provide information about brain and spinal cord development in the uterus, and the functions of these organs after delivery. This video was produced and entitled "A Brain is Born." It is currently available through The Upledger Institute. As I reviewed the video, it became clear that its value could be geometrically increased if it had a companion book to go with it. Clearly, the information provided would help the patients, the parents, the significant others, the caregivers, and involved therapists from a wide range of disciplines.

I began writing this "simple" companion book. Two years later, the book *A Brain is Born* was born, and you are presently holding it before you. The fields of genetics, embryology and neurology, as well as all the related basic sciences, such as neurophysiology and biophysics, are absolutely ablaze with progress. What started out to be a simple manual based on an information video turned into a two-year piece of work. *A Brain is Born* is a labor of love. It is reasonably up to date as of mid-year 1995. It crosses many disciplinary boundaries, and I have tried to make it comprehensible to non-medically trained persons and, at the same time, useful to those with backgrounds in the healthcare sciences.

This book is one of my efforts to dispel myths about brain and spinal cord dysfunction problems. Its goal is to help interested persons begin to apply "common sense" to these problems so that higher levels of functional potential can be reached, and the suffering related to guilt can be rationally alleviated.

I do hope you find the reading pleasurable and worth the effort.

John E. Upledger, D.O., O.M.M.

Section I

The Preliminaries

The Ovum

The ovum is the egg. It is supplied by the female participant in the sexual union (**Fig. 1-1**). The male participant in such a sexual union provides the sperm. In order for a sexual union to take place, the sperm must overcome a series of obstacles. First the sperm must find the ovum. Then "he" must penetrate the protective outer layer of the ovum in order to be received and to fertilize the ovum so that the creation of another member of the species can begin. When we see fertilization occur we are doubtless witnessing yet another of nature's miracles.

Let's back up a bit and take a closer look at this ovum or egg, as it is often called. First off, it is rather interesting to note that, under normal circumstances at the time of the first menstrual cycle in the human female, all of the ova or eggs that will be released during the entire reproductive life of that female have been formed and are present within the ovarian tissue. These eggs are usually released at a rate of one each month from alternate ovaries. Thus, each of the two ovaries releases an ovum/egg every other month.

The typical ovum/egg for humans is about .14 millimeters in diameter. The ovum is enclosed within a tough and transparent membrane which encases an area of clear, non-cellular material

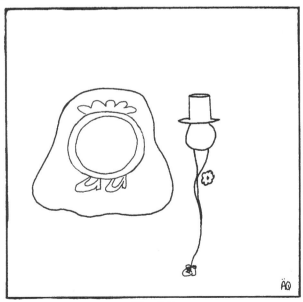

Fig. 1-1
Sexual Union:
This is the story of a bride and a groom and how they
became a mama and a papa.

about 12 microns thick, called the zona pellucida (**Fig. 1-2**). The ovum/egg cell itself has within it a spheroidal nucleus and a surrounding area of cytoplasm. Both the nucleus and the cytoplasm have visible structures located within them.

The nucleus is bounded by a nuclear membrane. This nucleus, which is within the ovum/egg, contains within it organelles, nucleoli, chromatin and nucleoplasm.

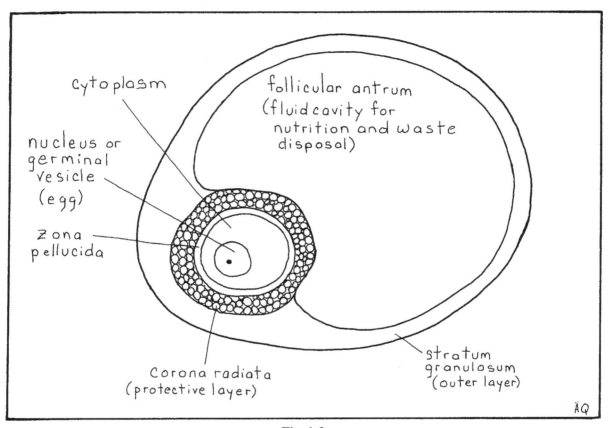

Fig. 1-2
Graafian or Ovarian Follicle with Ovum/Egg:
This diagram illustrates the follicle as it appears within the ovary prior to ovulation. The ovum/egg is well-protected and cared for by the various component parts of the follicle.

An organelle is a structure that does specialized work. Organelles are located within the nucleus as well as within the cytoplasm of the ovum/egg. Organelle is sort of a generalized word that is used to describe such things as mitochondria, Golgi complexes, lysosomes, endoplasmic reticulum, ribosomes, centrioles, and many more microscopically visible structures (**Fig. 1-3**).

A nucleolus is a rounded refractile body. In this case refractile means that the direction of light waves is diverted by a nucleolus. The nucleolus within the ovum's/egg's nucleus serves as the site where RNA is manufactured or synthesized. RNA is ribonucleic acid, a complex organic chemical compound which is concerned with the manufacture of the protein molecules that we find to be essential for life.

Chromatin is the "stuff" from which chromosomes are made. Chromosomes are the structures that contain DNA (deoxyribonucleic acid). DNA is the complex chemical compound that gained fame as a double helix. The DNAs are the compounds or structures that transmit genetic information from parent to child through the generations.

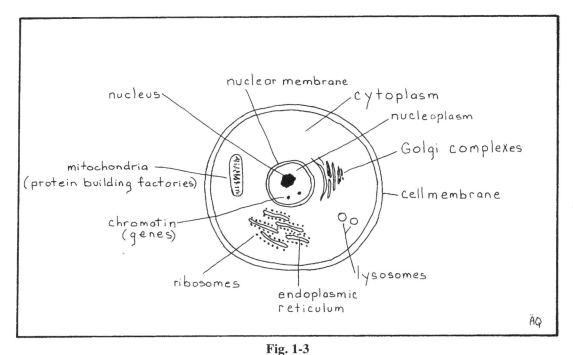

Fig. 1-3
Cell Anatomy:
This drawing illustrates some of the various microscopic structures that are found within living cells.

The mother's chromatin contains a single set of chromosomes before fertilization. This is called a haploid set. The sperm from the father furnishes another single or haploid set. At fertilization the ovum/egg receives the father's single set which, added to its own haploid set, makes a double set of chromosomes. This double set is called a diploid. The diploid set is required for cell division to occur. All body cells not involved in reproduction as ova/eggs or sperm have diploid sets of chromosomes **(Fig. 1-4)**.

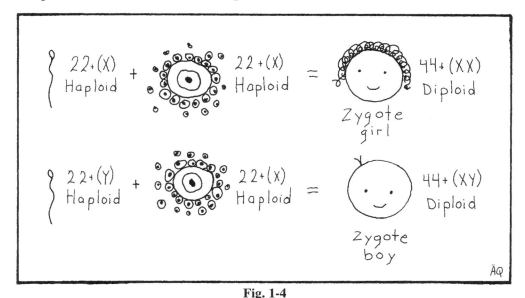

Fig. 1-4
Chromosomal Integration:
This is the way gender or sex is decided. We don't yet know the controlling factors,
but a single Y chromosome makes a male child.

Nucleoplasm is the subdivision of protoplasm which is found within the nucleus of the cell. Cytoplasm is the other subdivision of protoplasm that is found within the cell substance outside of the nucleus. Protoplasm, in general, is a rather viscous gel-like substance that transmits light and which is necessary for life as we know it.

The cytoplasm of the ovum/egg (that protoplasm which is outside of the nucleus of the ovum) contains centrosomes, mitochondria, a variety of granules, fat droplets, Golgi complexes and yolk material.

The centrosome is a specialized area of condensed cytoplasm which contains two centrioles. The centrioles play a very important role in cell division (mitosis). We will talk a lot more about centrosomes and centrioles a little later on.

Mitochondria (singular is mitochondrion) are structures within the cytoplasm of both plant and animal cells that carry out oxygen-dependent metabolism. They are the sites of the Krebs cycle and the electron transport chain activities. Granules in the cytoplasm of the ovum/egg perform a variety of functions. Most of these functions have to do with the secretion of substances that are necessary for the normal metabolic activity of the ovum/egg.

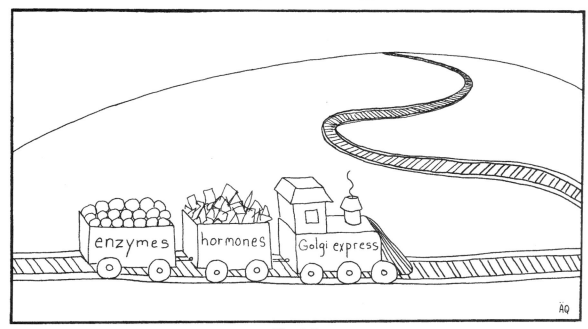

Fig. 1-5
Golgi Complex:
The Golgi complex is involved in the transport of enzymes and hormones, which in the ovum
are very much involved in the process of cell division.

Fat droplets are present in the cytoplasm of the ovum. These droplets can be high-energy fuel sources for metabolism or they may have other functions as yet unknown. I believe the function of fat droplets is open to conjecture because we are seeing a significant increase in the number of functions of various fat (lipid) molecules as biochemical research progresses.

Golgi complexes are assemblies of vesicles and folded membranes within the cytoplasm of cells. These Golgi complexes store and transport biochemical products such as enzymes and hormones. Quite often the Golgi complexes and their related materials contribute to the formation of cell walls. In the case of the ovum/egg, they seem to be involved in cell division **(Fig. 1-5)**.

Yolk material is the food stored in the cytoplasm which will be used by the embryo. It is a combination of protein and fat with little or no carbohydrate **(Fig. 1-6)**.

In the ovary, the mature ovum/egg that is getting ready to be sent out into the fallopian tube is contained within a vesicle in the ovary. This vesicle is about 1 centimeter in diameter. It is called the ovarian or the graafian follicle. We will discuss the process of ovulation after we look at the menstrual cycle and what makes it tick.

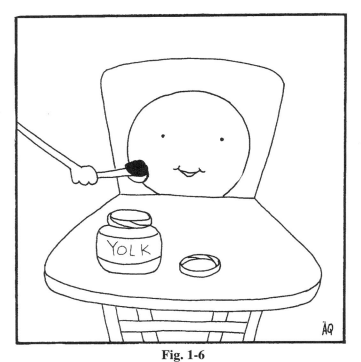

Fig. 1-6
The Baby Embryo:
Yolk material is stored in the cytoplasm of the cells. It is composed mostly of fat and protein. There is little or no carbohydrate in yolk material. It is used as nourishment by the embryo during its development.

The Menstrual Cycle

The menstrual cycle is initiated by the hypothalamus, which has a special connection to the anterior pituitary gland. The hypothalamus is a small part of the brain which is only about 1/300th of the total brain weight. For a structure so small it does an exceptionally large amount of work and performs a wide variety of functions. The hypothalamus is located above the pituitary gland about 2 1/2 to 3 inches directly into your head from a point on the midline where your two eyebrows would meet (if they haven't been plucked or separated by civilization in some

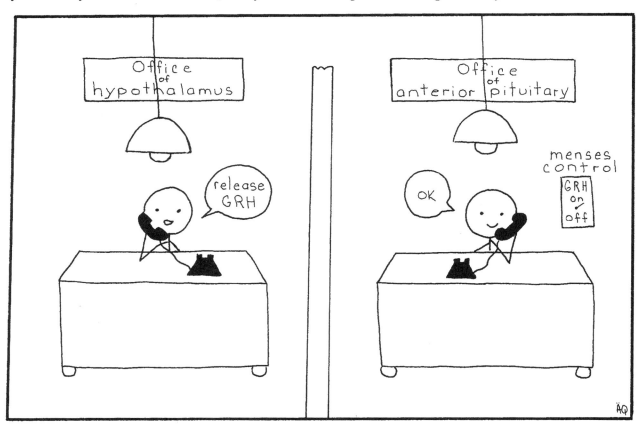

Fig. 1-7
Central Menstrual Control System:
The hypothalamus seems to be the highest control center for the menstrual cycle. It connects with the anterior pituitary gland by both nerve impulses and hormones. The principal hormone involved in this intercommunication center is G.R.H. (gonadotropic releasing hormone). The anterior pituitary gland, in turn, tells the ovaries and the uterus what to do and when to do it.

other way). The hypothalamus has its own private system which connects it to the anterior pituitary gland. This system is composed of both neural (nerve) connections and a specialized blood delivery system. The hypothalamus can send both nerve impulses and hormone secretions directly to the pituitary gland. It is by this system that the hypothalamus tells the anterior pituitary gland when to begin the menstrual cycles each month **(Fig. 1-7)**.

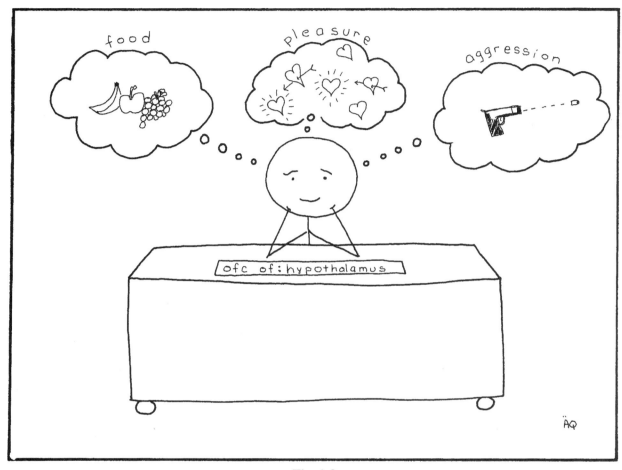

Fig. 1-8
Hypothalamic Functions:
The hypothalamus is extremely small yet its range of activity is very wide and powerful. It influences appetite, pleasure, aggression, and almost every other emotional feeling of which we are aware.

At the present time I am unable to tell you by what mechanism the hypothalamus triggers the human female's first menstrual cycle. I can tell you, however, that amongst the hypothalamic functions are things having to do with appetite, satiety, aggression, pleasure and a wide range of emotions **(Fig. 1-8)**. It seems reasonable that emotional states may have something to do with triggering the first hypothalamic signal to the anterior pituitary gland to begin the first menstrual cycle. It is also an enticing idea that the hypothalamus knows the percentage of body weight that is fat. When that percentage reaches a critical value the hypothalamus may decide that it is time to begin menstrual cycles, ovulation, and the rest of it that goes along with the urge to reproduce.

It wasn't until 1971 that Andrew V. Schally discovered that the hypothalamus releases a hormone into its specialized blood communication system with the anterior pituitary gland, which in turn triggers each menstrual cycle. The name that this hormone has been assigned is gonadotropic releasing hormone (G.R.H.). It is this hormone in both females and males that stimulates the anterior pituitary gland to produce hormones that activate both the ovaries of the female and the testes of the male. Schally was awarded a Nobel prize in 1977 for his ground-breaking work in this area of research.

In the female, the anterior pituitary gland's response to the gonadotropic releasing hormone from the hypothalamus is the production and release of two hormones into the blood stream which goes to the ovaries. The two hormones are: (1) follicle stimulating hormone and (2) luteinizing hormone.

When follicle stimulating hormone arrives at the ovary, it causes a follicle or cyst to be formed around one of the ova/eggs in that ovary. Remember that, at the time of the first menstrual cycle, all of the eggs that a woman will produce in her lifetime are present in the ovaries. One of the ova/eggs is selected for active duty by the follicle stimulating hormone. This ovum/egg then has a follicle or cyst formed around it in preparation for ovulation. How this selection is made I have no idea, but I do believe that nature has methods and purposes for everything that happens. Therefore, I would find it hard to believe that the ovum/egg to be follicalized or encysted was selected at random **(Fig. 1-9)**.

Once the follicle/cyst is formed it manufactures the hormone estrogen, which it secretes into the bloodstream. Once in the bloodstream the estrogen, among other things, goes to the anterior pituitary gland and tells it that the follicle/cyst has formed. Once the follicle has formed there is

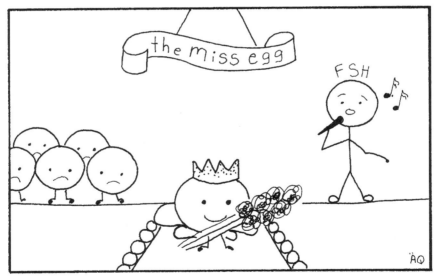

Fig. 1-9
Egg Selection:
We do not as yet know how or why a given egg is selected for
ovulation during any particular menstrual cycle, but somehow the
selection is made. All the eggs for the reproductive life of the woman
are present in the ovaries before the menarche (first menses) begins.
Occasionally, more than one egg is released at a time.
This may result in multiple births.

no further need for more follicle stimulating hormone during this menstrual cycle, so the anterior pituitary gland stops producing this substance. If there is a communication breakdown and follicle stimulating hormone remains in production, more cysts may be formed around more

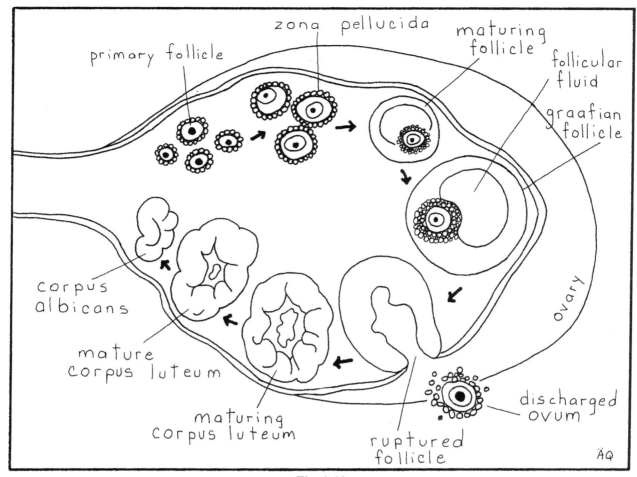

Fig. 1-10
The Ovarian Cycle:
As you move clockwise around the drawing beginning with the primary follicle, the stages before ovulation, at ovulation and after ovulation are shown inside the ovary.

ova/eggs. We may then get more than one ovum/egg being released from the ovary at the same time. This could result in multiple births. The release of the ovum/egg from the ovary is called ovulation. We'll discuss ovulation in more detail soon. With its arrival at the anterior pituitary gland, the estrogen produced by the follicle/cyst reinforces the continued production of luteinizing hormone by the anterior pituitary gland.

Luteinizing hormone from the anterior pituitary gland causes the follicle/cyst to rupture and discharge the ovum/egg out of the ovary. This rupture occurs when that follicle/cyst is close enough to the periphery of the ovary to break through the side of the ovary and its enveloping membrane **(Fig. 1-10)**. Some ovaries have tough membrane coverings which are too strong for the follicle/cyst to break through. When this happens, the enlarged follicle/cyst is retained in the ovary. This condition is known as an ovarian cyst. It is painful, it is sometimes confused with appendicitis and it frequently requires surgical intervention. If the ovarian membranes are extremely tough and the follicles/cysts are frequently unable to rupture through these membranes, the result is the presence of many cysts in the ovary. This condition, called polycystic ovary, is often painful, causes infertility and may require surgery. It is often part of a larger syndrome known as the Stein-Leventhal Syndrome.

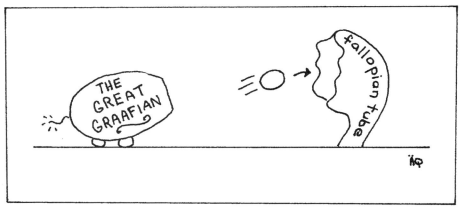

Fig. 1-11
Ovulation:
The extrusion of the egg into the abdominal cavity is such that it is propelled
into the fallopian tube for transport to the uterus. Nature hopes that
fertilization by a sperm will occur en route.

Under normal circumstances ovulation occurs 10 to 14 days after the follicle/cyst has formed around the selected ovum/egg. At the time of ovulation, the ovum/egg is released into the abdominal cavity of the woman (**Fig. 1-11**). The fallopian tube is very nearby and it has a cup-

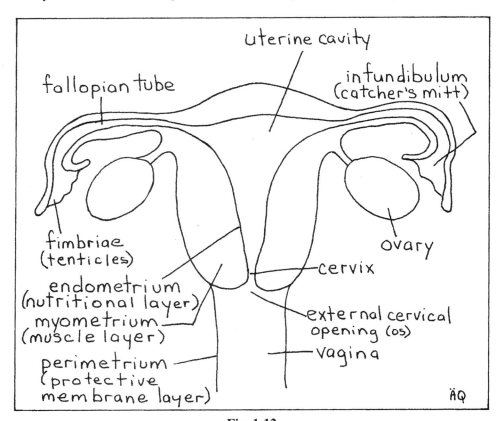

Fig. 1-12
The Female Reproductive System:
If all goes as nature has intended, the ovum, once discharged from the ovary,
will enter the infundibulum of the fallopian tube, become fertilized while moving
through the tube, and successfully implant into the wall of the uterus.
If the implantation is correctly done, a viable fetus will result.

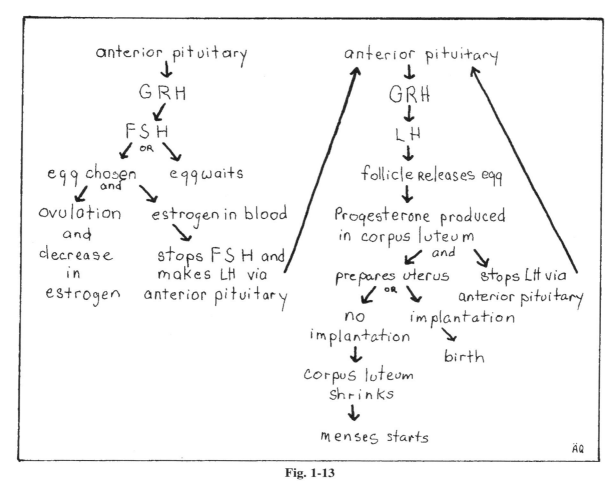

Fig. 1-13
Female Hormones:
This diagram illustrates both the complexity and the efficiency of the hormonal interactions and control of the human female menstrual cycle. See the text for more detailed explanation.

like receptacle with actively moving fimbria that are inviting the discharged ovum/egg into the tube **(Fig. 1-12)**. Should the ovum/egg not enter the fallopian tube for some reason, the ovum/egg is lost into the abdominal cavity. If a stray sperm manages to get all the way up the tube and exit via the fimbriated end near the ovary and then fertilize the displaced ovum/egg, the ovum/egg may implant in the abdominal cavity. This is known as an abdominal pregnancy. Most often this situation also requires surgical intervention.

After ovulation has occurred, the follicle/cyst that contained the ovum/egg changes into the corpus luteum. The corpus luteum is a yellowish glandular mass within the ovary. The luteinizing hormone from the anterior pituitary gland somehow causes the corpus luteum to begin producing progesterone. (That's what I call effective recycling.) Progesterone, in turn (and among other things), causes a very marked thickening of the wall of the uterus along with a significant increase in the blood supply to the uterine walls. In short, progesterone is getting the uterus ready for implantation of the ovum/egg should its fertilization occur. Also, the progesterone produced by the corpus luteum goes via the bloodstream back to the anterior pituitary gland and signals that gland to stop producing any more luteinizing hormone.

If there is no fertilized ovum/egg and hence no implantation in the uterine wall, or if a fertilized ovum/egg fails to implant in the uterine wall, the corpus luteum shrinks. Progesterone levels then

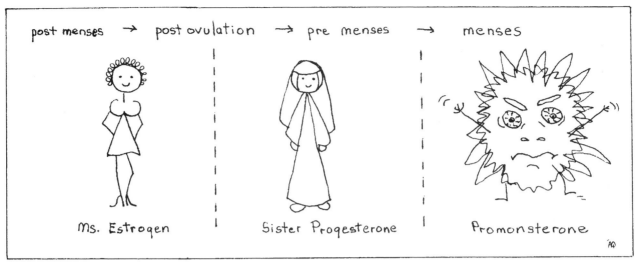

post menses → post ovulation → pre menses → menses

Ms. Estrogen | Sister Progesterone | Promonsterone

Fig. 1-14
Hormones and Libido:
Estrogen increases sexy feelings in women. Thus, it is most elevated when fertilization is a possibility.
Progesterone decreases sexy feelings. Therefore, it is most elevated when fertilization possibilities are past
and implantation of a fertilized ovum is the most important. If there is no implantation, the hormonal switch
often results in premenstrual tension (PMS).

drop and the thick, lush, highly vascularized uterine wall that was ready to receive a fertilized ovum/egg sloughs off. This is the menses that women experience on an almost monthly basis when pregnancy does not occur **(Fig. 1-13)**.

An additional point of interest about estrogen and progesterone that further illustrates the efficiency of nature is that estrogen seems to enhance the female's interest in sexual participation. Estrogen levels are most elevated subsequent to the menses up to the time just after ovulation. Progesterone elevates shortly after ovulation and drops before the menses. Progesterone causes the female to lose interest in sexual activity. Estrogen enhances libido when it could best result in pregnancy. Progesterone diminishes libido after ovulation has occurred and the potential for fertilization of the ovum/egg has passed. In other words, if the possibility of further fertilization is past, progesterone reduces the sex drive **(Fig. 1-14)**.

After ovulation the ovum/egg lives and is fertilizable for about 24 hours. Immediately before, during and after ovulation, the body temperature of the female goes up approximately half a degree. This temperature elevation lasts approximately two days.

Once the ovum/egg has been expelled from the ovary, if all goes well it will enter the fallopian tube. This ovum/egg will live about 24 hours as it begins to travel through the tube towards the uterus. It is within the tube that the ovum/egg normally encounters the sperm and fertilization occurs. If the encounter is later than 24 hours after ovulation, most likely the ovum/egg will be dead and fertilization cannot occur. Therefore, implantation in the uterine wall is not possible either. Consequently, the uterine wall is sloughed and the menses happens. It is of interest to note that sperm live about 24 to 48 hours after ejaculation. So, in order to obtain a pregnancy the timing has to be just right **(Fig. 1-15)**.

We have taken the ovum/egg to the point where it is fertilizable. Before we go on with the description of what happens after fertilization occurs, let's consider the life of the typical sperm before it fertilizes the ovum/egg as it moves towards its own immortality.

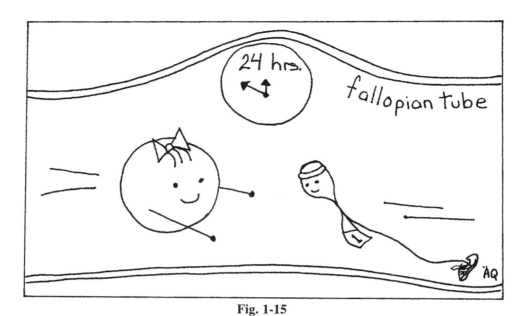

Fig. 1-15
Timing is Everything:
The egg lives about 24 hours after its entry into the tube. The sperm live between 24 and 48 hours after ejaculation. For a normal pregnancy, the sperm must fertilize the egg within the tube.

Topic 3

The Sperm

Sperm are manufactured or synthesized in the male testes or testicles. The average human male manufactures about 100 million sperm per day after puberty has been reached. As the male ages, sperm counts drop with great variability from one man to the next. Over a lifetime the average man manufactures about 400 billion sperm. In the average ejaculation, about 200 million sperm are released. So, clearly you can see that daily ejaculation reduces the sperm count significantly.

The testicles are descended out of the body because they require a lower temperature in order to do their work effectively. The cells that manufacture testosterone at the "request" of the anterior pituitary gland would seem to be able to function in higher (body) temperature. It is the cells that manufacture the sperm that seem to require a lower temperature in which to do their work. When the temperature goes up, the sperm count goes down. So much for the hot bath and the tight nylon briefs if you want to be a father (**Fig. 1-16**).

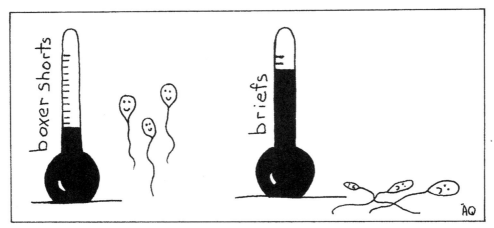

Fig. 1-16
Heat Kills:
When the temperature goes up in the scrotum, the sperm count goes down.
So, if you want to be a father, "stay cool."

Sperm are produced in seminiferous tubules by cell division. In the mature male about 200,000 sperm are produced each minute. That amounts to approximately 3,000 per second.

The average sperm has an oval head, a mid section and a tail. The head contains a nucleus (haploid) that contains a single set of chromosomes (**Fig. 1-17**). Actually, a half set depending on your perspective. These chromosomes contain the male's DNA contribution to the future child.

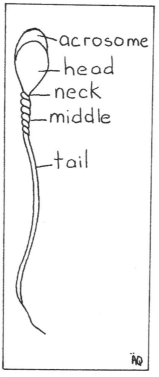

Fig. 1-17
Anatomy of a Sperm:
The sperm has an acrosome cap on its head which secretes enzymes that help it penetrate the egg. The head contains the chromosomes. The tail acts to propel the sperm towards its destination. The middle part contains mitochondria which provide energy to the tail and wherever else it is needed.

Remember, the fertilized ovum/egg requires a double set (diploid) of chromosomes. The other set will be furnished by the mother and will provide her DNA contribution to the future child. Also on the sperm head is an acrosome. The acrosome is a cuplike membrane that covers the anterior/front part of the head of the sperm. This membrane cap contains enzymes that help dissolve the protective membrane of the ovum/egg for sperm entry and fertilization. The middle section of

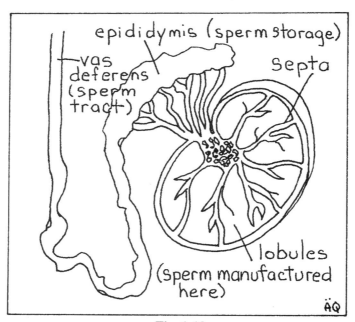

Fig. 1-18
Birth Place of the Sperm:
Sperm are formed in the testes and stored in the epididymis until they are moved through the vas deferens in preparation for ejaculation.

the sperm contains those little energy-manufacturing factories called mitochondria. The constant movement of the tail, which is used to get the sperm where it wants to go, requires a lot of energy.

Once manufactured in the tubules, the sperm are stored in the epididymis, which is an elongated structure attached to the testes (**Fig. 1-18**). It connects the seminiferous tubules where the sperm are manufactured to the vas deferens (of vasectomy fame). The vas deferens travels up through the scrotum as a part of the spermatic cord, and it ultimately joins with its partner from the opposite side and with the seminal vesicle within the prostate gland to form a part of the ejaculatory duct. Sperm that are not ejaculated from the epididymis (the storage corridor) are reabsorbed after about two weeks. Within the epididymis each sperm has a "private nurse" cell that protects and nurtures it as it matures and awaits its call to participate in the ejaculation (**Fig. 1-19**).

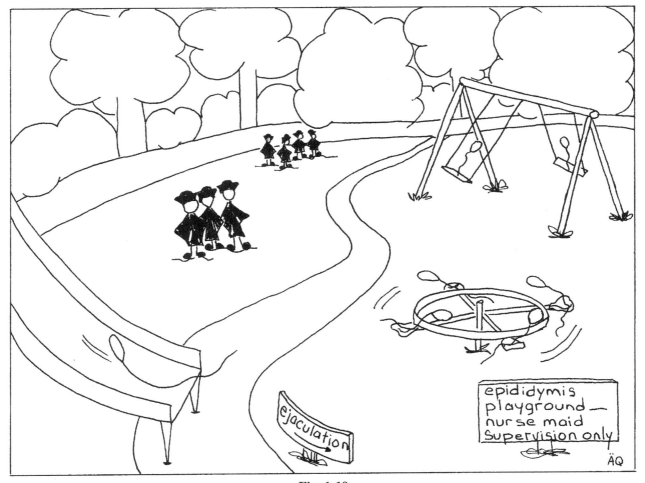

Fig. 1-19
Maturing Sperm with Nursemaid Cells:
Each sperm is cared for by its own private nursemaid cell as it waits in the epididymis for its call to ejaculation.

Sexual arousal and intercourse cause the sperm to begin their trek out of the epididymis into the vas deferens, which offers a very convoluted pathway up to the prostate and the ejaculatory duct. Within the prostate, alkaline seminal fluid is produced. Sperm require an alkaline fluid environment to survive. The average vagina has an acid environment. This acid is partially neutralized by the seminal fluid. There are also Cowper's glands in the same area that provide sugar (fructose) for the sperm to use as fuel before they depart the male host into the alien vagina (**Fig. 1-20**).

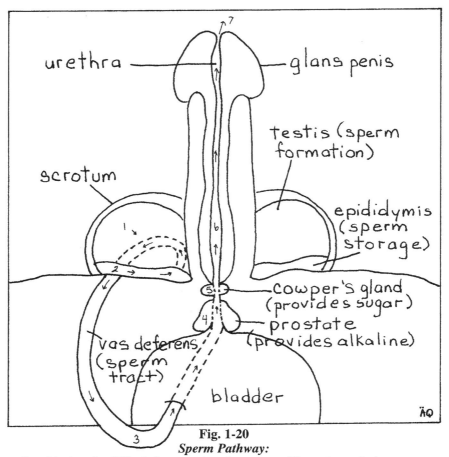

Fig. 1-20
Sperm Pathway:
Considering the difficult journey that the sperm will encounter in its attempt
to fertilize the egg, it is no wonder that only 40 or 50 sperm of the 200 million
in the average ejaculate reach the egg.

As we previously stated, there are about 200 million sperm in the average ejaculate. The obstacles are so severe that only about 40 or 50 sperm actually reach the ovum/egg in the female's fallopian tube. After leaving the male host, a sperm lives between 24 and 48 hours.

This preparatory process for sperm about to be ejaculated is almost like sending a hiker to cross a mountain range. You give them their supplies, wish them well and off they go. The sperm's mission is to get to the ovum/egg with its bundle of DNA so that it can fertilize and thus continue its march towards molecular immortality.

The usual acid environment of the vagina is life-threatening to the sperm. However, during ovulation the intravaginal and endocervical mucus provides conditions which protect the sperm to some degree from the acid. This mucus provides protective channels through which the "smart" sperm are able to swim and avoid the acid. The sperm must swim through the vagina, up the endocervical canal and arrive in the uterus. Now, after the sperm has done all of this, he has to guess which tube the ovum/egg is coming down. If he picks the wrong tube, he has simply done all that work for nothing because there is no ovum/egg in the tube (**Fig. 1-21**).

Once the sperm makes the tube selection, he has to swim up the tube from the uterus very much against the tide. There are little hair-like cilia that line the fallopian tubes. These cilia work to create a current towards the uterus in order to assist the ovum/egg in its journey from ovary to uterus. You might think of the sperm's plight as similar to a salmon swimming upstream to spawn.

It might also be considered a selective process so that only the strongest sperm get to reproduce. Is it any wonder that only about 40 or 50 sperm out of the 200 million ejaculated reach the ovum/egg with their dreams of immortality?

Once the 40 or 50 sperm reach the ovum/egg, several may try to penetrate, but only the very first one to arrive actually enters the ovum/egg. After one sperm is admitted through the protective membrane by the use of the enzymes in his acrosome, it seems that the enzymes are no longer effective and no more entries can be made. The first sperm to reach the inner membrane is drawn in and the others, even in the case of a photo finish, are rejected. Occasionally a second very determined sperm may penetrate the ovum/egg. In this circumstance the result may be identical twins.

Gestation begins at the time that the winning sperm is drawn into the ovum/egg.

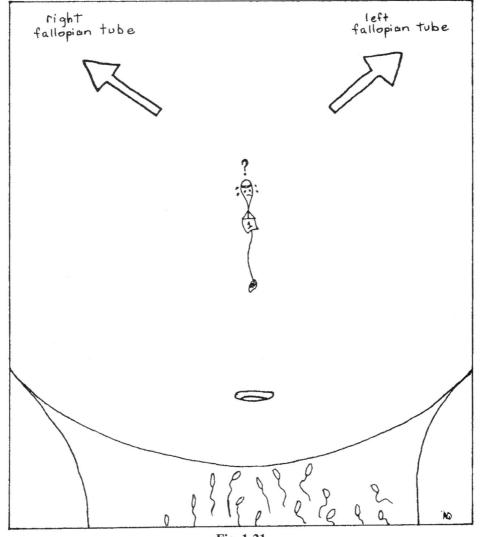

Fig. 1-21
A Chance of a Lifetime:
*After the strongest sperm have survived all of the adversities, they have only a
50-50 chance of choosing which tube has the egg and perhaps surviving to create
yet another generation.*

Section II

Conception and Gestation

Topic 4

Fertilization, Cell Division and Implantation

FERTILIZATION

Gestation is the moment in time when the sperm enters the ovum/egg. The age of the fetus is called the gestational age. Fetal age is calculated from the moment fertilization occurs. The amount of time from fertilization to delivery of the newborn under normal circumstances is 40 weeks. Usually, 38 to 42 weeks is considered within the normal range.

Once inside the ovum/egg, the sperm's tail drops off **(Fig. 2-1)**. The sperm's head swells up and appears to explode. This explosion releases the sperm's nucleus, which has been located in its head. The sperm's nucleus contains 23 chromosomes and is now located within the cytoplasm of the ovum/egg. These chromosomes are thread-like structures. They carry the genes that were contributed by the father's sperm. The genes are made up of DNA. It is the DNA (deoxyribonucleic

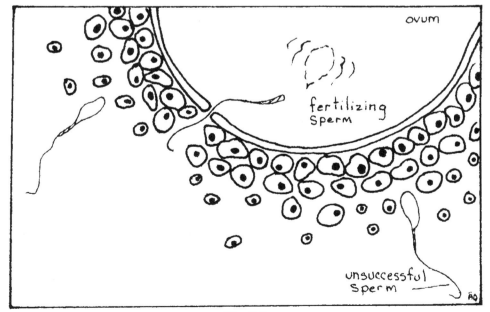

Fig. 2-1
Fertilization:
Once inside of the ovum, the fertilizing sperm's tail drops off and the head "explodes."
The explosion of the head releases the nucleus containing the 23 chromosomes, which
are the father's contribution to the future child.

acid) that somehow carries and passes on the genetic characteristics of the individual, such as eye color, hair color, body type, etc.

The nucleus of the ovum/egg also contains 23 chromosomes. All other body cells besides ova/eggs and sperm contain 46 chromosomes. The 23 chromosomes from the sperm will ultimately combine with the 23 chromosomes from the ovum/egg to make the 46 chromosomes contained in all other body cells. It is in this way that the child inherits characteristics from both mother and father. The 23-chromosome package is called a haploid. When the two packages of 23 chromosomes each combine to form the 46-chromosome-containing cell, it is called a diploid.

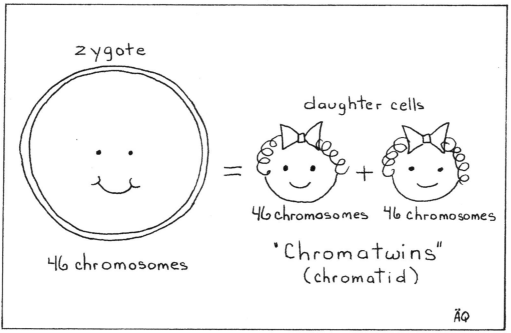

Fig. 2-2
Chromatid Set:
In the zygote the 46 chromosomes (23 from each parent) each divide in half, producing two sets of 46 half chromosomes. These half chromosomes are called chromatids. One set of 46 chromatids goes into each daughter cell. The chromatids then grow larger and become full-grown chromosomes which divide during the next mitosis.

Once the sperm's nucleus has been liberated by the explosion of the sperm's head, this nucleus finds itself more or less adrift in the sea of the ovum's/egg's cytoplasm. The "adrift" part doesn't last long. There seems to be some sort of magnetic attraction that draws the nucleus of the sperm and the nucleus of the ovum/egg together. As the two nuclei touch, they fuse together. As they fuse, they form a single nucleus. The individual nuclear membranes dissolve and the new cell with its 46 chromosomes is created. This miraculous creation is called the zygote. This is only a zygote for a short time because, when cell cleavage begins, the name zygote no longer applies. This first cell division occurs about 12 hours after the two nuclei have fused to form the diploid.

The zygote divides by mitosis. Mitosis means that each of the two cells derived from the division also has 46 chromosomes. The cells derived from mitosis are spoken of as daughter cells. The achievement of beginning in the zygote with 46 chromosomes and deriving two daughter cells with 46 chromosomes each is accomplished by dividing each of the zygote's 46 chromosomes in half. This division yields two sets of 46 chromosomes each. However, each daughter cell chromosome is essentially half the length of the parent cell's (zygote's) chromosomes at the time of mitosis. These half-length chromosomes are referred to as chromatids. Once in the daughter cell's nucleus, each chromatid set will be referred to as a chromosome set. And remember that, for both chromatid sets and chromosome sets, the magic number is still 46 (**Fig. 2-2**).

MITOSIS

Let us now take a rather detailed look at this miracle of cell division called mitosis (**Fig. 2-3**). As I indicated previously, mitosis is a method of cell division in which the two derived daughter cells receive the same number of chromosomes as the parent cell. Therefore, all derived daughter cells are genetically identical to the parent cell or zygote, and all of the future generations of daughter cells are genetically identical to each other.

There are four phases in the cell division called mitosis. These phases are:

1. Prophase
2. Metaphase
3. Anaphase
4. Telophase

(1) The prophase encompasses that time when the paired chromatids are formed from the chromosomes. The nuclear membranes of the sperm and ovum/egg disappear. The achromatic spindle fibers appear. These fibers are precursors of the microtubules that will form during the next phase (metaphase). The purpose of the microtubules is to guide chromatids to the correct position for mitotic cell division. Also, centrioles become apparent during prophase. The centrioles are the poles from which the achromatic spindle fibers radiate in order to form the fusiform network that connects them (the two centrioles). Prophase takes approximately one hour (**Fig. 2-3**).

(2) The metaphase is the time during which the chromosomes arrange in an equatorial plane considering the two centrioles as the poles. If you wish to use the earth as a model, the centrioles would be the north and south poles. The chromosomes would be located in the equatorial plane and spindle fibers, which have derived from the achromatic spindle fibers, would be comparable to the longitude lines of the earth. The chromosomes arranged in the equatorial plane are spoken of as a monaster.

Once the monaster has formed, the chromosomes divide into exactly similar halves. These chromosomes, by dividing, have become chromatids. They now oscillate back and forth in the

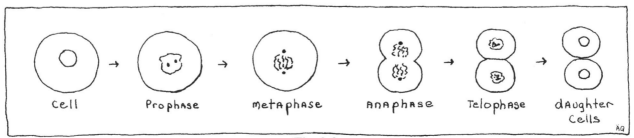

Fig. 2-3
Mitosis:
Diagrammatic representation of the stages of mitosis. These stages are described in more detail in the text.

equatorial plane as though they are being pulled first to one pole and then to the other. The metaphase takes approximately six minutes (**Fig. 2-3**).

(3) The anaphase is that time when the two groups of daughter chromosomes (chromatids) separate and move along the spindle fibers to one centriole pole or the other. At this time the centriole with its attached spindle fibers is called the aster. When we are considering both poles with the chromosomes approaching their preferred ones, the total unit is spoken of as the diaster. As the chromosomes approach the two poles of the dividing cell, the cell elongates and develops a groove or waistband at the equatorial plane. The anaphase takes approximately three minutes (**Fig. 2-3**).

(4) The telophase is the time when the equatorial groove or waistband sinks in deeper and deeper until the parent cell divides into two daughter cells by completely separating at the equatorial plane. Each daughter cell gets about half of the parent cell's mitochondria. You may recall that mitochondria are analogous to little energy-producing factories in the cytoplasm of the cell (**Fig. 2-3**).

The actual cell division takes only about three minutes, but the reorganization of the chromosomes, the formation of a nucleus with nuclear membrane in each daughter cell, may take several hours. During this time of daughter-cell organization, no further division can take place. That is, the daughter cell cannot divide until she is organized and ready to become a parent cell (**Fig. 2-3**).

To be strictly correct, cell division is the total process. Mitosis refers only to the division of the cell nucleus, and cytokinesis refers to the division of the cytoplasm between the two daughter cells.

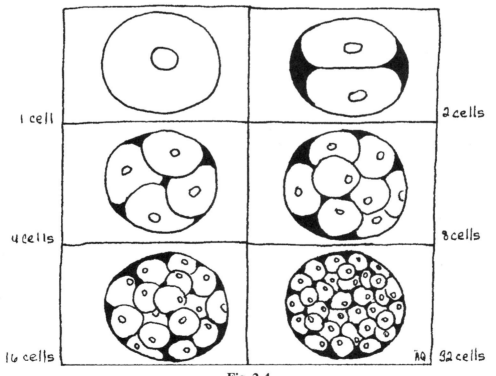

Fig. 2-4
Developing Zygote:
Illustration of zygote cell division and subsequent division
of daughter cells until 32 cells are present.

After the first cell division is completed, the daughter cells each divide in the same way as the zygote or parent cell divided. Thus, one cell produces two cells. Two cells produce four cells. Four cells produce eight cells. Eight cells produce 16 cells. Sixteen cells produce 32 cells. It takes approximately five days to reach 32 cells from the single zygote by mitotic cell division (**Fig. 2-4**). The actual volume or size of the 32-cell package is not much larger than the original parent cell. The cells are more numerous, but in these early stages of development the daughter cells remain much smaller than their parent cells for quite awhile.

During the five days when the zygote remains about the same size, it continues its descent through the fallopian tube to the uterus. This continuation of the journey through the tube after fertilization is probably the reason that nature decided to keep the 32-cell package small. Otherwise, it might get caught in the tube. When it does get caught it can develop into a tubal pregnancy which cannot go to completion, hurts like the dickens, and will usually require surgical intervention (**Fig. 2-5**).

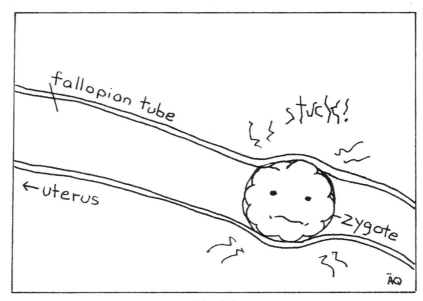

Fig. 2-5
Tubal Pregnancy:
If the zygote becomes too large to pass through the tube to the uterus,
it may remain in the tube and grow. This is a tubal pregnancy.
This condition is quite painful and may require surgery.

The five days does include a safety factor because the zygote usually enters the uterus at about three days gestation, and with about eight cells in its package. When cell division within the zygote reaches the magic number 32, a cavity forms inside of it. This cavity is appropriately named the central cavity. Once the cavity is formed, the cell package is properly named a blastocyst (**Fig. 2-6**).

The blastocyst is usually formed at five days gestational age. Another five days may be required to achieve implantation in the uterine wall. A blastocyst that has not implanted by 10 days after fertilization by the sperm (gestational age) has significantly reduced chances of survival.

I feel compelled to digress at this juncture and share with you a most interesting case that seems almost impossible to have happened unless you were there to witness it. The patient was a divorced woman in her mid-thirties. The problem was that she had a great deal of difficulty in trusting anyone. She was always suspicious. She had tried hard to really and truly feel trust but she was unable to get rid of that little seed of suspicion.

We decided to try some Therapeutic Imagery and Dialogue along with the bodywork that we call SomatoEmotional Release℠, in an attempt to discover the cause of her problem. We developed a dialogue with her "Inner Physician" and enlisted the cooperation of the image. We asked that she be allowed to go back in time to a place or situation that preceded the experience that resulted in her inability to trust. The image that ultimately presented itself to her was that she

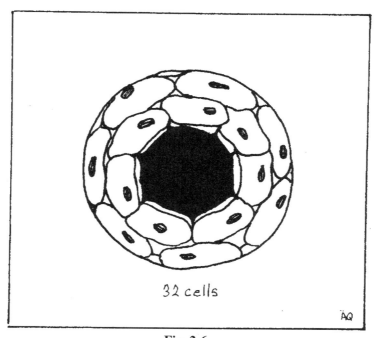

32 cells

Fig. 2-6
Blastocyst:
When the zygote reaches 32 cells by means of cell division, it becomes a blastocyst. The blastocyst has a cavity in its center.

was a very happy little zygote made up of 16 cells. Then she became a blastocyst of 32 cells. She stated that she felt happy, safe, content, and trusted that everything would be wonderful. Suddenly, as she exited her mother's nice, safe and snug fallopian tube and entered the vast cavity which was her mother's uterus, she panicked. She didn't know what to do. She completely lost her trust in those that were caring and watching over her.

We honored her image. We assumed that what she was imaging was valid (at least to her). So we took her back into the mother's fallopian tube and restored the feelings of safety and trust. Then we told her what it would be like when she reached the end of the tube and entered the uterus. I asked if I could be with her during her entry into the uterus. She agreed that that would be helpful. As we entered the uterus I told her to make a sharp right turn, feel the lush, receptive uterine wall, and go ahead and implant. In her image she did this with little or no fear because she was being accompanied and guided. After implantation, she was fine. Now it is about a year later and she continues to be able to trust much more fully. She is much happier.

Whether the image and the cellular consciousness that it implies are valid or not matters very little to me. What does matter is that, for whatever reason, this patient is much better and happier now.

IMPLANTATION

Implantation is also called nidation (**Fig. 2-7**). It occurs as the blastocyst enters the uterine cavity and makes contact with the wall of the uterus. Recall that the hormone progesterone has as a part of its function the thickening and increase of blood supply to that uterine wall. So, the uterus is ready for implantation. Some of the outer cells on the blastocyst's surface are now specialized. These outer cells are called trophoblasts. These trophoblasts have the ability to dissolve the superficial, or surface layers of the lining of the uterus. Trophoblasts do their work and a cavity forms in the uterine wall into which the blastocyst sinks and makes itself at home. The trophoblasts will ultimately form the placenta.

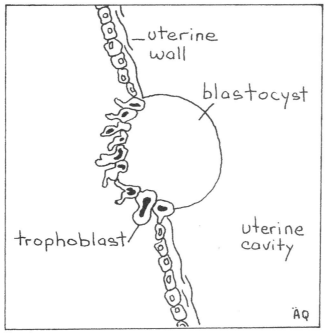

Fig. 2-7
Implantation:
The blastocyst enters the uterine wall with the assistance
of some of the trophoblast cells located on its outer
surface. These cells are able to dissolve the uterine
lining and allow the blastocyst to enter the uterine wall.
This entry is called implantation or nidation.

When implantation occurs and the trophoblasts form the placenta, progesterone is then manufactured by this placenta. There is a safety factor in that the corpus luteum in the ovary continues to produce progesterone until the placenta is well established and producing lots of progesterone. The pregnancy cannot survive without a plentiful progesterone supply. After about three months gestation, the placenta takes over progesterone production and the corpus luteum shrinks. During the pregnancy progesterone also serves to prevent ovulation, and therefore acts to prevent a second pregnancy from occurring after an initial pregnancy has already started. Occasionally, there may be an ovulation after an implantation has occurred. This apparently happens because there is not sufficient progesterone to prevent ovulation. Progesterone is a key ingredient in birth control pills.

After implantation has occurred, the uterus takes over the nourishment of the blastocyst. The trophoblasts form the placenta and the pregnancy becomes well established. Occasionally, the cavity in the uterine wall that is formed by implantation does not heal immediately. This may be the source of a little bleeding. This is the irregular spotting that sometimes occurs after a pregnancy is established. It is sometimes mistaken as a menstrual period. This mistake often throws the expected date of delivery of the newborn off by a month.

Section III A

The Embryo

Topic 5

The First Four Weeks

The first eight weeks of gestational life (after fertilization) are termed the embryonic period. This period of eight weeks is the time during which all organs, systems and tissues are put in place. The remaining 30-34 weeks spent in the mother's uterus are for growth, development and refinement of these organs, systems and tissues. Therefore, if something goes wrong during the first eight weeks, it may result in a defectively designed structure or system whereas, if the problem occurs after the eighth week of gestation, it will more likely result in a failure of growth, development or refinement of the involved structure or system. The latter situation is more amenable to treatment.

Once implantation has occurred and the rudimentary placenta is established, some of the cells within the blastocyst flatten out to form a disc. This is called the embryonic disc. This disc first grows in two distinct layers, then a third layer is formed between them. This three-layered disc extends out from the wall of the blastocyst into its cavity. The part of the disc that remains attached to the wall of the blastocyst will become the tail end of the embryo. The part that protrudes out into the cavity will become the head end of the embryo (**Fig 3-1**).

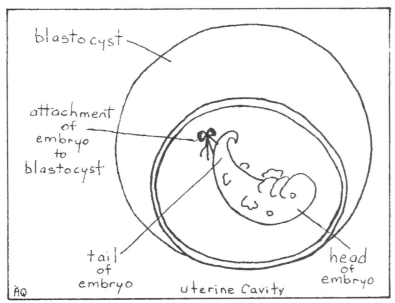

Fig. 3-1
The Embryonic Disc:
The future head of the fetus protrudes out into the blastocyst cavity.
The tail end remains attached to the wall of the cavity of the blastocyst.

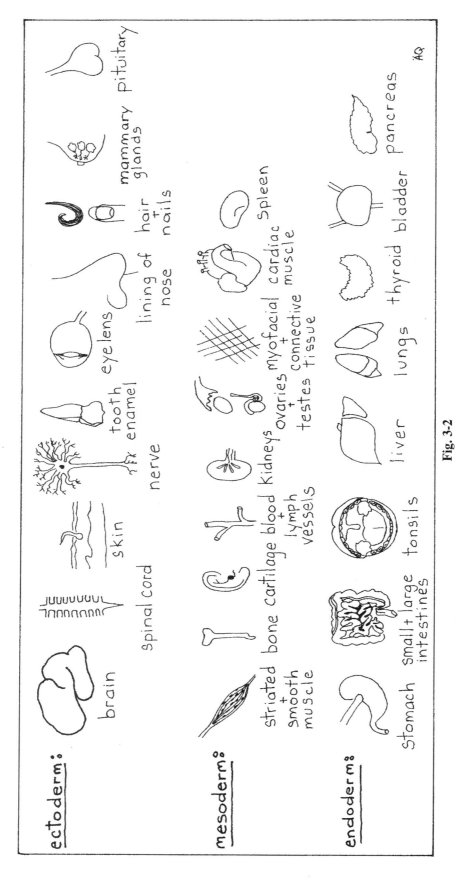

Fig. 3-2

Embryonic Disc Layer — Precursors of Various Organs and Tissues:
Chart of embryonic origin for several body tissues and organs. See text.

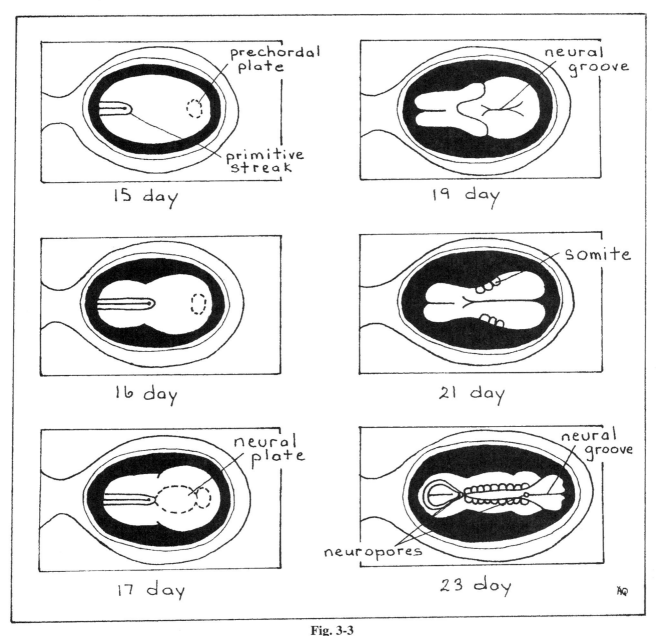

Fig. 3-3
Top View of Primitive Streak Development on the Embryonic Plate:
These drawings demonstrate the rapid development of the nervous system between days 15 and 23 of gestation. See text.

The layers of the embryonic disc are ectoderm and entoderm initially, then the third layer called mesoderm forms between them in very short order.

The ectoderm becomes the source of the brain, spinal cord, skin, nerves, tooth enamel, lens of the eye, the lining of the nose and so on. The mesoderm layer gives origin to the muscles, bones, cartilage and other connective tissues, and all of the blood vascular system. The internal organs such as the stomach, intestines, liver, lungs and all of the rest are derived from entoderm (**Fig 3-2**).

Next the embryonic disc has a streak develop on it. This streak runs from the attachment of the disc to the inner wall of the blastocyst out to the edge that protrudes the furthest into the blastocyst cavity. This primitive streak, as it is called, is actually a line of very rapidly proliferating cells at the bottom of a groove that has formed in the embryonic disc. The proliferation of the primitive streak cells contributes to the mesoderm layer that interposes between the ectoderm and the entoderm (**Fig. 3-3**).

As the primitive streak proliferates, a protective plate forms across the head end of the embryonic disc. This plate is called the prechordal plate. The prechordal plate will prevent primitive streak mesodermal cells from passing beyond it into the head end of the embryonic disc. The plate will also become the source of many of the tissues of the mouth and throat (**Fig 3-3**).

At about two weeks of gestational age, the embryo is about 2 millimeters long, about one-twelfth of an inch. Its tail end is attached to the placenta that is blended with the wall of the mother's uterus, and its head end protrudes out into the uterine cavity. This protrusion of the embryo out into the uterine cavity is enclosed in tissue derived from the blastocyst. You might say that the two-week-old embryo has its own private apartment in the uterine cavity of the mother.

The aforementioned neural groove is still present (**Fig 3-3**). At about this time a solid but elastic line of cells develops deep to the bottom of the neural groove, but not so deep that it would touch the entoderm. This line of cells will be called the notochord. The notochord now induces the further development of the brain and spinal cord, the vertebral column, and the muscles and ligaments related to the vertebral column. This notochord is only the inducer of these developments. Once the development of the brain, spinal cord and vertebral column is begun, the notochord simply disappears (**Fig 3-4**). But it is important to note that it is the notochord that initially determines the future axis of the newborn's body. It seems reasonable to me that some distortion in the notochord during this early time of gestation might be responsible for some forms of scoliosis at a later time in life.

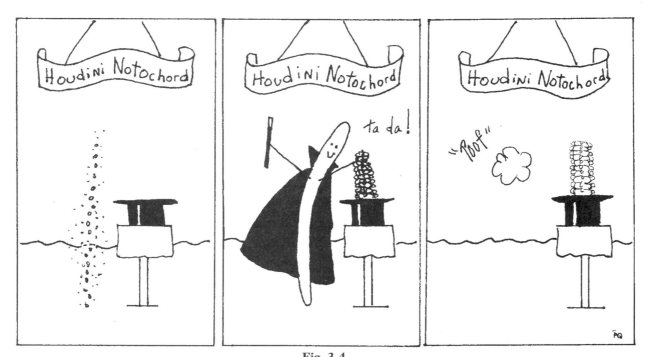

Fig. 3-4
The Disappearing Notochord:
The notochord appears. It then induces development of the spinal column and its related muscles, as well as the brain and the spinal cord. Once these developments have begun, the notochord simply disappears. However, without a notochord to start the process, we would have no brain, no spinal cord and no vertebral column.

NEURULATION

I have gotten a little ahead of myself talking about the neural groove and the notochord. Let's go back and look at this series of events in detail. The process to which I refer is called neurulation. (Everything has a fancy name.) Neurulation refers to the process by which the precursors to the brain and spinal cord are formed and do their work. The first thing that happens is that a thickened area of ectodermal cells running from future tail end to future head end of the embryo appears on the embryonic disc. This is called the neural plate. The neural plate then develops the aforementioned neural groove in it. It is in the bottom of this neural groove, which is still made up of ectodermal cells, that the primitive streak develops. The cells proliferated by the primitive streak are mesodermal cells, which as they develop will spread out and interpose between the entoderm and the ectoderm. Between the primitive streak and the entoderm the notochord forms. It seems that the presence of the notochord is necessary for the further development of the neural groove into the neural tube, which will then develop into the brain and spinal cord (**Fig 3-3**).

THE NOTOCHORD

Let's take a quick but more in-depth look at notochord formation. Near the cranial or head end of the primitive streak, a primitive node of cells occurs in the ectoderm layer. This node may be called Hensen's node as well as the primitive node. Next, a strand of cells grows as an extension of the primitive node towards the head end of the primitive streak in between the layers of ectoderm and entoderm. This strand of cells extends forward until it encounters the prechordal plate which, as we mentioned above, selectively blocks mesodermal cells from extending into the head end of the embryonic plate.

This prechordal plate blocks the passage of the strand of cells extending from the primitive node. The extension cells from the primitive node to the prechordal plate is called the notochordal process. It delineates the axis of the embryo. Since further growth towards the embryonic head is blocked, the primitive streak diverts its growth towards the tail end of the embryo. This growth of the primitive streak carries the primitive node with it. In this way the notochordal process also begins to extend towards the tail of the embryo as the primitive node draws this notochordal process along with it.

As the notochordal process extends towards the tail, its cells also begin to extend laterally, first forming a plate which becomes a groove and ultimately a tube. This tube is called the notochordal canal. This canal then develops an opening in its floor. This opening communicates with the yolk sac of the embryo. The yolk is a temporary food supply to the embryo. Via the notochordal canal, food from the yolk sac is distributed to the rapidly multiplying cells that are geographically related to it (the notochordal canal).

A little further towards the tail, the yolk sac and the amniotic cavity communicate to form the neuroenteric canal. As the name implies, this canal offers communication between nerve tissue (neuro) and the alimentary canal (enteric). Since ectoderm is the precursor of nerve tissue and entoderm provides the origins for the alimentary canal (mouth to anus), in this primitive state of development the neuroenteric canal provides communication between ectoderm and entoderm.

Very soon the notochordal canal will fill in and become the notochord. This occurs when the placenta, with its system of arteries and veins, has become fully competent to supply the embryo with nourishment and the yolk sac is no longer needed. The amnionic sac and its fluid persist throughout embryonic development because they will become the reservoir for embryonic urine.

Since the notochord has formed between ectoderm and entoderm, it is classified as mesoderm. (Meso means middle in Greek.) Now the notochord, by some mysterious means, will induce the development of the neural groove which becomes the neural tube and, finally, the brain and spinal cord. The notochord also induces the formation of the vertebral column, the related muscles and the base of the skull. Once the induction of these structures is established, the notochord, per se, simply disappears. Its cells do not participate in these structures; they are only involved in the induction of their formation.

NEURULATION, CONTINUED

At about the 18th day of gestational age, the neural plate development is complete. The neural plate thickens in two parallel lines that are oriented with the axis of the head-tail ends of the embryo. These thickenings become the neural folds. These folds elongate as the primitive streak elongates towards the tail of the embryo. The neural folds will extend over the neural groove, reaching towards each other so that when they join on about the 21st day, a neural tube is formed. At first the neural tube does not close completely. Pores are maintained until about the 25th day of gestational age. The last pores to close are at the head and tail ends of the embryo, and these two pores close on the 26th or 27th day of gestational age. The closure of the neural tube and its pores makes use of protein bridges that are bound together by calcium.

Failure of pore closure is the cause of spina bifida, meningocele, myelocele, anencephaly and pilonidal cyst. So as you see, a problem with the pregnancy at days 25, 26 or 27 may result in spinal bifida or one of the other aforementioned conditions. It makes one suspicious that calcium and/or protein deficiency of the mother during the first four weeks of gestation may be contributing factors. Also tentatively incriminated as causes of spina bifida are zinc and folic acid deficiencies. At the time of this writing (August 1993), the experts are considering the addition of folic acid, a B vitamin, to bread in order to correct deficiencies that may lead to spina bifida or other neural tube related birth defects. There are about 2,500 neural tube closure defects seen in newborns each year in America. These problems can be devastating.

THE NEURAL CREST

The neural crest is formed as the cells within the neural folds specialize. These specializing cells then migrate across the top of the neural tube as it is formed. The neural crest then is located between the ectodermal surface and the neural tube. These neural crest cells form all of the nerve cell ganglia, which are located alongside the spinal cord and in the head. Neural crest cells will also migrate all over the body to form other nerve cell ganglia, which are located near the various internal organs, glands and blood vessels. Nerve cell ganglia are masses of nerve cell bodies aggregated together. These ganglia serve as relay stations for the nerve impulses that are generated either in the central nervous system or in the sensory receptors of the body. Ganglia are essential for effective function and integration of the total nervous system. It is also my personal opinion that some ganglia possess decision-making abilities that obviate the necessity for sending the input sensory information all the way to the central nervous system before appropriate action can be taken by the body.

Neural crest cells also give origin to the myelin-producing glial cells of the nervous system: from glial cells which do not conduct nerve impulses but which do perform a myriad of ancillary functions for the nervous system, to melanocytes, which provide the melanin pigment to the skin and thus help you get a suntan. Neural crest cells, in addition, contribute to the formation of the bone and cartilage of the face and the skull.

THE SOMITES

During the third week of gestation as the neural folds grow, a multitude of mesodermal cells present themselves along the sides of the notochord and the neural folds **(Fig. 3-5)**. This expanding mass of mesoderm organizes into paired blocks that lie on either side of the neural folds and the notochord just underneath the ectoderm. These paired blocks are initially called primitive body segments. The cells making up these primitive body segments are called epithelioid cells. Ultimately, these primitive body segments will give origin to somites. The somites are paired blocks of mesodermal cells (epithelioid cells) arranged in segments alongside the neural tube and the notochord. These somites will eventually produce or become the vertebral column and its related musculature.

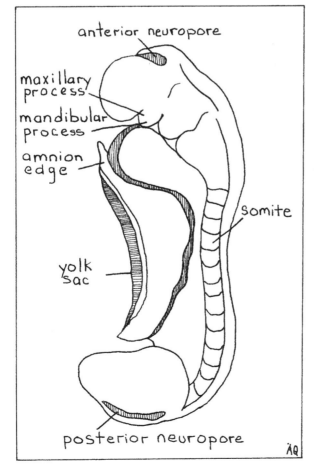

Fig. 3-5
Embryo at Three Weeks Gestation:
At the early age of three weeks, the embryo has several somites developed. It has a definite head and a tail with large neuropores at each end. The jaws and face are beginning to form.

On about the 20th day of gestational age, the first pair of somites will have developed from the primitive body segments at the head end of the embryo. New pairs of somites appear sequentially from the head end to the tail end. This process should be complete by the end of the fifth week of gestation. If all goes well there will be four pairs of occipital somites, eight pairs of cervical somites, twelve pairs of thoracic somites, five pairs of lumbar somites, five pairs of sacral somites and eight to ten pairs of coccygeal somites.

Later on in humans, the first pair of occipital somites and the lower three or four pairs of coccygeal somites will disappear. The remaining somites will ultimately produce most of the axial skeleton, the associated muscles and the dermis (skin and all of its specialized glands, follicles, etc.).

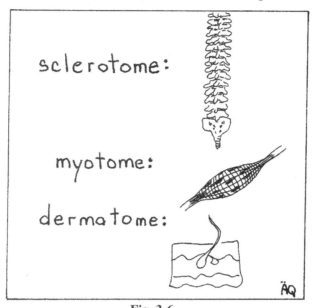

Fig. 3-6
The Three Specialized Divisions of the Somite:
The sclerotome produces bone, cartilage and tough connective
tissues. The myotome produces the muscles which support
and move the bones. The dermatome produces the skin.

Each somite produces three divisions of derived tissue system. Each member of a somite pair has the mirror image of itself on the opposite side, with the exception of those somite-produced structures that relate to non-symmetrically distributed internal organs. The three divisions produced by each somite are called: (1) the sclerotome, (2) the myotome, and (3) the dermatome **(Fig. 3-6)**.

The sclerotome becomes the vertebral column. Cells of the somite migrate towards the notochord. The cells, which are essentially generic mesenchyme originally, appear to be affected by the notochord. This notochordal effect causes the non-specialized mesenchyme cells to differentiate and specialize into: chondroblasts, which then manufacture cartilage; osteoblasts, which produce bone; and fibroblasts, which produce ligaments, fascia and other tough connective tissues **(Fig. 3-7)**.

The myotome division of the somite produces the muscles that move and support the axial skeleton. A given myotomal muscle group receives its nerve supply from a given segment of the spinal cord.

The dermatome is that part of the somite which produces the skin. A given dermatome represents that section of skin that receives its nerve supply from a single spinal cord segment.

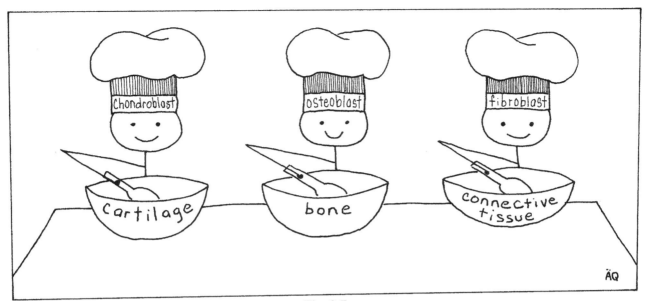

Fig. 3-7
Mesenchyme Chefs:
As you can see, our chefs are highly specialized. The mesenchyme cells differentiate into chondroblasts, osteoblasts and fibroblasts which then produce cartilage, bone and connective tissue, respectively.

Thus, the nerves to related sclerotomes, myotomes and dermatomes are all mainly derived from the same spinal cord segment. I say "mainly" because there is overlapping of spinal cord segmental innervation. The somite's innervation above and below a given somite will offer some "back-up" nerve supply to the structures within that somite and/or its derived sclerotome, myotome and dermatome.

The spinal cord has horizontal crossover nerve fibers, which means that a somite on the left, for example, will have a close working relationship with its partner on the right via this crossover nerve network. In clinical practice we frequently make use of this crossover network, which we call "reciprocal innervation." In practical terms it means that if a given muscle on one side of the body is in chronic spasm, this spasm may often be relieved by asking the patient to contract the same muscle on the opposite side. If this can be done successfully it may well relax the chronically spastic muscle. It is as though the excess nerve impulses going to the spastic muscle are diverted to the other side of the body by asking the mirror-image muscle to contract **(Fig. 3-8)**.

SPINAL CORD SEGMENTS

It is convenient and common to think of the body as divided into horizontal segments which are related to horizontal segmental divisions of the spinal cord. It is less commonly realized that the spinal cord also has vertical or longitudinal connections running from head to tail and vice versa. These longitudinal connections pass through the aforementioned series of horizontal or transverse segments. Impulses going up and down the spinal cord might be thought of as elevators going up and down within a tall building **(Fig. 3-9)**. The floors of the building may be considered analogous to the horizontal or transverse segments of the spinal cord. If a passenger gets off of the elevator on a given floor, that passenger can then go to any subdivision on that floor, just as a nerve impulse can go to a selected muscle or other end organ. If a lot of passengers

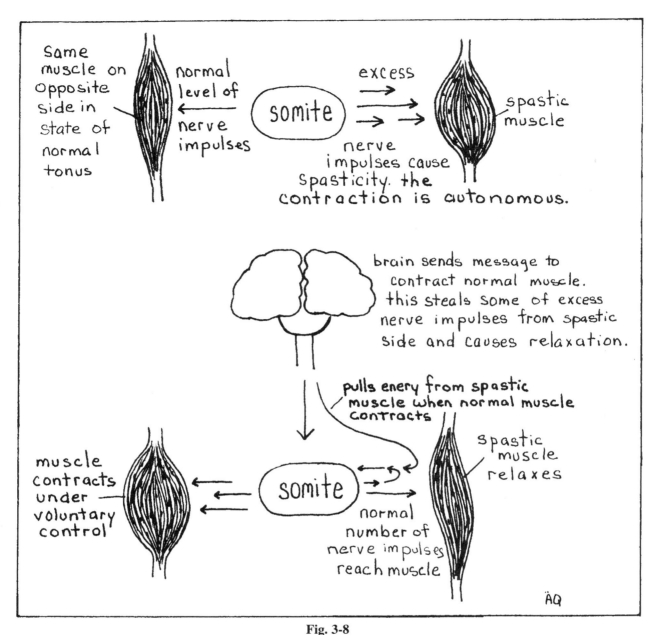

Fig. 3-8
Reciprocal Innervation:
Reciprocal innervation principles can be used both by a therapist and as a "do-it-yourself"
method of treatment for chronic muscle spasm.

go to the same floor, the crowd may overload and affect everything on that floor. The same sort of overload of nerve impulses occurs within a given spinal cord segment. When this kind of spinal segment impulse overload occurs, we call this segment "facilitated." A facilitated spinal cord segment loses some of its innervational specificity and control. For example, when there is a pre-existing crowd or overload of impulses present, one more impulse intended for a specific muscle may cause an overload. The crowd of impulses are no longer correctly directed by the spinal cord segment. The impulse outflow then goes to all muscles innervated by that segment of the spinal cord, and the result is a generalized cramping or spasm of a group of muscles rather than the specific muscle which was intended to contract in a controlled fashion.

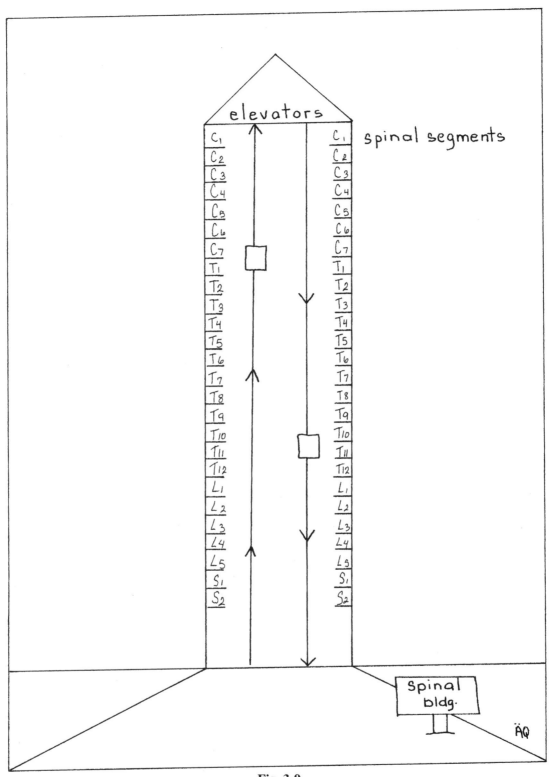

Fig. 3-9
__Longitudinal Spinal Connections:__
The spinal cord sends messages up and down through the segments much as the elevators in a tall building travel through all of the floors of that building. The spinal segments may be thought of as analogous to the floors of the building. Thus, messages are transmitted between segments much as elevator passengers are transported from one floor to another.

AMAZING GROWTH

By the end of the third gestational week of embryonic life, a lot has happened. There are certain flexures that have occurred in the embryo that signify the beginnings of brain formation. The primary divisions of the brain are now visible. These are precursors of eyes and ears, and are spoken of as ocular and auditory vesicles, respectively. A primary system for blood circulation is established and a rudimentary heart is starting to beat. The mouth to anus alimentary canal is formed. It connects with the yolk sac as a source of nourishment. The ends of arms and legs are present. There is a diverticulation in the primitive oral cavity called Rathke's pouch, which appears during the third week. By the end of the sixth week of gestation, Rathke's pouch will have become the anterior division of the pituitary gland. A failure of Rathke's pouch to do its thing and become part of the pituitary gland often results in a tumor of the oral cavity called a craniopharyngioma. Brachial arches are present, which in fish will become gills, but in the human embryo they will form many of the structures of the head and neck. Excretory organs of the embryo in the form of Wolffian bodies are present. These Wolffian bodies, also called mesonephros, are the beginnings of the urinary system. This is a great deal of work and development that has happened in just three weeks (**Fig. 3-10**).

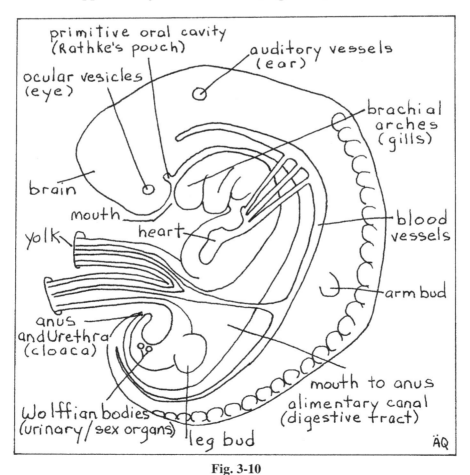

Fig. 3-10
The Embryo at the End of the Third Week:
This illustration serves to show the remarkable development that has occurred
in only three weeks since the egg was fertilized. See text for further details.

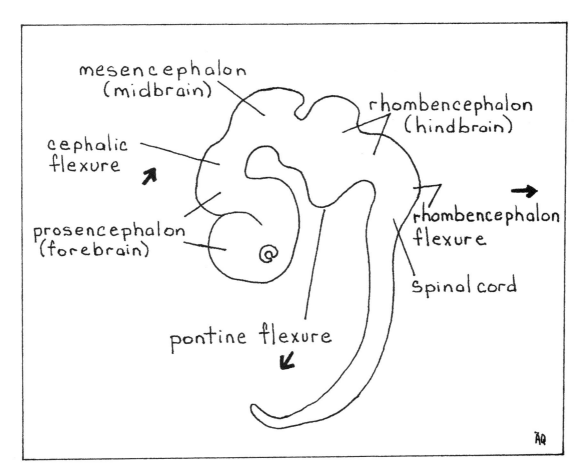

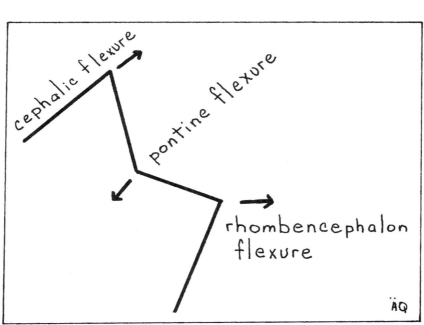

Fig. 3-11
Flexures in the Developing Central Nervous System:
The flexures that occur during the third and fourth week of development of the central nervous system are shown more anatomically in the top drawing and more diagrammatically below.

During the fourth week, more rapid development takes place. The embryo is about 3 to 4 millimeters long (about 1/8 to 3/16 of an inch). The beginning of an umbilicus or belly button is present. The arms and legs are growing rather rapidly. The anus and rectum, called a cloaca at this stage of the game, are developing. During this fourth week the rudimentary heart divides into right and left sides. It began as a two-chambered pump and now it becomes a four-chambered pump. Lungs and the pancreas develop. The face develops and the openings for the nose become apparent. Special nerve ganglia and motor nerve roots from the spinal cord are now visible. Things are moving very, very quickly.

THE BRAIN AND SPINAL CORD

Now let's look in more detail at how the brain, spinal cord and nervous system are coming along in their development.

During the third and fourth weeks, the flexures of the embryo go almost to completion. The significance of these flexures are that they will strongly influence how the brain develops into its specific regions, as you will soon see.

The first flexure that we consider is the cephalic flexure **(Fig. 3-11)**. This flexure allows the forebrain (forward part of the brain) to bend forward over the front end of the notochord. Recall that the prechordal plate prevents extension of the notochord all the way to the head end of the embryo. Now the forebrain simply wraps itself around this head end of the notochord. This flexure actually occurs more in the midbrain area which is right behind the forebrain.

At about the same time, a second bend called the rhombencephalic flexure occurs at the juncture between the brain and the spinal cord **(Fig. 3-11)**. This bend goes to about 90 degrees, allowing the brain to more or less tilt forward on the spinal cord. There is a third flexure called the pontine flexure that bends backward **(Fig. 3-11)**. It occurs just a little after the first two flexures. It helps to compensate for the two forward flexures that occur initially.

During the third week, three vesicles develop at the head end of the neural tube. A vesicle is simply a small sac or cyst filled with fluid. The three vesicles will very quickly become the: (1) forebrain or prosencephalon, (2) midbrain or mesencephalon, and (3) hindbrain or rhombencephalon.

Two of these three brain divisions will further subdivide as follows. The forebrain (prosencephalon) will become the telencephalon, which is the forwardmost division, and the diencephalon, which is the posterior division of the forebrain. The midbrain (mesencephalon) will not further subdivide. The hindbrain (rhombencephalon) will further subdivide into the metencephalon and the myelencephalon.

Some of the more commonly known parts of the brain that are derived from the five major divisions given above are:

I. Forebrain (prosencephalon)
   A. Telencephalon (forward part of the forebrain)
      1. Cerebral Hemispheres
      2. Terminal Lamina
      3. Two lateral ventricles and part of the third ventricle of the brain's ventricular system
      4. Foramina of Monro that connect the lateral ventricles to the third ventricle

B. Diencephalon (posterior part of the forebrain)
 1. Thalamus
 2. Hypothalamus
 3. Metathalamus
 4. Epithalamus
 5. Subthalamus
 6. Part of the third ventricle

II. Midbrain (mesencephalon)
 A. Tectum (rooflike structure)
 B. Cerebral Peduncles (anterior part of the midbrain)
 C. Tegmentum
 D. Crus Cerebri
 E. Cerebral Aqueduct of Sylvius (connects third and fourth ventricles of the brain)

III. Hindbrain (rhombencephalon)
 A. Metencephalon
 1. Pons
 2. Cerebellum
 B. Myelencephalon
 1. Medulla Oblongata
 2. Fourth Ventricle of the Brain

Before we get into details with the functions of these various brain structures, we will take a look at concurrent developments in the skull, the spinal cord and the vertebral column.

SKULL FORMATION

During the third and fourth weeks, the notochord induces the formation of chondroblasts in the surrounding mesoderm at the head end of the embryo. As you recall, chondroblasts make cartilage. These chondroblasts make a cartilaginous basal plate which forms a floor, a base for the skull. Ultimately, this cartilage will calcify and the bones of the floor of the skull will be the result. Actually, four somites contribute to the formation of this skull base between the sella turcica (where the pituitary gland drops into the skull floor) and the back part of the occiput. The forwardmost occipital somite disappears and the other three occipital somites fuse together to form the continuous piece of cartilage called the basal plate.

Two lateral cartilage-producing areas extend around the notochord. Somehow the notochord's presence seems to cause the cartilage to keep its distance from it (the notochord). In this way the foramen magnum is formed. The foramen magnum is the big hole in the occiput that allows the spinal cord to pass through and become one with the brain.

Ordinary growth of the cartilage then provides the total floor of the skull. The outer surface or vault of the skull comes from the membrane that encases the primitive brain. The membrane calcifies and forms the bones of the skull vault. This calcification process goes on almost throughout the whole pregnancy. And it continues until the fontanelles are closed during infancy (**Fig. 3-13 and 3-14**).

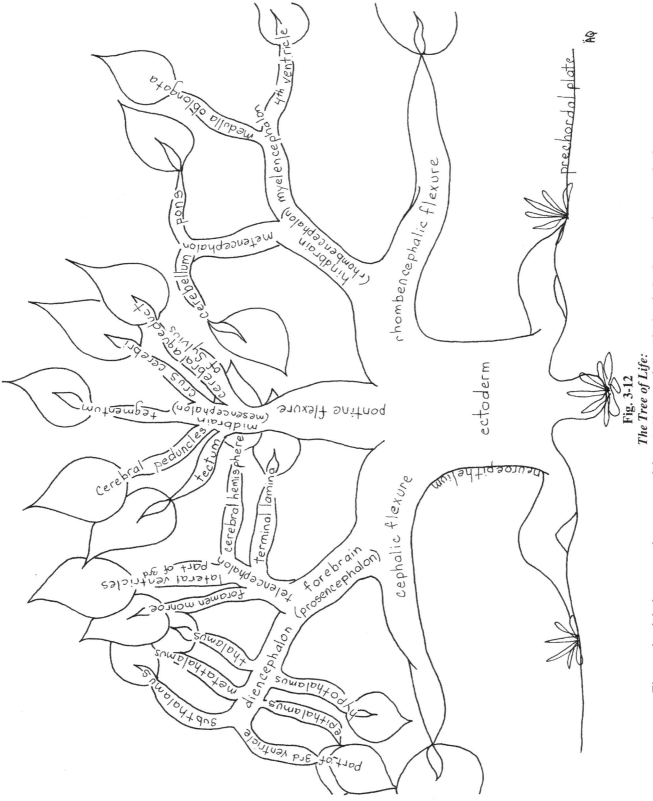

Fig. 3-12
The Tree of Life:

The prechordal plate stops the progress of the primitive streak into the head. It also contributes to the formation of the mouth and the throat. Ectoderm is the embryonic tissue source of all of the central nervous system tissues. It is derived from neuroepithelial cells. This drawing is the artist's conceptual presentation of the dividing and subdividing which occurs as the human brain develops from the embryonic ectoderm.

SPINAL CORD DEVELOPMENT

The development of the spinal cord during the third and fourth weeks of gestational age is a wonderful example of a developmental process which we call induction. Recall that the notochord develops from mesoderm just underneath the ectodermal layer of tissue in the embryonic plate. The notochord induces or causes the line of overlying ectoderm to form the thickening that we call the neural plate. The neural plate then develops two parallel ridges called

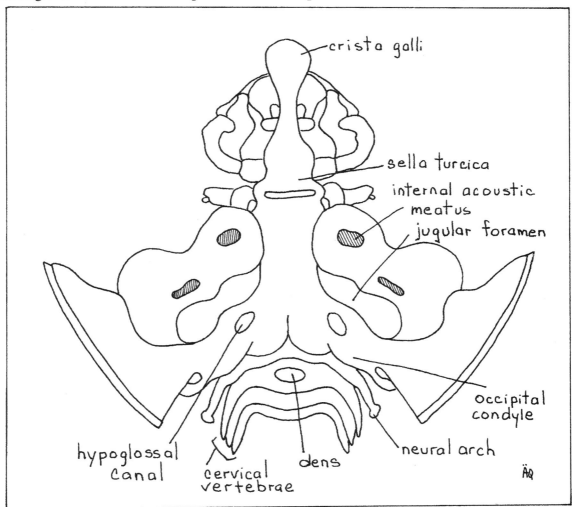

Fig. 3-13
The Chondrocranium at Six Weeks Gestational Age:
The chondrocranium forms the floor of the skull cavity. It is formed from cartilage. The crista galli is a thick, bony prominence that projects upwards from the floor of the skull near the front. The sella turcica is a depression in the sphenoid bone on the midline of the skull which houses the pituitary gland. There is an internal acoustic meatus in each of the temporal bones near their junctions with the occiput. These meatuses connect the inside of the skull with the hearing apparatus. The occipital condyles are the joint surfaces between the skull and the upper vertebra of the neck (atlas). The jugular foramina are on each side between the temporal bones and the occiput. They afford passage to the large veins that drain blood from within the skull (the jugular veins) and to the IXth, Xth and XIth cranial nerves as they exit the skull to innervate many of the body's internal organs and some muscles. These nerves are discussed in detail in Topic 36. The hypoglossal canals pass the hypoglossal nerves through the occiput en route to the tongue from the brain. The dens is an upright bony projection from the second cervical vertebra, about which the first cervical vertebra (the atlas) rotates. The neural arches are the embryonic precursors to the cervical vertebrae.

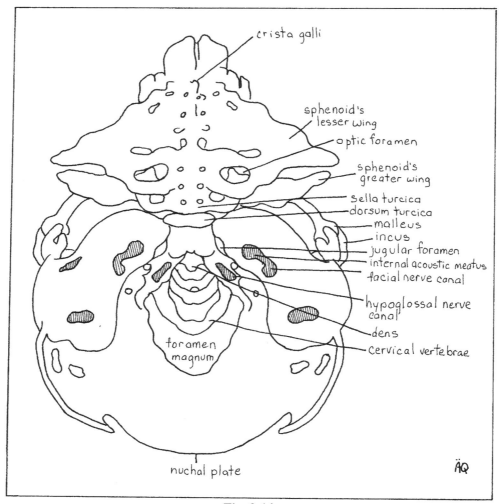

Fig. 3-14
Chondrocranium at 11 Weeks Gestation:
By comparison with Fig. 3-13, it is amazing what can happen in five weeks. The foramen
magnum affords passage for the spinal cord to exit the head and enter the spinal canal.
The malleus and incus are tiny bones in the inner ear that conduct sound. The sphenoid
bone is taking shape. The optic foramina pass the optic nerves to the eyeballs
from inside the skull cavity.

neural folds. These neural folds have a groove between them. The groove is named the neural groove and it lies directly over the notochord that is located in the mesoderm. The neural folds then grow together much like a roof over the neural groove so that a neural tube is formed. The neural tube is the future spinal cord (**Fig. 3-15**). Once the neural tube is a reality, the notochord simply disappears. Research with vertebrate animals (possessing a spine and spinal cord) has demonstrated that experimental interference with a normal notochord will result in deformity of the spinal cord and vertebral column, or it may even result in incomplete or even a complete lack of development of these structures. The notochord just seems to appear, induce the spinal cord and vertebral column to develop and then, having done its job, it disappears.

Now let's look at the details of the spinal cord as it develops. The neural tube will become the spinal canal. The cells which surround the neural tube will give rise to the spinal cord. There is a lot of spinal cord tissue development that goes on during the fourth week of embryonic development.

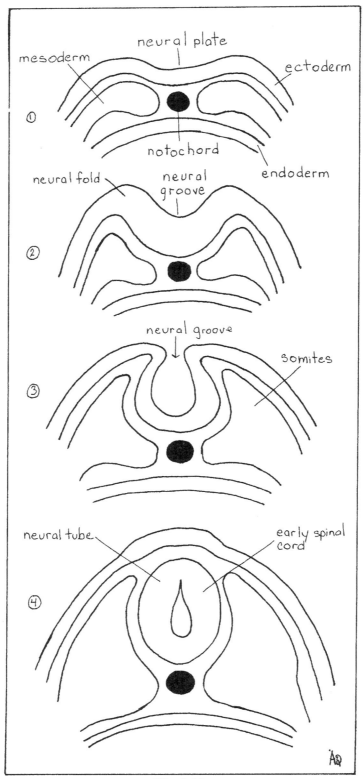

Fig. 3-15
Stages of Spinal Cord Development:
*Notice how the progression of the neural plate to neural groove
and finally to neural tube occurs. The neural tube is the early
spinal cord. The drawings represent cross-sectional views.*

There are actually three layers of cells or tissue that develop around the spinal canal. The layer of cells that are right next to the spinal canal are called the neuroepithelial cells. This layer of cells becomes the neuroepithelial layer. Moving outward from the spinal canal and through the neuroepithelial layer, we encounter the mantle layer and then we meet the marginal layer.

In very short order a very precise and specific process of specialization occurs. Within the mantle layer a very rapid proliferation of neuroblasts occurs. You may recall that the neuroblast is the cell from which a full-fledged neuron (adult nerve cell) will develop. Once the neuroblast is produced, it will no longer undergo cell division (mitosis).

This proliferation of neuroblasts thickens the mantle layer of the developing spinal cord significantly. At the same time a limiting membrane called the sulcus limitans develops in a vertical, transverse direction (left to right or vice versa as you prefer) across the developing spinal cord in such a position that cuts across the midsection of the spinal cord. Since the spinal cord is situated longitudinally in the embryo, the sulcus limitans essentially divides the spinal cord into an anterior (front) longitudinal half and a posterior (back) longitudinal half. The front half will function as the motor or outflow part of the spinal cord. The back half will serve as the sensory or input part of the spinal cord **(Fig. 3-16)**. And as we described previously, there are lots of nerve cells that will connect the left side to the right side and vice versa at every segmental level of the spinal cord. These are called internuncial neurons. There are internuncial neurons that connect the two sides or the two somites (if you wish). There are also internuncial neurons that connect spinal cord segments for short distances above and below.

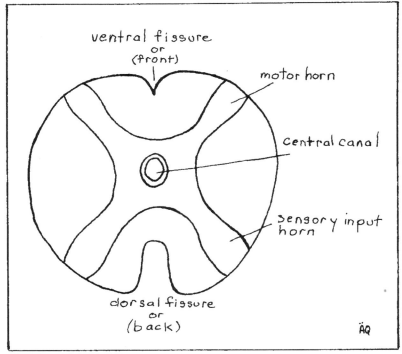

Fig. 3-16
Cross-Section of the Spinal Cord:
The motor and sensory horns represent the segmental outflow
and input nerves that service the somites at a given transverse
level of the body. The central canal is full of cerebrospinal fluid.
The rest of the area shown is taken up by vertical nerve tracts,
which conduct impulses up and down the spinal cord.

By the end of the fourth week the marginal layer nerve fibers appear. This layer begins to accept fibers of ganglion nerves that are sent in to them from the peripheral ganglia. I know this all sounds very confusing and complex, and it is. Please see the illustrations. Especially in this case, a picture is worth a thousand words (**Fig. 3-17**).

The aspect of this process that I find absolutely astonishing is that, during this developmental process, we have millions and perhaps billions of young neurons discovering just where they belong anatomically. They go to the correct destinations with a very high degree of accuracy, and once there they send out connecting fibers that are often three or four feet in length. These connecting fibers travel through a maze of other fibers and tissues to their assigned destinations.

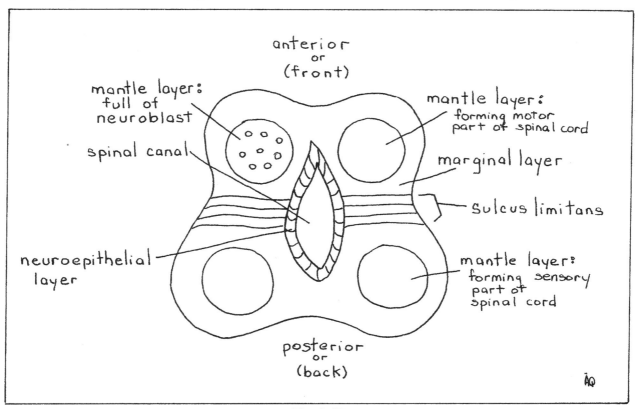

Fig. 3-17
Embryonic Spinal Cord Cross-Section at Four Weeks Gestation:
This is a cross-section of the embryonic spinal cord at about four weeks gestation. The sulcus limitans divides the front half of the spinal cord from the back half. In doing this it separates the nerve impulse outflow in the front from the nerve impulse inflow into the back half. These are called motor and sensory systems, respectively. During this developmental and organizational stage, the sulcus limitans prevents cross talk between inflow and outflow of impulses. See text for further explanation of neuroepithelial, mantle and marginal layers. The spinal canal contains cerebrospinal fluid.

They then begin to function correctly. This is probably the most effectively engineered process that one can imagine. There is presently a tremendous research effort being put forth to help us understand how this works. I will cover some of the fascinating results of these efforts a little later on.

The final result of all of this development is a spinal cord that conducts messages up, down and across itself. The messages almost always seem to get to the right place. The mature spinal cord also has the ability to respond in a reflex manner so that information coming in can be acted upon without waiting for the message to go up to the brain and back. This nervous system of ours, how it got there and how it works places me in a state of awe!

SPINAL CORD SEGMENTATION

Before we move along I should like to discuss the segmentation of the spinal cord and what it means. Segmentation may be considered as the repetition of structural patterns at successive levels in the spinal cord. This pattern of segmentation is found in the spinal cord of all vertebrates. It is apparent very early (third week) in the human embryo. The spinal cord segments furnish nerve supply to each somite according to their individual assignments. Thus, each somite has its own set of segmentally unique spinal nerves.

This segmental relationship to the components of each somite is actually the basis for spinal manipulation and its effect upon organs and tissues other than the manipulated bones. It is via the segmental relationship that a proper manipulation of a specific vertebra or pair of vertebrae can have a beneficial effect upon an internal organ that shares the segmental relationship with the vertebra in question. For example, an effective and correctly applied spinal manipulation of the fourth thoracic vertebra can increase the blood flow to the heart muscle and thus help reverse the effect of lack of oxygen to that heart muscle, perhaps reversing the course of heart disease. This beneficial effect occurs because the heart and the fourth thoracic vertebra share the same spinal cord segment and perhaps the vertebra was "stuck." This stuck condition may cause an excessive input of nerve impulses into that spinal cord segment. As a result, everything that shares that segmental nerve supply becomes hyperactive and irritable. For the heart muscle, this means that the arteries that deliver its blood supply may be contracted so that they are unable to deliver the required amount of blood. Also, the muscles through which they pass may be tight and cause partial obstruction of blood flow.

As the segments of the spinal cord are developing, they are called neuromeres. These neuromeres appear as thickened areas of the spinal cord, thus giving the cord a beaded appearance.

The vertebral column grows faster and attains a greater length than the spinal cord. At the sixth month of gestation the spinal cord actually reaches the top of the sacrum within the vertebral canal. At birth, the spinal cord only reaches the level of the third lumbar vertebra within the vertebral canal. And in adulthood, the spinal cord reaches the disc between the first and second lumbar vertebra (**Fig. 3-18**). This means that the roots of the spinal cord must compensate for its shortness within the vertebral canal. The roots that extend from the end of the spinal cord to the exits from the vertebral canal down at the lower lumbar and sacrum are called the cauda equina. This is Latin for horse's tail.

THE VERTEBRAL COLUMN

During the fourth week of embryonic development (gestational age), the cells of the sclerotome begin to migrate so that they surround the newly forming spinal cord and the notochord. You should recall that the sclerotome is one of the three derivatives of the somite. The other two are the myotome and the dermatome. You should also keep in mind that the notochord

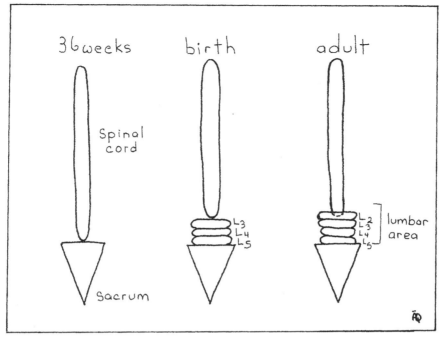

Fig. 3-18
Spinal Cord Length:
This illustration shows the growth and final length discrepancies
between the spinal cord and the vertebral/spinal column. At 36
weeks gestation there is no discrepancy. At birth the spinal cord
only reaches to the level of the third lumbar vertebra, and in the
adult the spinal cord ends at the top of the second lumbar vertebra.
The nerve roots compensate the length discrepancies.

serves as an inducer to stimulate the development of the spinal cord, the somites and the vertebral column. Once the developmental process is established, the notochord disappears.

During this "surrounding process" by the sclerotome cells, the segmental pattern discussed previously is also observed by these sclerotome cells. Soon, hard cell blocks develop in each segment. These hard cell blocks are destined to become the bony vertebrae. Between the hard cell blocks is a softer, less-dense tissue which interconnects these hard cell blocks. This softer interconnecting tissue contains intersegmental arteries.

A little later, the upper and lower parts of adjacent segments unite to form the bodies of the vertebrae. By this method of vertebral body formation, the intervertebral disc, which lies between each two vertebral bodies, becomes located in the middle part of each sclerotome. Therefore, each bony vertebra is intersegmental. It connects two somites or sclerotomes. It is the intervertebral disc that occupies the center of the sclerotome, not the vertebral body as is commonly believed.

The notochord induces the formation of the center (nucleus pulposus) of each intervertebral disc. As this formation continues it is inevitable that the continuity of the notochord is interrupted by each bony vertebral body. This is the beginning of the disappearance of the notochord.

By the end of the fourth week of gestation, the entire blueprint and foundation for the vertebral column, its discs, supporting soft tissues, vascular system and nerve supply are in place. Maturation and refinement of this system then continue throughout the remainder of the pregnancy.

The Fifth Week of Embryonic Life

GENERAL DEVELOPMENT

By the end of this fifth week of embryonic life, the embryo achieves a length of 5 to 8 millimeters from crown (top of the head) to the rump (the tail bone) **(Fig. 3-19)**. This is approximately 1/5 to 1/3 of an inch. The measurement is made from crown to rump because the legs are flexed and pulled up at the hips, making a total length measurement on a live embryo almost impossible from an x-ray or ultrasound image.

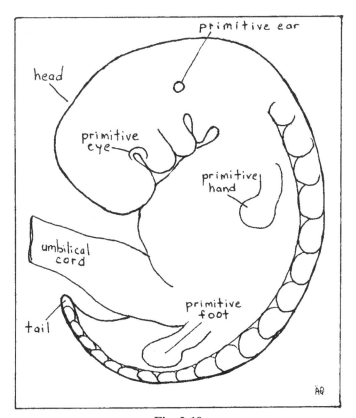

Fig. 3-19
The Embryo at Five Weeks Gestation:
At five weeks of age the embryo is 5-8 millimeters long from crown to rump.
The beginnings of some of the anatomical parts are labeled on this side view drawing.

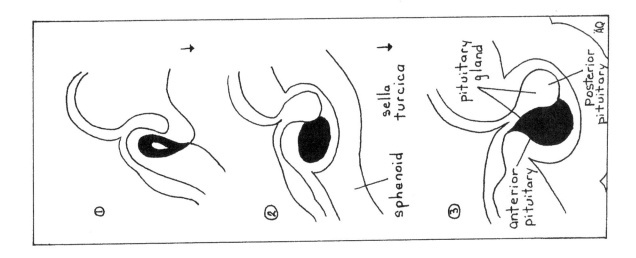

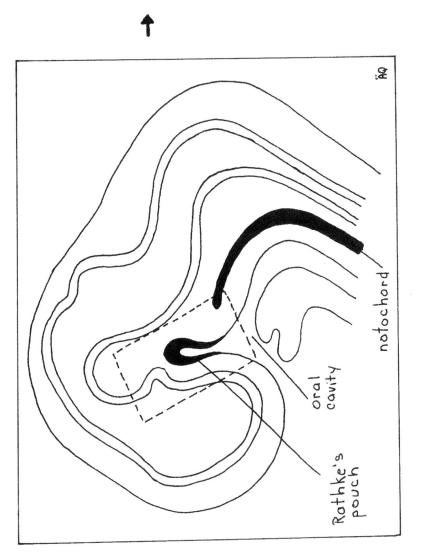

Fig. 3-20
Formation of the Pituitary Gland:
Rathke's pouch is shown in the larger drawing. The three steps of its development in the formation of the pituitary gland are shown in the drawing on the right. See text for further detail.

Previously, we saw the arms and legs begin to develop in their rather primitive form. During this fifth week we see the beginnings of hands and feet starting to show up at the ends of the arms and legs. The arms grow more rapidly than the legs.

Concurrently, there is a rather extensive development of the head region going on which involves the early nose, eyes and ears becoming apparent. Formation of that very important master gland, the pituitary, begins during this fifth week. There is a little pouch called Rathke's pouch that has formed from the oral cavity. This pouch closes during the fifth and/or sixth week in order to form the sella turcica, a sort of cave-like depression in one of the bones that form the floor of the skull cavity above the mouth. This bone that houses the sella turcica is the sphenoid bone **(Fig 3-20)**. The sella turcica houses the pituitary gland. Failure of Rathke's pouch to close during the fifth and/or sixth week of embryonic life results in a tumor called a craniopharyngioma. The craniopharyngioma is really a cystic mass that develops along the route of the Rathke's pouch that has failed to close. The unclosed pouch actually forms a canal that connects the embryo's oral cavity with its sella turcica. There may be more than one craniopharyngioma that develops in the canal that is formed when Rathke's pouch fails to close.

Also during this fifth week, the blood vessels that connect mother to embryo are developed in one of the membrane layers that surround the embryo. This is the allantois membrane. The primitive aorta, which is the main artery coming from the heart, divides into the aorta and the pulmonary artery. This division accommodates the division of the initially formed two-chambered heart into the more sophisticated four-chambered heart **(Fig. 3-21)**.

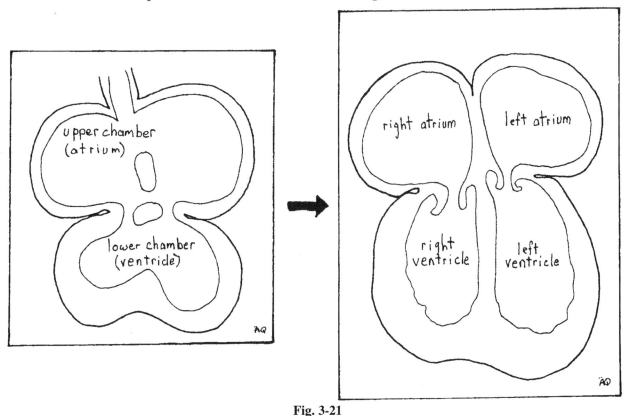

Fig. 3-21
Development of the Two-Chambered Heart into the More Complex Four-Chambered Heart:
During this fifth week of gestation the vertical system that separates the right side of the heart from the left side develops. In this way the heart actually becomes two separate pumps. The right side pumps blood to the lungs. The left side pumps blood to the rest of the body.

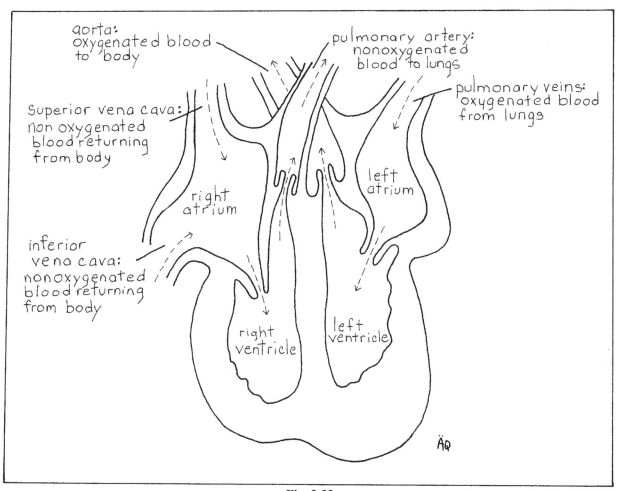

Fig. 3-22
Blood Flow Through the Four-Chambered Heart:
The four-chambered heart is in action by the end of the fifth week of gestation. However, the lungs do not act as oxygenators for the blood until the fetus is delivered and begins to breathe air outside of the uterus, as illustrated in this adult heart.

The right side of the four-chambered heart receives blood from the veins of the body into its upper chamber (auricle). This venous, oxygen-poor blood then passes through the tricuspid valve into the lower chamber (ventricle), which then pumps this blood into the pulmonary artery for circulation through and future oxygenation by the lungs. The lungs will begin to function later on as oxygenators at the time of delivery. The upper chamber (auricle) on the left side of the heart receives the oxygenated blood from the lungs and passes it through the mitral valve into the lower chamber (ventricle) on the left side. This ventricle then pumps the oxygenated blood into the aorta, which distributes this "rejuvenated" blood to the arterial system of the body **(Fig. 3-22)**. You can see this system developing as the two-chambered heart becomes a four-chambered heart, and the primitive aorta divides into a pulmonary artery that sends blood to the lungs and the more-mature aorta that distributes blood to the rest of the body.

There is a duct that connects the aorta and the pulmonary artery called the ductus arteriosus **(Fig. 3-23)**. This duct is necessary until the lungs become functional oxygenators. The fetal lungs do not actually put oxygen into the blood until that first breath after delivery. Sometimes the ductus arteriosus does not close when the lungs begin to function. This condition may require surgical correction.

Other events that are taking place during this jam-packed fifth week of embryonic life include the visible development of the genital glands (ovaries and testes). The duct of Müller is visible also. This duct is the beginning of the kidney-bladder system that will ultimately be used to excrete urine. Bony development of the lower jaw (mandible) and the collar bones (clavicles) also becomes apparent.

The brain and spinal cord are developing very rapidly during this fifth week of gestation. In those ganglia, which are known as dorsal root ganglia and which will serve as sensory input conductors for stimuli coming in to the central nervous system from the body, young nerve cells are sending fibers into the spinal cord. These fibers will be known as sensory dorsal nerve roots. They enter the back or posterior part of the spinal cord. In the front or anterior part of the spinal cord, young neurons are sending out nerve fibers that will connect up mostly with muscles. This anterior development is the beginning of the motor nervous system that tells these muscles when to contract, when to relax and so on. It enables my hand to write these words. It enables your hands to turn these pages as you read these words.

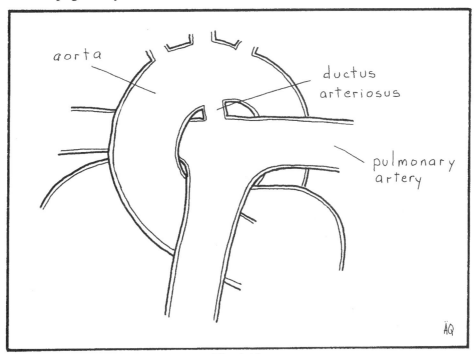

Fig. 3-23
Ductus Arteriosus:
The ductus arteriosus is shown in this drawing. This duct must remain open until the lungs become functional after birth, then it must close. Failure of closure is known as patent ductus arteriosus. This condition may require surgical correction.

THE AUTONOMIC NERVOUS SYSTEM

The part of the nervous system called autonomic, which functions largely beneath your level of awareness, is also beginning to lay out its foundation. Neural crest cells have migrated out from their original position between the neural groove and the surface ectoderm on the embryonic plate and formed (sympathetic) autonomic ganglia that are adjacent to the spinal cord on both sides. These ganglia are connected to nerve cells within the spinal cord. Now the ganglion nerve cells begin to send out nerve fibers that enter the adrenal glands, the heart muscle, many of the blood vessels and so on. In short, these sympathetic ganglia innervate organs and tissues that are called upon to help your body respond to increased levels of stress and the many demands of life's adversities.

THE BRAIN

The brain also grows very rapidly during this fifth week of embryonic life. At the beginning of the week the cerebral hemispheres make their appearance known as two rather rapidly growing out-pouchings at the forward or head end of the neural tube. This, of course, happens at the forebrain ahead of the lamina terminalis which separates the most forward or head end of the brain from the other or lower parts. As we said previously, the forebrain produces by its division the telencephalon and the diencephalon largely during these fourth and fifth weeks of development.

The midbrain lies immediately behind the lamina terminalis. It (the midbrain) does not further subdivide as do the forebrain and the hindbrain. The midbrain becomes a part of the brain stem. It also becomes a significant part of the motor-control system of the brain, and it contains within it the nuclei or control centers for the cranial nerves that control and coordinate eye movement, pupil dilation and constriction. The midbrain also participates in systems that control our hearing reflexes and the function of our internal organs. In addition, it is a significant participant in the receipt of sensory input information. Within the part of the neural tube's central canal, or lumen, that passes through the midbrain, the aqueduct of Sylvius is formed. This aqueduct is the connection between the third and fourth ventricles of the brain through which cerebrospinal fluid passes. It is a malformation of this aqueduct of Sylvius that accounts for the majority of hydrocephalus problems. This aqueduct is first developed during this fifth week of embryonic life (gestation).

Also during this fifth week of gestation, the hindbrain is very busy. As we have said before, it further subdivides into the metencephalon which gives us the pons and cerebellum, and the myelencephalon which becomes the medulla (oblongata). Also, the lumen of the neural tube that runs through the hindbrain will dilate during this week to become the fourth ventricle of the brain.

Because the brain is growing much faster now than its container (the skull), certain flexures become much more exaggerated in the hindbrain area. First is the pontine flexure between the metencephalon and the myelencephalon. This flexure (pontine) has its acute angle facing towards the back. The second flexure in the hindbrain is the rhombencephalic flexure, which has its acute angle facing forward. It is located between the medulla oblongata and the spinal cord (**Fig. 3-11**).

The hindbrain also houses the nuclei, or subsidiary, control centers for the eighth, ninth, tenth, eleventh and twelfth cranial nerves. The eighth, the vestibulocochlear nerve, controls equilibrium, balance and hearing. The ninth, the glossopharyngeal nerve, controls taste, secretion of saliva, sensation from the back part of the tongue, pharynx, tonsils, tubes to the ears, and carotid arteries in the neck, as well as some motor control of swallowing and the pharyngeal muscles. The tenth, the vagus nerve, offers a wide motor supply to muscles of the larynx and pharynx. It also provides some controlling nerve supply to the heart, blood vessels, trachea, bronchi, gastrointestinal tract from the pharynx to the colon (except for its last two or three feet), and to all the associated glands. The tenth cranial nerve also controls sensory sensations from parts of the meninges, the ear and the eardrum, some taste, the soft palate, and a small amount of motor control to major neck muscles (trapezius and sternocleidomastoideus muscles). Clearly, this is an important and very major nerve. The tenth nerve (vagus) is sometimes entrapped and receives undue pressure at the base of the skull during obstetrical delivery. This problem will often result in a colicky baby, or a baby who doesn't breathe or swallow very well. The eleventh, the accessory nerve, is exclusively motor in function. It services the pharynx, larynx, soft palate, and some of the major neck muscles, namely the trapezius and the sternocleidomastoideus muscles. Control of these muscles is shared with the vagus nerve. The twelfth, the hypoglossal nerve, is also exclusively motor in function. Its major function is to move the tongue. Some of its branches go to the smaller muscles of the upper neck.

The sulcus limitans divides the front part (motor) from the back part (sensory) of the spinal cord. This sulcus limitans, which is really a fibrous barrier, extends from the spinal cord forward through the hindbrain and into the midbrain, where it continues to act as an insulator as it segregates the motor neurons from the sensory neurons **(Fig. 3-24)**.

You can see the tremendous amount of development that has occurred during this week, not only in the brain and spinal cord but in the whole embryo...and remember, it's only between 1/5 and 1/3 of an inch long.

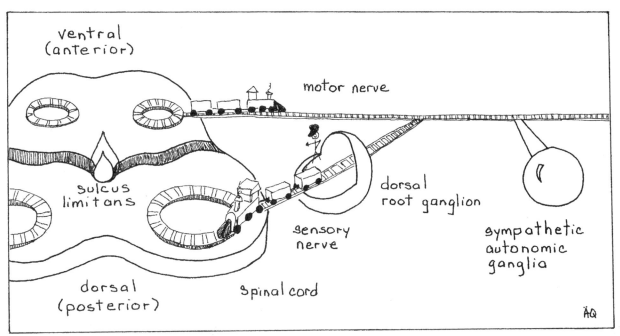

Fig. 3-24
The Sulcus Limitans:
The sulcus limitans, by acting as an insulator between the sensory and motor divisions of the spinal cord, prevents short circuiting of nerve impulses. It forces the use of the internumerical neurons and helps maintain order in the spinal cord.

Topic 7

The Sixth Week of Embryonic Life

During this sixth week of embryonic life, or gestation (as you prefer), the embryo usually achieves a crown-rump length (remember, this is top of head to tailbone length) of between 10 and 14 millimeters (3/8 to 5/8 of an inch). The primitive arms and legs continue their development. The umbilical vesicle, which relates to the yolk feeding system, ceases to develop and begins to atrophy **(Fig. 3-25)**.

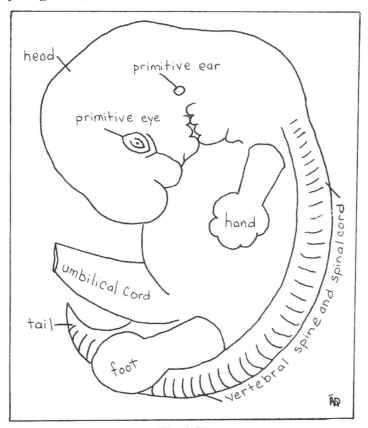

Fig. 3-25
The Six-Week-Old Embryo:
The embryo is much more detailed now. But its crown-rump length is only about 3/8 to 5/8 of an inch. The hands are developing primitive fingers. The eyes and ears become much more apparent this week.

Also, the pharyngeal or branchial clefts disappear. (In fish these clefts would become the gills.) Cartilage development in the spinal (vertebral) column, the skull and the ribs is visible. By the end of this sixth week, the tongue, the larynx (voice box), the germs that will become the teeth, the rudimentary thyroid gland, the kidneys, the bladder and the beginnings of the genitals are all present.

The growth of the nervous system and brain includes the continuation of the development of the dorsal (sensory inflow) nerve roots of the spinal cord. The nerve roots began their development during the fifth week of gestation as the dorsal root ganglia began sending fibers into the spinal cord. This process continues as these dorsal roots become quite prominently developed. In addition, during this sixth week of gestation these same dorsal root ganglia begin sending fibers out into the periphery of the body towards their assigned organs and structures. How these fibers find their proper destinations amidst all of the seemingly chaotic development that is going on is a wonderment. However, these dorsal ganglion nerve fibers do indeed find their assigned destinations within their myotomes, sclerotomes and dermatomes **(Fig. 3-26)**. Ultimately, they will relay information from the peripheral organs and structures to which they connect centralward to the spinal cord. This information, be it pain, temperature, pressure, touch, "warm glow," etc., will then be relayed to the proper place in the brain where it will be screened, interpreted, acted upon and perhaps sent into our conscious awareness. Much of this sensory input (sensation) does not reach our conscious awareness. If most of it did invade our awareness we would probably break down from the overload. Imagine feeling what goes on in your right kidney compared to your left kidney, your liver and your gall bladder, the arteries to your legs, your stomach and intestines 24 hours a day. Add to it every sensation in your skin, your muscles, your bones and so on all day long. Could you handle it? I know I couldn't. So, screening and censoring of input information is of vital importance to our thought process and perhaps to our sanity.

By the end of the sixth week the rudimentary development of the five brain vesicles is complete. Recall that the hindbrain vesicle further divides into the myelencephalon and the metencephalon. The midbrain vesicle, or mesencephalon as it is more formally named, does not further subdivide. The forebrain vesicle divides into the diencephalon and the telencephalon. These divisions are all completed during this sixth week, and the development of the derived brain parts is well-established in a rudimentary fashion.

There is an isthmus, or non-widened area of brain apparent now which separates the hindbrain from the cerebrum. This isthmus actually contains the midbrain.

The cerebral hemispheres, which began formation during the end of the fourth or early fifth week of gestation, have grown very rapidly during this sixth week. By the end of the sixth week, they cover or overlay the diencephalon, the midbrain (mesencephalon) and the cerebellum, which has begun its development this week. This means that the cerebral hemispheres now overlay about three-quarters of the brain beneath them. Because of their rapid growth, the two cerebral hemispheres begin to contact each other at the midline, causing them to flatten on their medial or midline sides. As the two hemispheres flatten against each other, it is the dural membrane (falx cerebri) that separates them. They now grow outwards. This outward growth, along with the medial side flattening, creates a deep fissure between them. This fissure is known as the longitudinal cerebral fissure **(Fig. 3-27)**. The membrane that separates the two hemispheres and

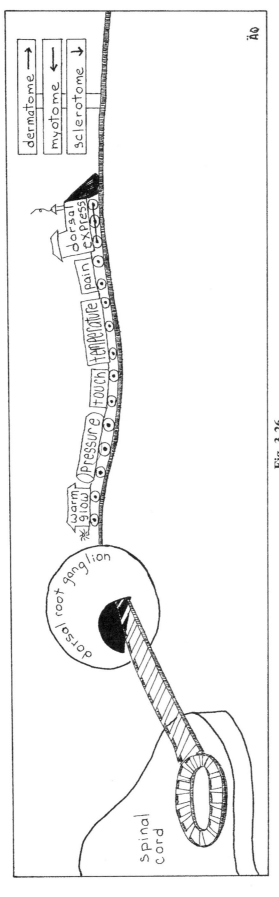

Fig. 3-26
The Dorsal Root Ganglia Make Their Connections:

It is nothing short of miraculous that the dorsal root ganglia are able to send out sensory receptors to the peripheral body to exactly the right places, and at the same time make-proper connections within the spinal cord so that this information will get on the correct tract that goes to the right place in the brain.

occupies the fissure is known as the falx cerebri. The falx cerebri is made up of dura mater, which is the proper name for the outer layer of the three layered meninges that cover the brain and spinal cord. This system of meningeal membranes is very apparent by the end of the sixth week. We will discuss the meningeal membrane system in great detail at the time of the delivery, because it is of great importance to brain and spinal cord development and function throughout life.

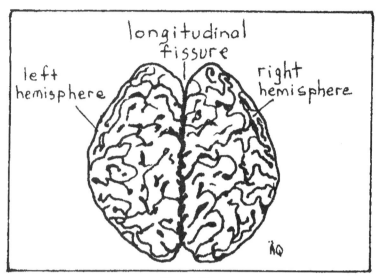

Fig. 3-27
The Longitudinal Fissure:
This is a top view of the developing brain, which illustrates how the two hemispheres are divided by the longitudinal fissure.

Topic 8

The Seventh Week of Embryonic Life

During this seventh week of embryonic life, the embryo will achieve a crown-rump length of 3/4 to 1 inch (**Fig. 3-28**). Using the ultrasound we can begin to see the beginning of movements of the hands and newly formed fingers. The internal organs are quite visible during this week, as are the differentiated genital organs. It is true that the chromosomes that determine the physiological sex of the child are present at the time of fertilization. However, the developing sex organs of the female or male are grossly the same until this seventh week. Now they begin to show the male-female differences.

During this week, ossification (formation of bone) from cartilage becomes perceptible in the skull as well as in the ribs, the scapulae (shoulder blades), the bones of the arms and the legs, and the hard palate of the mouth.

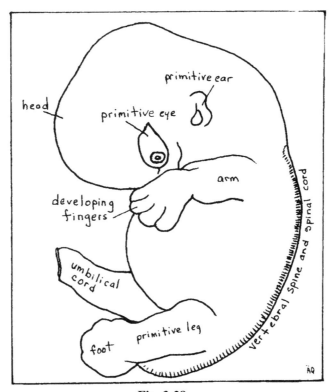

Fig. 3-28
The Seven-Week Embryo:
The seven-week-old embryo is about 3/4 to 1 inch in crown-rump length. The newly formed fingers are beginning to move. The internal organs are visible by ultrasound examination.

The nervous system makes giant strides during this seventh week. Neuroblasts are hard at work creating the grey and the white matter of the brain. The grey matter is essentially made up of nerve cell bodies, and the white matter is composed largely of the axons (nerve fibers) that are the communication extension lines between neurons. The white matter is what is seen on the surface of the brain hemispheres.

At the same time that all of this brain and spinal cord development is going on, the muscles, which will take their orders from the motor part of the nervous system, are perceptible. Movements of these muscles begin during the seventh week of embryonic life.

The spinal cord differentiation into input or sensory afferents and outflow, or motor efferents, is well-established during this seventh week. As you recall, the sensory input comes into the dorsal (back) part of the spinal cord, and the motor outflow goes out the anterior (front) part of the spinal cord. These sensory and motor parts of the spinal cord are clearly divided, but keep in mind that there are nerve fibers developing that will provide direct communication between the sensory input part of the spinal cord and the motor outflow. These interconnecting fibers are the means by which we have spinal reflexes.

These spinal reflexes provide the means by which our body can react to something before our brain gets the message. The classic example is touching a hot object with your finger and having your hand jump back before your brain receives the message and issues the order to pull your finger back. It is as though you watch your hand do something of its own volition and you are just an observer, except that you become aware of the burning sensation somewhere around the time that you see your hand move. I am often amazed at the way in which I watch my body do things without a conscious order from my brain. Going a step further, there have been a few studies done that show that pianists' and violinists' hands do things with their instruments in a reflex manner without orders from the brain or even the spinal cord. Even without these "brainy" directions, the result is oftimes beautiful music.

The spinal ganglion nerve cells began development earlier in the sixth week of embryonic life. During the seventh week they are sending out a multitude of sensory nerve fibers to the peripherally located end organs. This process continues in earnest through the rest of the embryonic period, which ends at the close of the eighth week.

Also during this seventh week, the pupil of the eye forms. The nose becomes more prominent. However, the nostrils are directed forward. The upper lips are formed and will be completed by the end of the eighth week. Interference with this process during the seventh and eighth weeks by disease, toxicity, emotional upset and the like may result in a harelip. The hard palate will complete its fusion a little later. Failure of this fusion results in a cleft palate (**Fig. 3-29**).

Also during this seventh week of embryonic life, the eyelids and the ears are showing themselves. The previously mentioned flexures of the brain begin decreasing in acuteness and the embryo's neck begins to lengthen.

The brain itself is going through remarkable development on several fronts during this time. The forwardmost part of the brain, the telencephalon, produces the olfactory lobes which will ultimately produce the limbic lobes, also called the rhinencephalon. This brain area, in conjunction with the sensory receptor system, gives us our sense of smell. Smell is not so simple. The perception of smell is very closely tied to memory and emotion. We will discuss this vital area and its interrelationship with the limbic system and the "mammalian brain" a little later.

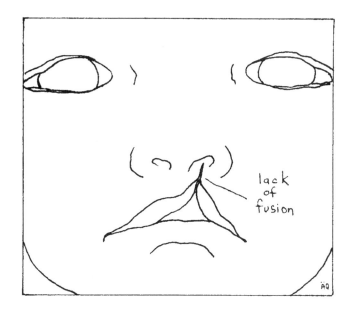

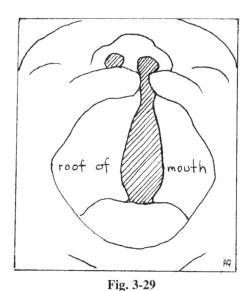

Fig. 3-29
The Harelip or Cleft Palate:
The harelip and/or the cleft palate result from
some problem during the seventh or eighth
week of pregnancy that interferes with the
midline fusion by the fetus. These congenital
deformities often require surgical correction.

Concurrently, the roof of the diencephalon (the posterior subdivision of the primitive forebrain) forms many of the nuclei and structures which become the thalamus (thalamic system) and the hypothalamus. The thalamic system becomes a very complex relay station for nerve impulses coming up from the sensory system of the spinal cord. It is largely the thalamic system that sorts these incoming messages and decides which brain area should receive which message. This thalamic system also sees to it that brain orders being sent out, which require that action be taken, go to the correct nerves that will send appropriate impulses in order to initiate action by appropriate muscles and other effector organs.

Also during this week, the roof of the diencephalon (the posterior or back subdivision of the primitive forebrain) forms the pineal gland. The pineal gland is highly controversial even today. Some believe that it has a lot to do with our circadian rhythms. Some believe it to be very much involved in the immune system. Others believe it to be part of a magnetic system that keeps us oriented within the magnetic field of the earth. Still others believe it to be the "third eye." And there are the skeptics who believe that it does nothing. Take your choice.

The choroid plexus is a system that extracts cerebrospinal fluid from blood. This system relies largely upon the principles of osmotic pressure and selective conduction mechanisms. Cells located in the roof of the diencephalon form the choroid plexus largely during the seventh and eighth week. The specialized cells from which the choroid plexus is formed are called the ependymal cells. These ependymal cells are a specialized subdivision of the epithelial cells.

Sometimes there is an abnormal formation in the roof of the diencephalon. It sags and causes an obstruction to the flow of cerebrospinal fluid from the lateral into the third ventricle of the brain. This is called a paraphysis. If this problem presents after birth it can cause a form of hydrocephalus.

The Eighth Week of Embryonic Life

This eighth week of embryonic life, at its completion, marks the end of the embryonic period of gestation **(Fig. 3-30)**. The embryo will be about 1 1/8 to 1 1/4 inches in crown-rump length. All of the organ systems are established. From this time forward, these organ systems will develop and refine, but all the blueprints are laid out.

Well-defined finger and toe joints are present. The upper and lower divisions of both the arms and the legs are quite distinct, and the clefts between the fingers and the toes are present. There is visible ossification of the ulna and the radius (bones of lower arm), of the fibula and tibia

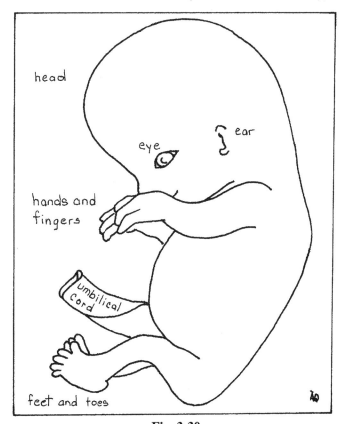

Fig. 3-30
The Eight-Week-Old Embryo:
The eight-week-old embryo has finally passed the 1-inch mark.
It is usually between 1 1/8 and 1 1/4 inches in crown-rump
length. Fingers, toes and much of the bony skeleton are now
present. It is astonishing to see a human being at this size.

(bones of the lower leg), and of the ilium (the hip bone). All of the bodies of the vertebrae are cartilaginous now, and the two halves of the hard palate are united by the end of this eighth week of gestation. A problem prior to the end of this eighth week may result in a cleft palate. The larynx (voice box and Adam's apple) is now formed in cartilage. Salivary glands are now present. The septa that divide the two upper and the two lower chambers of the heart are now well established. The spleen and the beginnings of the adrenal glands are present. The eyes begin to develop lenses, and the membrane which covers the pupil of the eye is present.

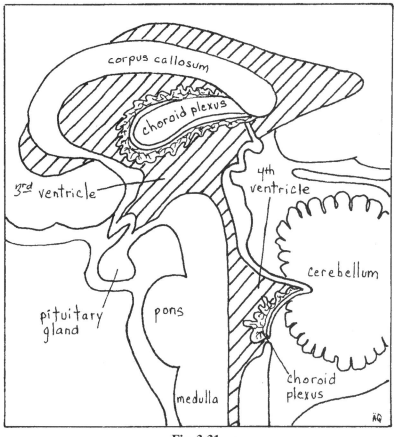

Fig. 3-31
The Beginnings of the Choroid Plexus:
The third and fourth ventricles are shaded. The rudimentary choroid
plexus is shown projecting into both of these ventricles.

By the end of the eighth week of embryonic life, the whole nervous system has undergone phenomenal development. The neuroblast production is completed. This means that, by the end of the eighth week, all of these cells (neuroblasts) that will form the nerve cells in the entire nervous system are present and no new neurons can develop. At least that is the present wisdom. I prefer to keep an open mind on this issue simply because I have seen things happen with patients, sometimes, that suggest the possibility that new neurons (nerve cells) may be formed later in life than our present body of knowledge would lead us to believe.

The neuroepithelial layer of cells, which lies next to the inner membrane lining of the neural tube, has changed or differentiated into cells called glioblasts. The glioblasts will become neuroglia cells a little later on. These neuroglia cells will then migrate to all parts of the body where nerves go. This means all through the body. The neuroglia cells then further differentiate into astrocytes and oligodendroglia gliocytes. These cells serve to support the nerve cells. Some of them help to guide the nerve cell projections to their proper destinations throughout the body. Some of them produce the myelin sheath that surrounds nerve fibers. They also play a role in the healing process in the case of injury to the nerve or neurological disease. A single layer of cells (the ependymal cells) do not migrate away from the membrane. This layer of ependymal cells remain behind and form the choroid plexus.

The meningeal membranes, which are the three layers of membrane that enclose the brain and spinal cord as well as some of the major nerve roots, are well formed by the end of this embryonic phase of development. These membranes have been derived as follows: the pia mater from neural crest cells; the arachnoid membrane from neural crest and mesenchyme cells; and the outermost membrane, the dura mater, strictly from mesenchymal cells.

In the brain itself the ventricular system is well formed by the end of the embryonic phase of development. The choroid plexus develops as tiny tuft-like projections into the ventricular system of the brain **(Fig. 3-31)**. The choroid plexus interacts with the blood vascular system in the brain tissue and filters out the cerebrospinal fluid from the blood. The constituency of the cerebrospinal fluid is quite different from blood, in that normal cerebrospinal fluid contains no cells that originate in the bloodstream. There are a few cells that originate within the ventricular

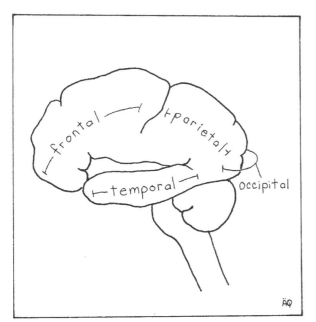
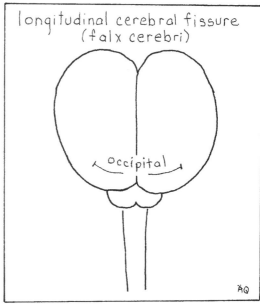

Fig. 3-32
Early Development of the Major Lobes of the Brain:
The frontal lobes are the first to appear. Next we see the parietal lobes. The temporal and the occipital lobes appear concurrently and last.

system itself and which are discharged into the fluid. Also, the cerebrospinal fluid glucose (sugar) level is about 50-75 milligrams per hundred milliliters of fluid whereas, in the blood serum, the normal fasting level of glucose is 80 to 100 milligrams per 100 milliliters. One other important difference is that the level of total protein substances in cerebrospinal fluid is only 15 to 45 milligrams per 100 milliliters whereas, in blood serum, the total protein concentration is sometimes 200 times greater. That is, 6000 to 8000 milligrams (6 to 8 grams) per hundred milliliters. These comparisons offer testimony to the efficiency of the filtration abilities of the choroid plexus, which extracts the cerebrospinal fluid from the blood as this blood circulates through the capillary system adjacent to the brain's ventricular system.

By the end of this embryonic phase of development a most remarkable growth has occurred in the cerebral cortex. By its growth and folding, it now provides a cap over about two-thirds of the subcortical brain. It is coming down over the sides and posterior (back) part of the brain. First the cortex forms the frontal lobes of the brain. Next it forms the parietal lobes, and last, the temporal and occipital lobes form concurrently **(Fig. 3-32)**. It is also noteworthy that the limbic or mammalian brain development is well underway at the end of this eighth week. We will discuss this in much greater depth later on, in Section V, Topic 20. For the present simply know that this system is all set up in this 1 1/8- to 1 1/4-inch-long embryo.

Clinically the significance of the end of this embryonic period of development is simply that problems during the first eight weeks of pregnancy usually result in a defective design or the absence of a part or structure within a given system in the newborn. Since after the eighth week all of the building blocks for all of the systems are present, problems that appear in the second phase (fetal phase) of the pregnancy result in lack of growth and or development for the affected part of the system. The latter situation offers greater hope of remediation by treatment than does the former.

Section III B

The Fetal Period of Growth

The Third Month of Gestation

The third through the ninth month of the pregnancy is known as the fetal phase. The embryo, as if by magic, suddenly becomes the fetus. You may wonder whether the third month begins with the beginning of the ninth week, which would be the 57th day of gestation, or whether we have switched to 30- and 31-day months (or 28, 29 for February). In our discussion we will accept the inexactitudes of the biological sciences and call this the beginning of the third calendar month.

THE THIRD MONTH OF GESTATION

During this third month the fetus will usually achieve a crown-rump length of about 3 inches. It grows about 1/2 of an inch per week. At the end of this month, the fetal legs will be about an inch long. The fetus may also begin the third month with the stump of what was a 2-inch tail. This tail will disappear by the end of the month. It leaves only a coccyx, or tailbone.

During this month facial changes occur that make the fetus look much more human. The eyes now face forward and are on the front of the face. Previously, they were more on the sides. However, the upper and lower eyelids are fused together and will remain that way until about the end of the sixth month. The ears are now correctly placed on the sides of the head and some of the inner structures of the ears, such as the ear drums (tympani) and the vestibular apparatus are recognizable. The tympani help us with hearing and the vestibular apparatus helps us with balance and equilibrium.

During this month the arms grow so that they are proportionate with the rest of the body. However, the legs will remain disproportionately short by comparison. We will also see tiny fingernails and toenails about now.

The genital structure becomes well-differentiated during this third month of gestation so that sex determination of the child is now easily possible. Mammary glands, prostate gland and testes are now present. Also, the pericardium, which is the protective covering for the heart, makes its appearance. All of the intestines, some of which were in the umbilical cord until now, move into the fetal abdominal cavity. And the primitive cloaca, which houses the urethra and the anus together, divides so that these two structures are separated from each other. Hence, urine and feces will be eliminated via separate orifices from now on. Also, we see a gall bladder if you can imagine such a thing in a three-month-old product of conception.

It is important to note that the union of the two sides of the hard palate must be complete by about the 10th week of gestation at the latest, or else the chances of a cleft palate at delivery are almost 100 percent (**Fig. 3-29**). A lot more ossification (bone formation) goes on during this third month of pregnancy. Almost all of the bones of the skull are now showing points of ossification from which bone formation will spread. Also, the ischia (bones you sit on) are showing ossification points as are the bones of the hard palate (roof of the mouth). Ossification points are simply the areas in a future bone where the cartilage or membrane begins to calcify and form bone. The bone then spreads out radially from the point of ossification.

Also, the cartilage arches of the spine, down as far as the bottom end of the rib cage, close during this month. As this process progresses, the canal in which the spinal cord is housed and protected is formed. This canal is called the vertebral canal or sometimes, less correctly, the spinal canal.

THE NERVOUS SYSTEM

Within the developing nervous system there is a lot of activity during this third month of pregnancy. The communication lines between the brain and the periphery of the body are called the cortico-spinal tracts. These tracts begin forming during the end of the embryonic phase. They develop very rapidly during the beginning of this fetal phase and will be largely completed by about the end of the seventh calendar month of gestation.

During this month the olfactory (smell) bulbs grow forward from the underside of the cerebral hemispheres and begin developing the connections with the smell receptors in the lining of the nose. Many of the fissures and gyri of the brain tissue become apparent as the cerebral cortex works to develop more surface area (**Fig. 3-33**).

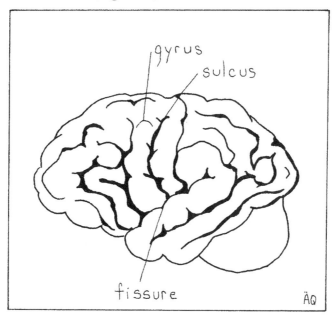

Fig. 3-33
Surface of the Brain:
In order to increase the surface area of the brain fissures,
sulci and gyri develop. The fissures and sulci are the
acute grooves in the surface, and the gyri are the folds
which protrude out from between the fissures and sulci.
This system of "peaks and valleys" increases brain
surface area many fold.

COMMISSURES

During this third month the commissures develop **(Fig. 3-34)**. Commissures are nerve fiber tracts that cross over from one side of the brain to the other and thus function to integrate right and left-side brain activities **(Fig. 3-35)**. The first crossover fibers that appear are in the forwardmost (anterior) part of the brain. These fibers, called the anterior commissure, connect the right and left olfactory bulbs and the right and left temporal lobes of the brain. The second group of crossover nerve fibers are called the fornix commissure. This commissure connects the right and left sides of the hippocampus in the diencephalon area of the brain. In advanced mammals, like people, the hippocampus is highly developed. It seems related to the expression of emotional responses like fear and anger. More about this later.

The third crossover section is probably the most well-known. It is called the corpus callosum. This is a large right-left side crossover structure that connects much of the right and left brain, excluding the olfactory (smell) system. As the corpus callosum develops, the aforementioned fornix commissure recedes somewhat.

Another crossover structure is the optic chiasm that sends some of the visual messages from the right eye to the left side of the brain and vice versa. This system helps us to integrate the total picture that we look at with both eyes. Without it we would see two slightly different visual images and probably suffer from double vision, depending on the ability of the occipital cortex to compensate.

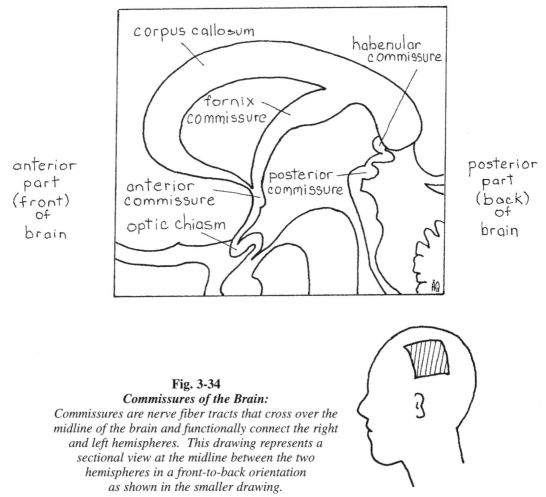

Fig. 3-34
Commissures of the Brain:
Commissures are nerve fiber tracts that cross over the midline of the brain and functionally connect the right and left hemispheres. This drawing represents a sectional view at the midline between the two hemispheres in a front-to-back orientation as shown in the smaller drawing.

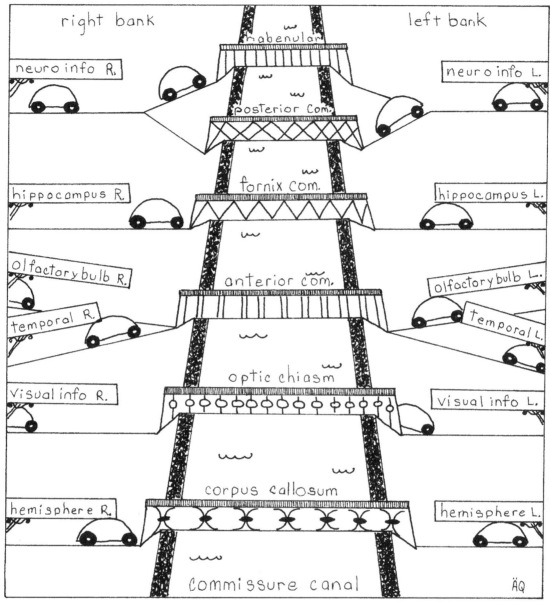

Fig. 3-35
Commissure Functions of the Brain:
*This diagrammatic representation shows the bilateral brain structures that are
connected to each other by the various commissures. The commissures are shown
as bridges across a canal. See text for further details.*

There are two other rather small crossover structures that work largely in conjunction with the thalamus. These are the habenular commissure and the posterior commissure. The thalamus, as you recall, is largely a sorting out and triage part of the brain that decides which information should go to which region of the cerebral cortex for consideration, decision and action. Then when the brain orders the action, the thalamus works on getting the orders to the right body parts to carry out the action.

All commissures are derived from the lamina terminalis. You may recall that the lamina terminalis prevented mesenchyme from entering the head very early on in the embryonic phase of development.

MYELINATION

Myelination of nerve fibers in the brain begins in this third month. The first myelination occurs in the cranial nerves that arise from the midbrain and the medulla oblongata. The medulla, as it is most frequently called, is the end of the brain that connects to the spinal cord. These cranial nerves are largely involved in sucking and swallowing. This myelination probably begins first in preparation for the feeding of more solid food. As you may recall, myelination is done by some of the glial cells, which act in a more or less ancillary fashion to support the neuronal growth, development and function. In the brain and spinal cord, the cells that do the myelination are called oligodendroglia. In the peripheral nervous system the myelination is carried out by the Schwann cells **(Fig. 3-36)**.

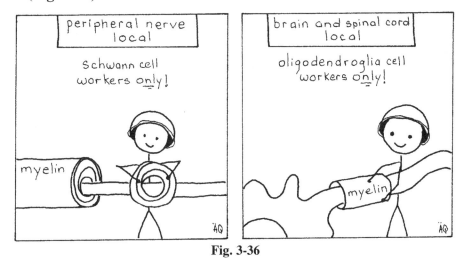

Fig. 3-36
Myelination Union:
In the peripheral nervous system, myelination is carried out by the Schwann cells.
In the central nervous system, myelination is carried out by the oligodendroglia cells.

THE VENTRICULAR SYSTEM

The ventricular system of the brain is fairly well laid out during the embryonic phase of development. In this the third month of gestation, the ventricular system of the brain develops rather fully. It is now appropriate to discuss this system and its functions in greater detail.

The ventricular system is composed of four ventricles, all of which are interconnected via ducts or openings called foramina **(Fig. 3-37)**. The hindmost ventricle connects to the central canal of the spinal cord. Thus, the four ventricles are within the skull and, of course, the central canal of the spinal cord is within the vertebral canal, which is formed by the spinal vertebrae.

All of the four ventricles and the central canal of the spinal cord are derived from the neural tube, which began way back at about the end of the third week of gestation. The forebrain divides into two hemispheres. Hence, the ventricular derivatives of the neural tube within the forebrain duplicate, and each of these hemispheres gets one ventricle. These two paired ventricles are called the lateral ventricles. Incidentally, in biological science a ventricle is defined as a relatively small cavity or chamber. Thus, each hemisphere of developed brain has a "lateral" cavity or chamber (ventricle) within it. These two lateral ventricles connect by way of openings on their medial sides to a third ventricle which is at the midline of the midbrain. These connecting

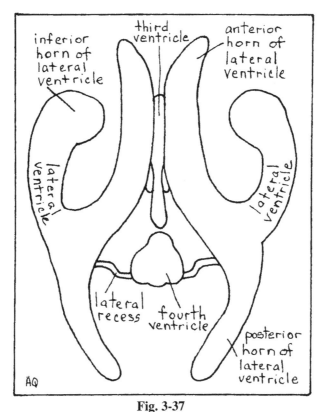

Fig. 3-37
Superior (Top) View of the Ventricular System of the Brain:
Cerebrospinal fluid is extracted from the blood mostly in the lateral
ventricles by the choroid plexuses. This fluid then travels from the two
lateral ventricles to the third and then the fourth ventricle. The fluid
is then released into the subarachnoid spaces and into the central
canal of the spinal cord. It is reabsorbed into the venous blood system
by the arachnoid granulation bodies. See text for further details.

openings are appropriately named the interventricular foramina. These foramina allow cerebrospinal fluid to drain from the lateral ventricles into the third ventricle. From the third ventricle at its lower and backward end is a duct called the aqueduct of Sylvius, which connects this third ventricle to the fourth ventricle of the brain. The fourth ventricle is located largely in the hindbrain. This Sylvian aqueduct allows the flow of cerebrospinal fluid to go from the third into the fourth ventricle.

At its lower end the fourth ventricle connects to the central canal of the spinal cord, which in turn allows flow of cerebrospinal fluid to go down through the center of the spinal cord.

The fourth ventricle also has some other openings in it that allow cerebrospinal fluid to drain into the subarachnoid space. I'll explain this space in just a minute. First, let's identify these other openings from the fourth ventricle. There is one opening on the midline called the foramen of Magendie. There is also a pair of openings, one on each side, that are known as the foramina of Luschka. Thus, the fourth ventricle actually has four openings for the passage of cerebrospinal fluid **(Fig. 3-38)**.

Now let's return to this subarachnoid space and then we will discuss the actual function and dynamics of this system that so effectively distributes cerebrospinal fluid. You recall that there are three membrane layers that encase the brain, the spinal cord, and some of the major nerve roots that exit from the brain and spinal cord.

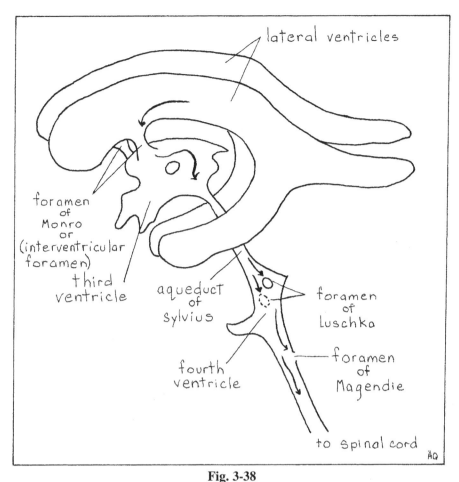

Fig. 3-38
The Ventricles of the Brain with their Interconnections (Side View):
The ventricular system is situated within the brain. The direction of flow of
cerebrospinal fluid is indicated by the arrows. See text for details.

These three membrane layers are, from the inside out (inside being closest to the brain and spinal cord): (1) the pia mater, (2) the arachnoid membrane and (3) the dura mater **(Fig. 3-39)**.

The pia mater is a very delicate membrane that follows all of the convolutions of the brain and spinal cord. It is full of blood vessels, and delivers a significant proportion of the required blood to the brain and spinal cord. This pia mater membrane adheres to the brain and spinal cord, and to the nerve roots for which it forms sheaths. It actually combines with the ependymal cells that have formed the choroid plexus and thus contributes to the formation of these plexuses. In the skull the pia mater is more delicate than it is in the spinal canal. As it covers the spinal cord, the pia mater is somewhat thicker, firmer, and has fewer blood vessels than the part of it that adheres to the brain.

The arachnoid membrane is separated from the pia mater membrane by a space which is called the subarachnoid space. Therefore, the arachnoid membrane does not follow the convolutions of the brain and spinal cord. It is into this subarachnoid space that the aforementioned foramina of Luschka and the foramen of Magendie pass the cerebrospinal fluid. The arachnoid membrane is also quite thin and delicate with lots of blood vessels. The pia mater and the arachnoid membrane are rather loosely connected by little anchoring strands of connective tissue called trabeculations. These trabecular anchoring strands allow for significant and necessary independent movement

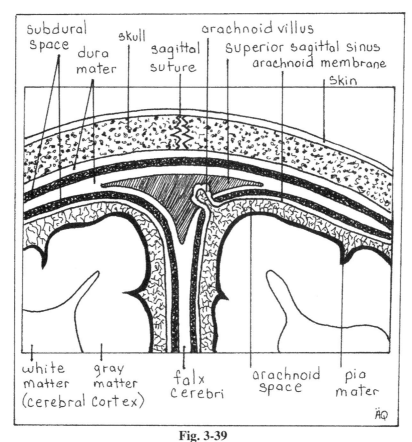

Fig. 3-39
Meningeal Membranes:
*This drawing illustrates the anatomy of the membranes and spaces in
cross-section through the sagittal suture and the superior sagittal sinus.
See text for further details.*

between these two layers of membrane. Without this independent movement we would be very stiff in the spine and have a lot of pain.

The dura mater is the outermost of the three membranes that enclose the brain and spinal cord. It is very tough and rather thick (as membranes go), and although it has lots of blood vessels, most of them supply blood to the bones of the skull and spine rather than to the nervous system. Within the skull the outermost layer of the dura mater (it has two layers) is actually the innermost lining of the skull bones. The dura mater is therefore manipulatable by using the bones to which it attaches as handles, be these bones in the skull, the spine or the pelvis. This is one of the anatomical situations that CranioSacral Therapists use to do their work. There is also a space between the innermost layer of dura mater membrane and the arachnoid membrane which is also fluid-filled. Although the fluid within this space (the subdural space) is not officially called cerebrospinal fluid, it differs little from cerebrospinal fluid in its constituents.

Let's look at how this system of ventricles, fluid, membranes, plexuses and arachnoid villi actually works. The cerebrospinal fluid is extracted from the circulating blood in the areas of brain tissue that lie essentially adjacent to the walls of the lateral and third ventricles of the brain. It is extracted by the choroid plexus which developed largely in this third month of pregnancy. The cerebrospinal fluid, which is extracted from the blood in the lateral ventricles, passes through the interventricular foramina into the third ventricle. If there is a problem with the patency (or openness) of either of these two foramina, the cerebrospinal fluid volume and pressure in the lateral ventricle rises because it is unable to drain. This rise in both cerebrospinal fluid volume and pressure may cause the related lateral ventricle to enlarge and perhaps to interfere with normal brain development in that hemisphere.

Assuming the patency of the two interventricular foramina, the cerebrospinal fluid, which is formed in the lateral ventricles, will drain into the third ventricle. This third ventricle also produces some cerebrospinal fluid which is added to the total volume thus far. The sum total of the cerebrospinal fluid must now drain through the aqueduct of Sylvius from the third ventricle into the fourth ventricle. A malformation of the aqueduct of Sylvius, which compromises this duct's competency, may result in hydrocephalus. This problem usually requires surgical intervention.

From the fourth ventricle we have the four outlets for cerebrospinal fluid to further circulate through this system. One outlet goes into the central canal of the spinal cord and the other three outlets (two foramina of Luschka and one foramen of Magendie) empty into the subarachnoid space. The cerebrospinal fluid that empties into the subarachnoid space can and does bathe the entire surface of the pia mater, the membrane which adheres to the brain and spinal cord in all of their convolutions and nooks and crannies. And there are hundreds, if not thousands, of these nooks and crannies. Recent studies have indicated that cerebrospinal fluid not only bathes the surfaces, but that it also penetrates through the pia mater and into the brain tissue. This is a new and rather revolutionary discovery.

The cerebrospinal fluid is reabsorbed back into the bloodstream by structures called the arachnoid villi. These arachnoid villi are located largely in a place called the sagittal venous sinus **(Fig. 3-39)**. This sinus runs directly under the top of the skull on the midline from front to back. The sinus lies directly beneath the sagittal suture, which is where two of the major bones (the parietal bones) of the top of the skull join together to form a slightly movable joint. This is a suture that CranioSacral Therapists make much use of during the treatment process.

The functions of cerebrospinal fluid still offer several mysteries to modern science. We know that it offers a hydraulic cushion for the brain so that it softens the blows of the delicate brain and spinal cord against their bony containers during accidents and so on. Also, it would seem that the cerebrospinal fluid supplies some nutrition, removes some waste, and perhaps provides some acid-alkaline balance stability for the brain and spinal cord.

Most practitioners of CranioSacral Therapy witness results in patients by working with cerebrospinal fluid and its dynamics, which seem to go far beyond those mentioned in the preceding paragraph. We can conjecture but scientifically acceptable proof is very difficult to obtain when you are working with living, suffering human beings. In any case, the work is done and the results are appreciated even though we cannot as yet offer an impeccable explanation as to what exactly has happened that yields the desired results.

The Second Trimester

THE FOURTH MONTH OF GESTATION

During this fourth calendar month of gestation or pregnancy, as you prefer, the fetus achieves a crown-rump length of 12-13 centimeters, which is about 4 1/2 to 5 inches. The legs lengthen to about 4-8 centimeters, which is about 1 3/4 to 3 1/2 inches. The weight will reach about 500 grams, or about 1 pound and 1 or 2 ounces.

About halfway through this fourth month, the fetus can usually be seen to bring its hands together and turn within the uterus. This corresponds to the beginning of motor function of the nervous system.

Some hardening of the dura mater membrane in the region that overlies the brain occurs. This is the beginning of the skull vault. These are the skull bones that will form the roof and walls of the vault. These bones are formed by ossification or hardening of the outermost membrane layer. This ossification begins during this month and is pretty well completed at the time of delivery except for the fontanelles (soft spots in the newborn baby's head) and the sutures. The sutural development is such at the time of delivery that it allows for some overriding of skull bones upon each other in order to reduce the circumference of the newborn's head as it passes through the birth canal. They also enable a shaping or molding of the newborn head when needed **(Fig. 3-40)**.

During this fourth month all of the spinal arches close. However, the closure is with cartilage which will later change into bone. Points or centers of ossification (bone formation) occur in the upper sacrum (S-1) and the pubic bone. Also, ossification begins in the bones of the ankles and feet. The cartilage of the eustachian tubes and the ring around the ear drums appears. Tonsils are now present. In the male the scrotum forms and in both male and female the prepuce forms. The prepuce is the skin fold that covers the glans (head) of the penis in the male or the clitoris in the female. Eyebrows and head hair appear, and a fine hair called lanugo covers almost the entire body. The fetus is now inhaling and exhaling amniotic fluid through its mouth into and out of the developing respiratory system.

In terms of nervous system development, the outstanding features are the development of motor system function as evidenced by fetal movement in the uterus, and the fact that all rudimentary sensory input systems are ready to refine and develop. All the raw materials are in place. The brain and spinal cord are growing and developing at a very rapid rate.

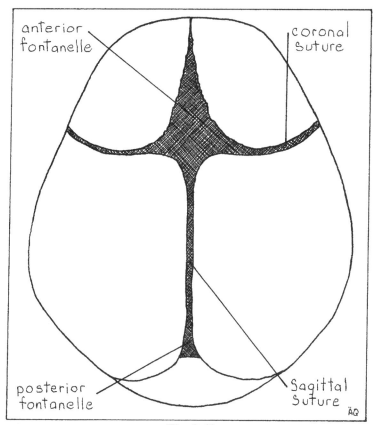

Fig. 3-40
The Fetal Skull (Top View):
Areas of the fetal skull that are not ossified are indicated by the
shaded areas in the drawing. The non-ossified areas allow for
reduction of head size as it passes through the birth canal at the
time of delivery. Also, one bone can override another if need be
without injury to the newborn. Occasionally bony override does
not self-correct. In these cases, CranioSacral Therapy is effective
as early as the first day after delivery.

THE FIFTH MONTH OF GESTATION

During the fifth calendar month of the pregnancy, the length of the fetus from crown to heel is about 5 1/2 to 6 1/2 inches. The mother is feeling lots of movements during this month. This increased movement signifies the further development of the motor nervous system. The development of vernix caseosa begins during this fifth month. This is an almost cream-cheese-looking substance made up of skin cells and sebum that covers the whole body. Sebum is the secretion of sebaceous glands that is composed of fat and cellular debris.

The germ buds of the future teeth become apparent during this fifth month. Ossification points for some of the upper cervical vertebrae and the bones of the base of the skull appear, as well as the bones of the middle ear. The organs of corte which are located in the inner ears appear. These organs are involved in the sense of hearing. They are a part of sound-pitch discrimination. At this time the eyelids remain closed, the nose is plugged, and the mouth and lips are formed. All important physiological systems are now formed. The female uterus differentiates from the vagina.

In the nervous system, rapid development continues. Myelin formation in the spinal cord begins. This myelination process also begins in the dorsal nerve roots which carry sensory input to the spinal cord from the periphery. Myelination also begins in the ventral motor nerve roots, which carry command messages out from the central nervous system to the peripheral effector organs, such as muscles, etc. In addition, the nerve fiber tracts within the spinal cord are developing. These tracts, which transmit messages from the brain, are called the corticospinal fiber tracts. They will carry commands from the motor cortex of the brain to the various muscles and other effector organs of the body.

THE SIXTH MONTH OF GESTATION

During this sixth month of pregnancy, the fetus may achieve a crown-heel length of about 10 inches. And although the nervous and respiratory systems are not fully developed as yet, should the fetus be delivered during this month there is a chance for survival outside the uterus.

Several general maturational characteristics are seen. The fingernails and toenails now project slightly beyond the ends of the fingers and toes. The aforementioned fine body hair (lanugo) persists and covers the whole fetus. The glands of the skin are now apparent (sebaceous glands). Developing lymph follicles will help protect the fetus from noxious substances which may be swallowed not only in the uterus but throughout life.

Also, more ossification points appear in the spinal vertebrae and in the sacrum. The sternum, or breastbone, also now begins to appear as its ossification points develop. The angle that contributes to the upright stance of human beings at the juncture between the lowest lumbar vertebra and the sacrum also becomes apparent.

The central nervous system continues its remarkable development during this sixth month of pregnancy. By now the cerebral hemispheres cover the whole top and sides of the brain, including the cerebellum. Cerebellar development begins during this sixth month of pregnancy, but will not be complete until 1 1/2 to 2 years after delivery. Drugs which affect DNA during cerebellar development may well contribute to cerebellar dysfunction. The cerebellum contributes powerfully to balance, equilibrium and motor coordination. It is this belated cerebellar development that determines when an infant learns to walk, how its sense of balance works and so on.

Within the cerebral cortex, we now have the development of six rather discrete layers. In order to get more surface area with the volume of the skull, the cerebral cortex continues to develop its system of sulci and gyri. Ultimately about two-thirds of the mature cerebral cortex cells will be buried in the walls of the sulci and fissures. The sulci and the fissures are the grooves, and the gyri are the folds formed by the grooves (**Fig. 3-33**). Almost all of the neurons within the central nervous system are present by the end of this sixth month. These neurons formed from neuroblast cells. By the end of the second year after delivery, almost all of the original first layer of cerebral cortex neurons will have died.

This is how brain function develops. At the beginning of development there is an overabundance of nerve cells. Those cells that are not used *initially* then die, which is perhaps why it is more difficult to learn things like piano playing and second languages as you get older. The body builder's saying, "use it or lose it," seems quite appropriate here. Further, this method of development of specialization of neural circuits supports the benefit of varied and generous stimulus input for newborns and infants. It also explains how easily isolation of newborns can inhibit brain development and function. Apoptosis is the official name for this type of neuronal cell death that occurs during the development of neural circuitry.

The Third Trimester

THE SEVENTH MONTH OF GESTATION

The seventh month of the pregnancy is marked by the appearance of many new osseous (bone-growth) points. The osseous growth points in the sacrum are almost all present except for the fourth and fifth segments of that bone. The fetus may well achieve a crown-heel length of about 12 inches. In the male the testes descend into the scrotum. The membranes over the pupils of the eyes disappear and the eyelids open now. Meckel's cartilage totally disappears. This completely eliminates the chance that the infant will be born with fish gills. And if the seven-month fetus is delivered prematurely, he or she has a much better chance for survival outside of the uterus.

In the brain, the sulci and gyri (convolutions) of the cortex are becoming much more prominent so that surface area of the cortex of the brain is greatly increased. Within the brain the insula and tubercula quadrigemina are formed.

The insula is also known as the central lobe. The insula lies deep in the brain and can be seen from either side of the cerebrum only if you separate the lips of the lateral cerebral sulcus so that

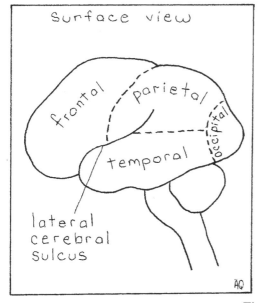
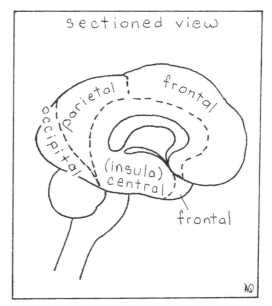

Fig. 3-41
The Insula (Central Lobe):
The insula, or central lobe as it is also known, cannot be seen on the surface of the brain.
You must separate the "lips" of the lateral cerebral sulcus and look into its depths.

you can see into its depths **(Fig. 3-41)**. It relates to both the frontal and the parietal lobes of the brain and to the limbic system via the amygdala.

Essentially, this seventh month of pregnancy is characterized by rapid growth, development and organization.

THE EIGHTH MONTH OF GESTATION

During this eighth month of pregnancy the fetus may achieve a crown-heel length of 16+ inches. It may grow to a weight of 4 1/2 to 5 1/2 pounds. The fine body hair (lanugo) disappears. But the amount of vernix caseosa, sebum and skin cells that are sloughed off increases significantly.

The amount of subcutaneous fat reduces so that, although the skin is pink, it presents a wrinkled appearance.

All of the additional ossification points of the spine are present except for two at the very end of the sacrum.

There is not much new in this eighth month except for growth and strengthening of the body **(Fig. 3-42)**. Also, the nervous system continues making its connections so that the fetus is increasingly receiving more sensory input, and is gaining more control of its movements and organ functions.

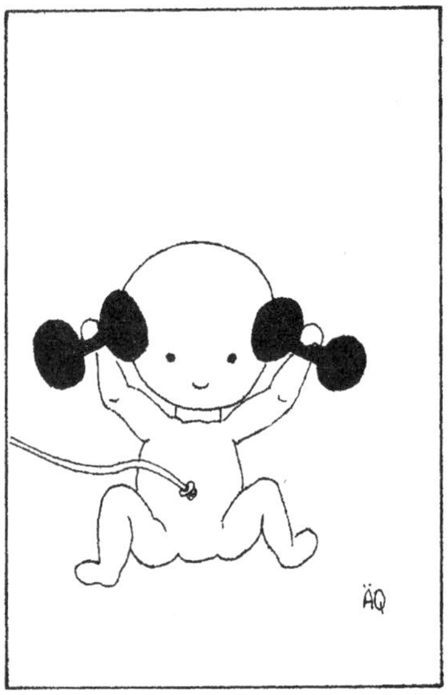

Fig. 3-42
Strengthening at Eight Months:
Most things are in place at eight months of gestation. This is now time for strengthening and development.

THE NINTH MONTH OF GESTATION

During the ninth month the fetus will achieve a crown-heel length of 20 or more inches. It will gain weight up to 6 1/2 to 8 pounds on the average, but there are very many gross variations from these ranges of length and weight.

All ossification points are now in place. The male testes are completely in the scrotum under normal circumstances. The lanugo (fine body hair) is all gone. The umbilicus (belly button) is in the middle of the body. The nine-month fetus is normally very active.

In our present body of knowledge, it says that no new neurons are added after the delivery, so all brain cells must be there by the end of the ninth month. Research has shown that new neurons can form after delivery in animals. But does this generalize to people? We do know that the neurons form new interconnections throughout life. And we know that these new interneuronal connections occur in response to demand. As these new interconnections are formed, we are able to perform new brain functions or improve on some that we already have. It has been shown that a single nerve cell may receive input from over 100,000 different connections. It is the interneuronal connections that give you the intelligence or new skills. It is not the number of neurons involved. Thus, it is never too late to learn to read or to do math. It may take longer as you age, but interconnections related to these demands (or requests if you wish to be more courteous) will occur, and you can learn something new no matter how old you are.

Since the spinal column outgrows the spinal cord, at delivery the spinal cord only reaches to the level of the third lumbar vertebra. When we started this development during the embryonic period, the spinal cord reached all the way to the bottom of the fifth lumbar vertebra. In the full-grown adult the spinal cord reaches to about the bottom of the first lumbar vertebra or perhaps halfway down the second lumbar vertebra. At the time of delivery, the spinal cord usually reaches the level of the third lumbar vertebra. The compensation of the difference in length between the shorter spinal cord and the longer vertebral column is accomplished by longer nerve roots from the spinal cord as one descends from the head towards the tail (bone). These longer nerve roots descend more vertically to get to their proper exits (intervertebral foramina) from within the vertebral canal **(Fig. 3-43)**.

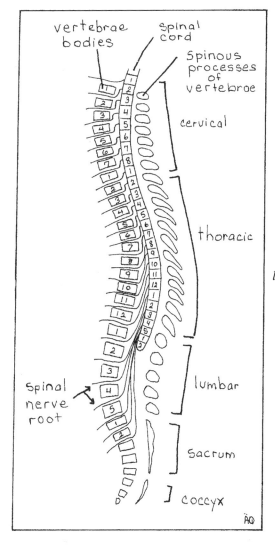

Fig. 3-43
The Adult Spinal Cord and Vertebral Spinal Column:
This cutaway side view shows the discrepancy between spinal cord length and vertebral spinal column length in the adult. Note how the spinal nerve roots compensate for the difference in lengths.

Section IV

Inside To Outside - The Journey

Topic 13

Labor and Delivery of the Newborn

What factors come together that signal a mother's body to begin the uterine activities that result in the delivery of the newborn child? This is still one of those mysteries of life for people. However, research with animals is shedding some light on this subject.

A research team at the University of Auckland in New Zealand (Gluckman, et al) and investigators in Ithica, New York, at The Cornell University College of Veterinary Medicine (Nathaniels, McDonald, et al), have concurrently observed an apparent mechanism that initiates labor and delivery of the fetus in sheep. Both teams of investigators have discovered that it is the sheep fetus that gives the mother the signal that it is ready for the transition from intrauterine to extrauterine life.

The model put forth by these investigators goes like this. By signals as yet to be identified but presently under investigation, parts of the fetal hypothalamus known as the paraventricular nuclei receive signals from the fetal organ systems that they are ready to begin life independent from the maternal placental and intrauterine systems. When all organ systems have communicated their readiness for the transition, the hypothalamus sends a signal to the anterior pituitary gland which responds by secreting adrenal corticotropic hormone (ACTH) into the fetal bloodstream. The ACTH in the fetal blood arrives at the fetal adrenal glands, which then secrete cortisol into the blood. This hormone enters the maternal blood system where it stimulates maternal uterine contractions and the onset of labor. It also seems possible that the ACTH goes into the maternal blood supply and causes the maternal adrenal glands to secrete increased (maternal) cortisol, which initiates labor.

Evidence which supports this model comes largely from the fact that, when the fetal hypothalamic paraventricular nuclei are removed from the sheep fetus while inside the uterus, labor does not begin. However, when the same surgical procedures that were used to remove these paraventricular nuclei are carried out without removing the nuclei, the labor does begin on time. Also, labor is induced by injections of both sheep ACTH and sheep cortisol. These observations support the validity of the model.

Should this model be applicable to humans, it may explain how premature labor is often induced by stress and emotionally charged incidents. Both stress and emotion may result in increased maternal ACTH and cortisol production which may, in turn, induce the untimely onset of obstetrical labor. But remember folks, it's just a model for sheep. It is subject to modification as new data comes forward from the ongoing investigations. And even if it does hold true for sheep, it may not be applicable to humans. (Although at times we humans do sort of behave like flocks of sheep!)

THE BABY'S PERSPECTIVE

Now let's try to experience the labor and delivery process as the fetus-newborn. The description I shall present is a composite of the experiences related by patients, and of my own experiences which have occurred during the SomatoEmotional Release℠ with Therapeutic Imagery and Dialogue process.

Initially, we join our fetus inside of a very nice womb, sort of swimming and floating around in a warm sea of amniotic fluid. Sometimes, there seems to be a sort of red luminescence in the fluid. Gravity seems to be largely neutralized by the combination of the fluid and the fetal buoyancy. Sometimes it is quiet but often there are sounds to be heard. Voices and conversation is often perceived, as is the sound of music and so on. On occasion, the voices transmit emotions. Sometimes the conversations are loving and peaceful; sometimes they are angry, perhaps yelling, argumentative and the like. Our fetus is affected by both. Quite often we have rid adult patients of free-floating anxiety, low self-esteem, etc., that occurred as the result of statements made by persons outside of the womb before delivery. Most often, all that needs to be done is to have the patient re-experience the event. The patient is then able to put it in context and perhaps understand why mother and/or father, soon-to-be grandmother, etc., were arguing about the baby, the pregnancy or whatever. Resolution comes with acknowledgment and understanding. Resolution is accompanied by an end to the anxiety, the low self-esteem, etc. The lesson here is, please be careful what you say in the presence of an intrauterine fetus that may be listening and will usually take you at your word. I am also convinced that the feelings/emotions of the mother are contagious to the fetus. Don't sell that little person inside of the womb short.

Assuming that all is peace and love with the folks outside of the womb, the fetus lives in serenity until it perceives an increase in pressure upon its body surface. This pressure increase is resultant to the contraction of the muscular walls of the uterus. (I'm using uterus and womb almost interchangeably; womb seems more subjective and feeling, while uterus seems more scientific and detached.) This contraction reduces the intrauterine volume and the fluid inside the uterus does what all fluid does when it is compressed. It increases its pressure equally on all the surfaces with which it has contact. It also flows in the direction of least resistance. If we assume that mother's water has not yet broken, that is, the membranes are not yet ruptured, the amniotic fluid inside the membrane container will exert an increased hydraulic force on the inner side of the birth canal with each contraction of the muscular walls of the uterus. This occurs because the birth canal represents the path of least resistance to the fluid. It is by this means that some of the dilation of the cervix/birth canal is accomplished. The hydraulic force, which increases during uterine contraction, forces the membrane into the birth canal. These membranes that have entered the internal end of the birth canal form a cul-de-sac which fills with amniotic fluid. The volume/quantity of fluid within the cul-de-sac increases with each contraction of the uterus. In this manner it acts to open the birth canal from the inside out.

Ultimately, and under normal circumstances, the fetus feels its head entering the internal end of the birth canal once the fluid has partially opened this canal. We speak of this entry of the fetal head into the birth canal as engagement. At this time the fetus is hoping for the membranes to remain intact, because so long as they (the membranes) are intact they take the brunt of the increased pressure in the birth canal. This increased pressure occurs with each muscular contraction of the uterus. Now with the fetus' head in the birth canal there is a volume of fluid which precedes it through the canal. Soon the membranes rupture naturally or they are ruptured by the obstetrical delivery person and the fluid cushion is gone. Now that fetus' head becomes the "battering ram" that forces its way through this ever-so-tight birth canal. If mother can relax her pelvis it is much easier on the fetus. If mother has been anesthetized systemically, the fetus has also been anesthetized or "poisoned." This fetus will be very confused and disoriented about its delivery experience. This confusion and disorientation pattern often follows the fetus into adult life. It can be successfully corrected by the use of CranioSacral Therapy and SomatoEmotional Release℠ with Therapeutic Imagery and Dialogue, but it will require some work. We call it "Completion of a Biological Process."

In any case, let us assume that mother has not had heavy sedation or general anesthesia. The fetal head is pushing its way through the tissues that form the birth canal. The cushioning benefit of the fluid preceding the fetal head through the birth canal has been lost because the membranes have ruptured by one means or another. Now each uterine muscular contraction forces the fetus further out of the uterus. Some of the amniotic fluid is trapped behind the fetus in the uterus because the fetal head serves as a very effective "cork" in the birth canal. Therefore, the fetus is being forced into and through the canal not only by physical pressure as the uterine muscles literally push on its body, but by increased hydraulic pressure on its body from the remaining amniotic fluid.

In order to assist in accommodating the difference between fetal skull size and the circumference of the birth canal, the skull bones are not yet fully formed. They are actually bony plates seated in membranes. This construction allows for an overriding of the major bones of the skull during the passage through the birth canal so that the actual skull size and shape are flexible to some extent. This allows the various diameters of the skull to get smaller as the size of the canal demands that it be so. Once the fetal head has passed through the birth canal, it should expand to its full size. Fortunately, nature has not fully developed the fetal cerebral cortex at the time of delivery. Therefore, the changing volume within the skull during this passage through the birth canal seldom causes any damage to the newborn brain. Can you imagine how it must feel to have your skull bones slipping and sliding and overriding as you pass through the birth canal? I recall in one of my own birth re-experiences how the doctor was trying to rush the process of delivery. I really got upset by his hurriedness. I needed time as the fetus to allow my skull bones and, after that, my spine, to adapt at their own speed to the journey through this rather tight canal. I believe that babies were made to be pushed out by mother's uteruses. They were not made to be pulled out by overzealous obstetrical healthcare professionals.

Once the fetal head is out of the external end of the birth canal, we still have a body that has to complete its journey. This is a twisting, wringing sort of a trip that I believe actually gives the fetus its first spinal manipulation treatment. It would seem that, under ideal conditions, every joint in the fetal spine would be mobilized, as would each of the vertebrae in relation to the others. Further, all of the muscles and ligaments will be stretched and wrung out. It would be comparable, I'm sure, to a very extensive and complete whole-body massage. Also, the baby probably receives a thorough skin friction massage using the vernix caseosa as the oil. We probably shouldn't cut this process short except for emergency situations.

It takes time for the fetal body tissues to respond. They should be given that time so that this initial body treatment can be absorbed and offer its maximal benefit.

CAESAREAN SECTION

Now consider that this natural birth process is completely surrendered when the fetus is delivered into the outside world by Caesarean section. There is no molding of the skull, no spinal manipulation and no total-body stretch and massage. Frequently, the intrauterine pressure is significantly higher than the pressure outside the uterus. This statement is confirmed each time a pregnant uterus is incised with a scalpel and the intrauterine amniotic fluid geysers up in the air a few inches. Imagine how the fetus must feel when its first introduction to the outside world is one of abnormally rapid depressurization. Divers surface slowly or they get decompression sickness. On a smaller scale, wouldn't it be nice to allow the C-section fetus to depressurize slowly? It seems to me that it would be good both psychoemotionally and physiologically.

When I was still doing research at Michigan State University, one of our projects demonstrated that C-sectioned children had more craniosacral system dysfunctions than did vaginally delivered children. I blamed this on the rapid pressure change from inside to outside of the uterus causing a rapid expansion of the skull with some strain of the membrane system inside the skull. I also feel that the child has been deprived of the mobilizing effect of the birth canal journey upon the skull bones as these bones slip, slide and override in accommodation to this canal with its narrowness and its twists and turns. This deprivation probably leads to more craniosacral system problems.

Topic 14

What It Is Like Outside of the Birth Canal

You are the fetus. You have successfully passed through the birth canal. There are lots of bright lights. It is cold. Some person is holding you upside down by your feet and whacking you on the butt until you cry. (And you haven't even misbehaved as yet.) Once you cry, they put you on a table that is hard and they start sticking things in your nose and mouth. These things make scary, sucking noises. Then you get wiped off and, if you're lucky, you get to meet your mother after all this. Somewhere in all of this activity, your umbilical cord is cut and your dependence upon maternal blood for nutrition and other things is gone forever.

Luckily, this rather inconsiderate protocol is being modified into a more-humane modus operandi. We are now beginning to realize that fetuses and newborns are little people with sensitivities, memories and vulnerabilities that are not only physical but also psychoemotional. There are now lots of places (including at home) to have babies that respect the idea that nature knows best. Babies are caught as they exit the mother, rather than pulled. Harsh environments are toned down and warm, loving atmospheres are created. I would like this much better, wouldn't you?

Nature has created all of this birth process to give the newborn a better chance at a higher quality of life. Sometimes skull bone override or molding of the head does not self-correct. A competent CranioSacral Therapist can help nature to overcome these little obstacles in the first few days after delivery. If CranioSacral Therapy is done very early, many problems related to childhood brain function might be avoided. Included in these avoidable problems might be such things as dyslexia, attention deficit disorder or hyperactivity, some seizures, some cerebral palsy, some motor eye problems and so on. CranioSacral treatment is kind and loving. It should leave no emotional scars if administered in a reasonably correct manner.

Right after delivery the cerebral cortex begins more rapid growth because it can now more safely begin to occupy more of the space in the skull vault. Myelination of the spinal cord motor tracts may not be complete for about 18 to 24 months after delivery. This may be so that mothers don't have to chase their running children around the house during the earlier months. You need myelination of these motor tracts in order to walk, run, jump, etc. Thank you Mother Nature.

Section V

Inventory of Parts of the Central Nervous System

When the fetus has matured in the womb normally and all systems are working correctly, the baby is delivered to the outside world between 38 and 42 weeks gestation. Gestation begins with conception. A lot has happened since the sperm fertilized the ovum/egg.

Since we are focusing our attention primarily upon the central nervous system, it seems appropriate to take an inventory of the component parts of this system at this time. It is precisely now that the full-term baby must make its successful transition from life inside the womb to life outside of the womb. It must now enter the world with all of its various environmental challenges. The nervous system is of primary importance in meeting these challenges.

We will go through these component parts from the "tail" to the "head" as they contribute to the spinal cord, the hindbrain (myelencephalon and metencephalon), the midbrain and the forebrain (diencephalon and telencephalon), in that order. Topic 20 through the end of this section then considers more miscellaneous components of the nervous system. (At the end of this inventory, page 203, you will find an alphabetical index of these parts for your convenience should you desire information about individual central nervous system components.)

Keep in mind that almost all of the component parts of the central nervous system are originated by the end of the eighth week of gestation. From the end of the eighth week until delivery of the newborn, these components develop and integrate with each other as well as with the various other body parts and systems that interact with the central nervous system. Also, remember that the nervous system has a lot more developing to do after the delivery of the newborn. This situation mandates re-evaluation of this system's development on several occasions in order to keep track of that development. You will see in the next section on newborn evaluation that many reflexes and neurological signs change as this development continues.

Also, remember that problems of the pregnancy that occur before the end of the eighth week of gestation are more likely to result in the absence or malformation of the component parts of the central nervous system. We can't do much about these problems except to help the afflicted child adapt around the problem. On the other hand, problems of pregnancy that occur subsequent to the end of the eighth week of gestation have a better chance of responding to treatment. This is because the development has been impaired, but with luck the raw materials may be present. Therefore, the chances for inducing developmental progress are enhanced.

The Spinal Cord

Now, let's look briefly at the components of an essentially normal spinal cord in the full-term newborn.

The spinal cord is defined anatomically in the newborn as that part of the central nervous system that extends downward through the spinal or vertebral canal (spinal and vertebral are used interchangeably) from the foramen magnum at the base of the skull to the bottom of the spinal canal, which is in the sacrum. The sacrum is the "triangular" bone at the lower end of the spine. The sacrum is situated between the lowest (fifth) lumbar vertebra and the coccyx, or tailbone. The spinal cord is actually an extension of the central nervous system down from the medulla oblongata (which is the lowest brain component) to the lowest nerve roots, which exit the spinal canal down in the sacrum. In the human adult the spinal cord only extends down the spinal canal to about the level of the second lumbar vertebra. This discrepancy in length between the spinal canal and the spinal cord occurs because the growth of the vertebral/spinal column outstrips the growth of the spinal cord by several inches as we mature into adulthood **(Fig. 3-43)**.

From its top to its bottom, the spinal cord actually has 31 pairs of spinal nerves which enter and 31 pairs which exit. The incoming nerve messages (impulses) enter the spinal cord from the back via the posterior nerve roots. The outgoing nerve messages (impulses) exit the spinal cord via the ventral nerve roots. The nerve root sets are symmetrical on both sides of the spinal cord. There are eight sets of cervical nerve roots, 12 sets of thoracic nerve roots, five sets of lumbar nerve roots, and usually six sets down in the sacral region. There may be some variation at this lower end of the spinal cord. In the adult the lower spinal cord nerves have to descend from the spinal cord downward within the spinal canal to their appropriate exits out into the body. Those spinal cord nerve roots that descend within the canal after the spinal cord has ended are called the cauda equina. In Latin this means the horse's tail.

The spinal cord is comparable to a large cable that carries many smaller component cables to and from various destinations and origins. These component cables would be the cables that carry messages between the various brain regions and the parts of the body outside of the central nervous system. Some of these component cables within the spinal cord go away from the brain to the body, some go from the body to the brain, and some cross over and/or make short trips within the spinal cord without ascending up to the brain.

The spinal cord, therefore, may be considered as offering both longitudinal and transverse segmental connections. The latter connections correlate with the somites, the myotomes, the dermatomes, etc., that we discussed earlier.

In order to gain a better concept of the organization of some of the nerve tracts and interconnections that are present in the spinal cord, please see the accompanying longitudinal and cross-section illustrations. Once again, a picture is worth a thousand words (**Fig. 5-1 and 5-2**).

In general, it is important to note that the nerve tracts that are bringing information into the brain are located in the posterior region of the spinal cord. The motor commands to muscles and other end organs are sent out through nerve tracts located in the anterior part of the spinal cord. You can also see that some of the nerve nuclei for the sympathetic and parasympathetic divisions of the autonomic nervous system are located in the spinal cord (**Fig. 5-3**).

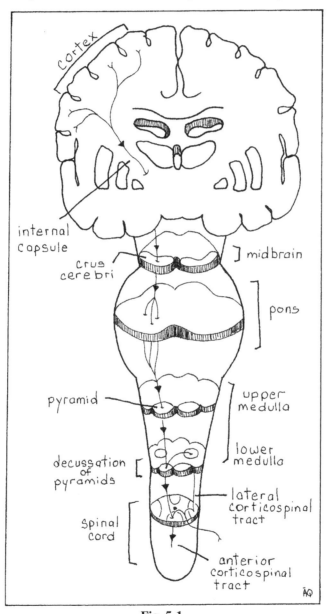

Fig. 5-1
Corticospinal Tracts:
Corticospinal tracts carry messages from the brain to the motor (outgoing) nerve roots. Many of these tracts cross over to the opposite side as they pass through the medulla oblongata. This is why a right-sided brain injury might paralyze the left side of the body, or vice versa. Direction of impulse flow is indicated by the arrows in the drawing.

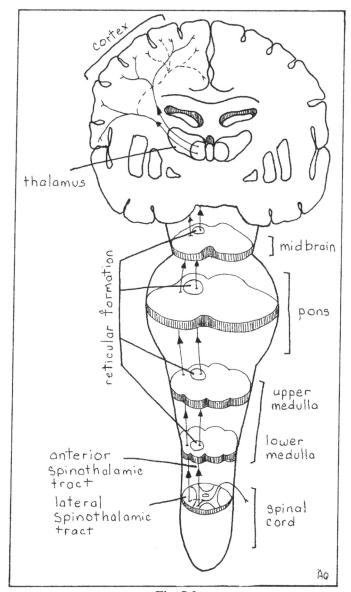

Fig. 5-2
Spinothalamic Tracts:
Spinothalamic tracts send messages from the sensory (inflow) system
up the spinal cord to the thalamus. The arrows indicate the direction
of flow. The thalamus then acts as a sorting and relay station which
forwards the incoming information to the proper brain areas.

Also, it may be helpful to realize that some, but unfortunately not all, of the longitudinal nerve tracts within the spinal cord are named for the structures or regions of the nervous system that they connect. For example, the vestibulospinal tract connects the vestibular nuclei in the brain with the spinal nerve roots that go out to the muscles which are activated in order to maintain balance. The spinothalamic tract connects the spinal nerve roots with the thalamus for triage and relay to higher brain centers. The corticospinal tract carries orders from the cerebral cortex to the motor nerve roots, and so on.

It is of interest to consider the role of the spinal cord in muscle tonus and spasticity. The muscles that receive the message to contract are called the agonists. Those muscles that oppose

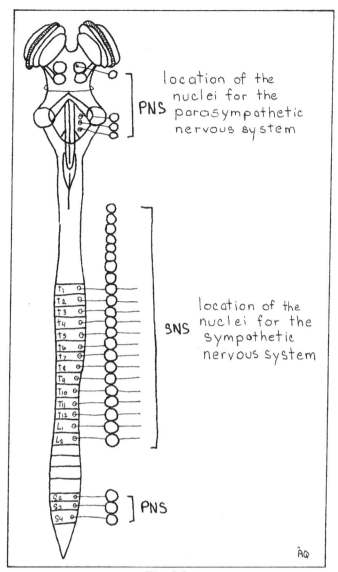

Fig. 5-3
Locations of the Autonomic Nuclei:
Most of the parasympathetic nuclei are located in the brain
stem and in the sacral region of the spinal cord. Most of the
sympathetic nuclei are located in the thoracic and upper lumbar
regions of the spinal cord. This latter design makes for quick
sympathetic response to the reticular alarm system. Both
systems have major influence from the hypothalamus.

the agonists are called the antagonists. Every agonist muscle has an antagonist muscle. Otherwise, the body part would move only in one direction. For example, if we had only a biceps muscle that flexes the elbow, but no triceps muscle to straighten the elbow again once it was flexed, we could only straighten the elbow by using an externally applied force. Also consider that the degree of flexion or straightening of the elbow at any given moment is governed by the balance of activity between the biceps and triceps muscles. (There are some other muscles involved, but I am not making my example all inclusive. I simply wish to illustrate the principle of agonist-antagonist action.)

From this example you can see that when the agonist muscle contracts, the antagonist muscle must relax enough to allow the agonist to successfully move the elbow joint without working against undue antagonist resistance. If the antagonist is not inhibited into an appropriate degree of relaxation, the result is a spasticity which interferes with smooth coordinated joint movement at best. At worst, the result could be a spastic paralysis which prevents joint movement entirely.

The role of the spinal cord in the inhibition of antagonist muscles is key to immediate and effective action between agonist muscle coordination and antagonist muscle inhibition (relaxation). The antagonist inhibition is carried out within the spinal cord via a direct inhibitory pathway. There are also influences from higher centers in the brain, but the immediate and reflexive response is carried out at the spinal cord level.

It works like this: when an agonist or effector muscle gets a message to contract, it does so. This muscle has certain stretch receptors in it that send a signal into the spinal cord as soon as the contraction is initiated. The signal that goes into the cord then synapses with both the motor nerve to the contracting muscle and the inhibitory nerve to the antagonist muscle. This message is continually modified on a fraction-of-a-second level to achieve the desired balance between agonist and antagonist muscles in order to obtain the desired movement. At the same time, messages are sent up to higher brain centers in order to gain further instructions and modifications of the movement.

The receptors in the muscles are called proprioceptors. These proprioceptors send in information about muscle contraction levels and tensions. All of this input is organized into what is called the proprioceptive system. It is this proprioceptive system that lets us know where our body parts are at any given moment without the benefit of looking at these body parts. And it is the proprioceptive sense that feeds into the spinal cord for immediate action and concurrently communicates with the brain for more general directions.

A couple of abbreviations that you may encounter in your reading are: IPSP = Inhibitory Post Synaptic Potential, and EPSP = Excitatory Post Synaptic Potential. They refer to the inhibition of the antagonist and the excitation of the agonist muscles, respectively.

Another little piece of information that you might find useful is that, as of June, 1994, research findings would indicate that the amino acid neurotransmitters aspartate and glycine have been found in higher concentrations in the motor areas of the spinal cord. Therefore, they probably have more to do with the motor function of muscles. Aspartate and glycine may prove to be helpful in muscle problems related to spinal cord injuries.

Acetylcholine is very abundant in the interneurons (of Renshaw) of the spinal cord. These are the interneurons that help spinal cord control of balanced muscle contraction and relaxation. Choline, one of the amino acids, may be helpful in re-establishing good agonist-antagonist muscle balance.

One more item on spinal cord injury. A neurosurgeon named Alf Brieg has published a book entitled "Adverse Mechanical Tension in the Central Nervous System." Dr. Brieg presently lives in Sweden, where he is in retirement from active practice. Dr. Brieg puts forth a model for post-traumatic spinal cord dysfunction that I find quite interesting and logical. His model has not, however, been considered seriously by the traditional medical community.

In brief, Dr. Brieg's idea goes like this. Consider that the spinal cord is about 95 percent (or more) water. This water is enclosed within the cellular, fibrous and membranous structure of the spinal cord. When a sudden blow is delivered to the spinal cord, even though there appears to be no significant damage to the traumatized area, this water is suddenly forced away from the blow or trauma by the sudden compression of the spinal cord at that level. Since this water is forced suddenly away from the sight of compression, it can cause microscopic ruptures of the spinal cord architecture in the areas that receive the water overload. These areas would be above and below the site of injury because the water would "squirt" in both directions.

These microscopic ruptures then heal with fibrosis, which may entrap excess water permanently within these spinal cord areas both above and below the original injury site. As long as the excess water is entrapped, the chances of the conduction of electrical impulses by neurons through these areas is almost nil. If the excess fluid can be liberated from its entrapment, the chances of re-establishing neuronal function are improved. However, the longer the fibrosis has been going on, the more it, too, may interfere with nerve conduction.

I am indeed heartened by Dr. Brieg's concept because we feel, in CranioSacral Therapy, that we do move/liberate entrapped fluids. Also, we do seem to be able to reverse fibrosis to some extent. So, for the spinal cord injured patient who has an intact but dysfunctional spinal cord, CranioSacral Therapy may be very helpful.

Topic 16

The Hindbrain

MYELENCEPHALON AND METENCEPHALON

Next we will consider the hindbrain, or rhombencephalon as it is known in scientific circles. The hindbrain is divided into the myelencephalon, which is its lower or backwardmost division, and the metencephalon, which is immediately forward of the myelencephalon.

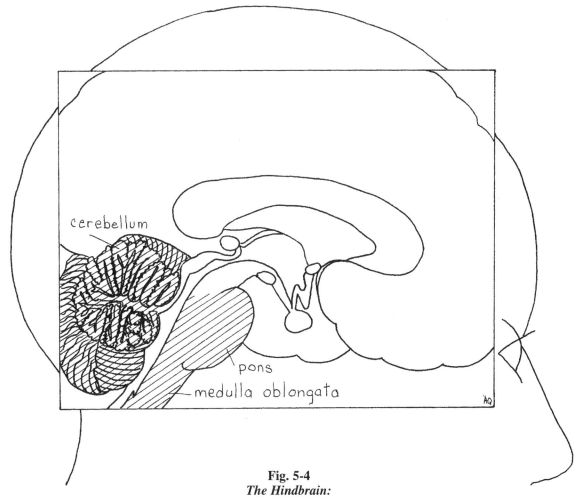

Fig. 5-4
The Hindbrain:
The hindbrain is the shaded area in the drawing. This is put in context by sketching in a side view of the head. The components of the hindbrain are the myelencephalon, which contains the medulla oblongata and the fourth ventricle, and the metencephalon, which contains the pons, the cerebellum, part of the third ventricle and the aqueduct of Sylvius.

The myelencephalon division of the hindbrain contains the medulla oblongata and the fourth ventricle of the brain. The metencephalon division includes the pons, the cerebellum, the aqueduct of Sylvius, and the hindmost or posterior part of the third ventricle. This third ventricle extends forward into the midbrain, or mesencephalon as it is more scientifically known. The midbrain is immediately forward of the hindbrain (**Fig. 5-4**).

THE MEDULLA OBLONGATA

The medulla oblongata is located in the myelencephalon division of the hindbrain (**Fig. 5-5**). It is about an inch long in the adult. It is perhaps 1/4 to 3/8 of an inch long in the newborn. The medulla oblongata connects the spinal cord below with the pons above. The decussation of nerve fibers occurs in the medulla oblongata. This decussation refers to the situation wherein the nerves from the right side of the brain cross over to control the left side of the body, and vice versa. The nerve tracts that cross over in the medulla are known as the pyramidal tracts (**Fig. 5-6**). There is also an extrapyramidal system of nerve fiber tracts that passes through the medulla oblongata. These fiber tracts do not cross over to the other side. That is, they do not "decussate."

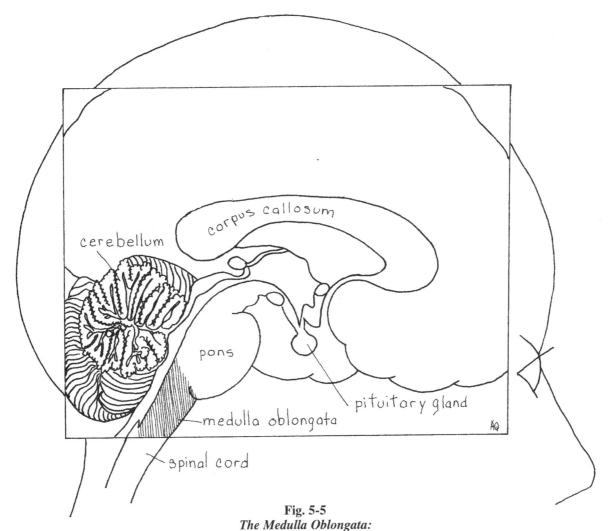

Fig. 5-5
The Medulla Oblongata:
This drawing has the medulla oblongata shaded to demonstrate its boundary with the pons.

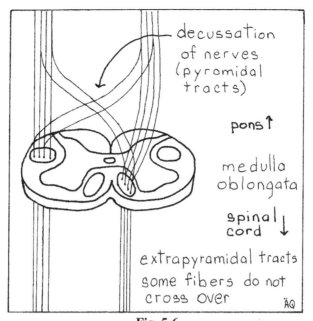

Fig. 5-6
The Decussation of Nerve Fibers in the Medulla Oblongata:
This drawing illustrates the crossover of nerve fibers in the
medulla. Some fibers cross. These are called the
pyramidal tracts. Those fibers that do not cross
make up the extrapyramidal system.

The medulla oblongata also contains several nuclei. These nuclei are mostly related to very basic physiological functions such as swallowing, breathing, blood pressure control, heart rate, and the evenness of heart rhythm. It also has a lot to do with vomiting (**Fig. 5-7**). If you cut across the lower end of the medulla oblongata, death is certain and quick. Needless to say, brain stem injuries that involve the medulla oblongata are *always* very serious, if not fatal.

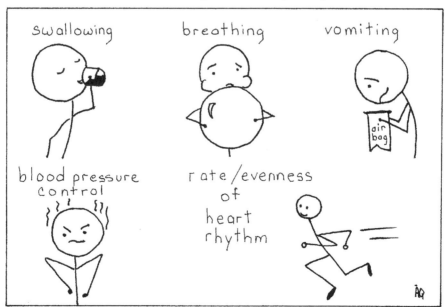

Fig. 5-7
Medulla Oblongata Functions:
The medulla oblongata has in it nuclei that control the functions shown in the above
illustration. Damage to the medulla oblongata is always serious, if not fatal.

In situations of extreme anger, fear, danger and the like, a neurotransmitter and hormone named norepinephrine takes over almost total control of our heart action, our breathing, our muscle strength and so on. The action of norepinephrine on heart and respiration is upon the medullary nuclei that control these vital functions, as well as upon the end organs.

The medulla oblongata also contains much of the sensory neuronal network that functions in the receipt of sensory input from the head and neck, as well as the sensory input from the special senses of hearing, seeing and proprioception. The medulla oblongata also acts as a relay station for nerve messages between the cerebral cortex motor control areas and the cerebellum.

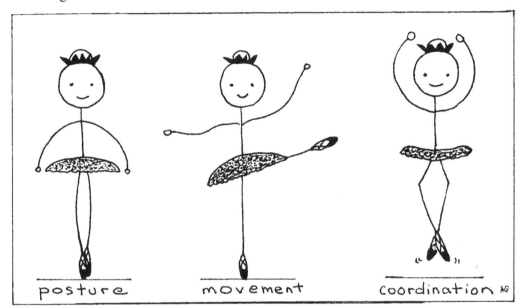

Fig. 5-8
Extrapyramidal System Functions:
The extrapyramidal system does not cross over/decussate in the medulla oblongata. It has a lot to do with posture, movement and coordination.

With all of this in mind, it becomes clear that the medulla oblongata has a great deal to do with bodily movements, especially those that occur almost as reflexes, of which we may or may not be aware. These reflexes occur in response to things we see, hear, feel and so on. The extrapyramidal system, which passes through the medulla oblongata, works in coordination with other neural structures in the medulla oblongata, and therefore has great influence and control over posture, movement and coordination (**Fig. 5-8**).

THE FOURTH VENTRICLE

The fourth ventricle is the lowermost ventricle of the brain. It receives cerebrospinal fluid from the third ventricle and distributes this fluid via the foramina of Magendie, Luschka and Monro to the subarachnoid spaces and into the spinal canal, which is located within the spinal cord (**Fig 3-38**).

THE PONS

The metencephalon division of the hindbrain houses the pons, the cerebellum, the aqueduct of Sylvius and the posterior part of the third ventricle.

The pons is the anterior or ventral part of the metencephalon. It is the bridge between the midbrain (mesencephalon) and the medulla oblongata. The pons contain several nuclei that are connected to the cerebellum, and it receives several nerve tracts from the cerebrum above. In Latin, pons means bridge. The pons is truly a bridge between higher brain centers, the cerebellum and the spinal cord. The spinal cord is the final relay station in the central nervous system that relays messages to the peripheral body.

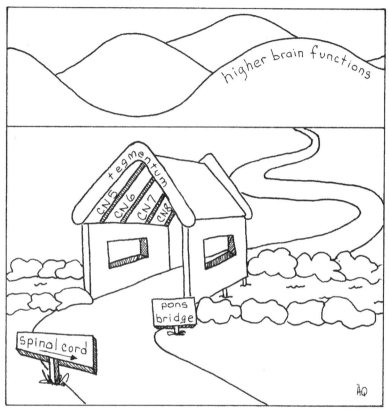

Fig. 5-9
The Pons is a Bridge:
*The pons is a very important bridge between higher brain centers and
the spinal cord. It also has in its "roof" the nuclei of the trigeminal
V, the abducent VI, the facial VII and the acoustic VIII cranial nerves.
These cranial nerves are discussed in detail in Section VI, Topic 36.*

The tegmentum, or roof of the pons is the more dorsal part. It is continuous with the tegmentum of the midbrain and the tegmentum of the medulla. Within this dorsal part of the pons are fiber tracts of the reticular formation and the nuclei of the Vth, VIth, VIIth and VIIIth cranial nerves. Thus, it has significant function in both motor and sensory systems of the head and neck. Clearly, the pons is a most important bridge or connecting link between the decision-making regions of the brain and the rest of the body **(Fig. 5-9)**.

THE RAPHE NUCLEI OF THE PONS

The neurons along the midline of the pons are called the raphe nuclei **(Fig. 5-10)**. One of the most important of the neurotransmitters in the entire central nervous system is called serotonin. Its highest concentration is located within the neurons that have their cell bodies within these

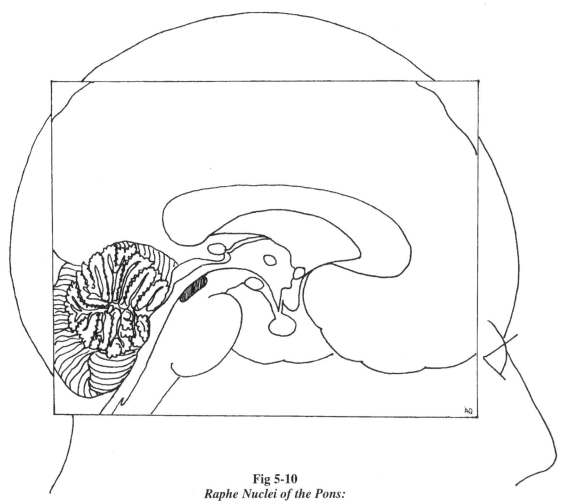

Fig 5-10
Raphe Nuclei of the Pons:
The raphe nuclei of the pons are the major producers of serotonin in the brain.
The shaded area demonstrates the location of these nuclei.

raphe nuclei. Serotonin distribution to the rest of the central nervous system is largely by way of the projections of the neurons of these raphe nuclei.

THE LOCUS CERULEUS OF THE PONS

The locus ceruleus is a very small pigmented structure in the pons where it forms a part of the floor of the fourth ventricle (**Fig. 5-11**). It contains only about 300,000 nerve cell bodies. This is a very small number by comparison to other brain structures. On the other hand, the locus ceruleus connects with most of the central nervous system via its nerve cell body projections.

The locus ceruleus manufactures the great majority of the norepinephrine that is made in the brain tissue. Therefore, the locus ceruleus has powerful influence in the process of emotional arousal. It appears to be a key factor in the sense of pleasure, in anger and in aggressive behavior. In addition, it is essential in learning, memory and sleep. Somehow it affects the balance between pleasure and anxiety. You might say it is the place where you learn to worry about impending trouble if things seem to be going too good.

Function of the locus ceruleus is depressed by alcohol and many of the popular mind-altering

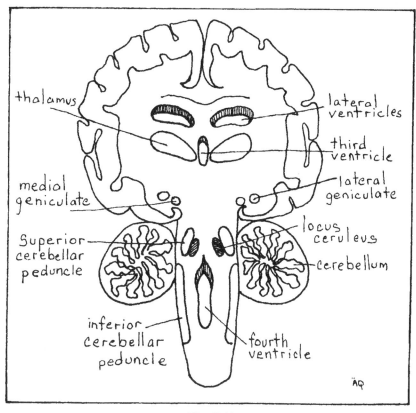

Fig. 5-11
The Locus Ceruleus:
The shaded areas in the drawing show the location of the locus ceruleus.
Each locus ceruleus contains only about 300,000 neurons. Yet these
structures connect with almost all brain centers, and they manufacture most
of the norepinephrine made in the brain.

drugs. It is also inhibited by serotonin and it is self-inhibited by a feedback loop involving its own product, norepinephrine.

The major locus ceruleus connections with other major central nervous system centers include the thalamus, the hypothalamus, the cerebral cortex and the cerebellum, as well as the spinal cord.

THE CEREBELLUM

The cerebellum is also a part of the metencephalon division of the hindbrain (**Fig. 5-12**). It is sometimes called the "little cerebrum." The cerebellum is located beneath the tentorium cerebelli, which is the more horizontally or transversely oriented part of the intracranial (in the skull) dura mater membrane system. It is the tentorium cerebelli membrane that supports the occipital lobes of the brain so that they don't rest their weight upon the cerebellum. The cerebellum is composed of two hemispheres, or halves. In the newborn each half is about the size of a walnut shell. In conjunction with the basal ganglia, which are higher up in the brain, the cerebellum modulates and coordinates all movements of the body that involve muscular activity. It is the cerebellum that remembers how to do things like walking, running, jumping, playing the piano, etc. It also smoothes out motor activities. It produces precise whole-body movements that are coordinated (**Fig. 5-13**). It also provides much of what is needed for fine/delicate motor

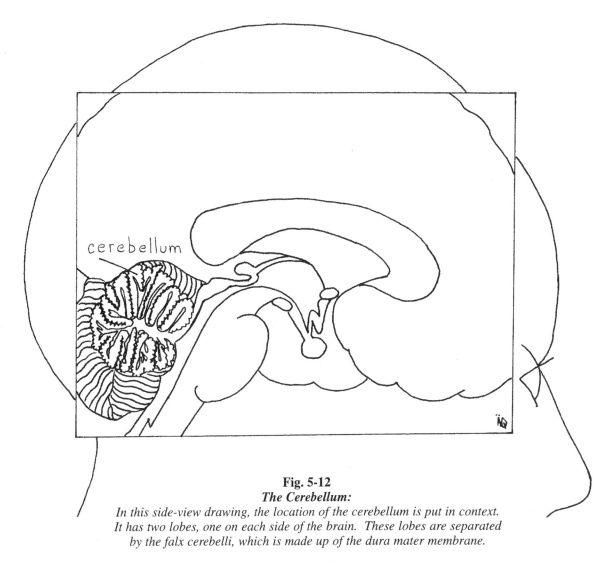

Fig. 5-12
The Cerebellum:
In this side-view drawing, the location of the cerebellum is put in context.
It has two lobes, one on each side of the brain. These lobes are separated
by the falx cerebelli, which is made up of the dura mater membrane.

activities, like threading a needle or flipping a coin. The cerebellum is actually analogous to an ancillary brain in that it contains its own complete sensory and motor representations of the body. It is closely connected to the cortex and the spinal cord. Cerebellar problems result in a lack of body movement, coordination and control. A person with cerebellar dysfunction may put a fork full of food in his/her eye while trying to put it in the mouth. Cerebellar patients appear drunk when they walk. Without a cerebellum, every body movement would have to process through your conscious mind. Imagine how difficult it would be to try to type this manuscript if you had to consciously tell each arm, hand and finger muscle, individually, what to do and when to do it.

THE THIRD VENTRICLE

In addition to the pons and the cerebellum, the metencephalon also contains the lower, or back part of the third ventricle of the brain and the aqueduct of Sylvius. The third ventricle receives cerebrospinal fluid from the two lateral ventricles and passes this fluid on into the fourth ventricle via the aqueduct of Sylvius. It is this aqueduct that, when it is malformed, is a very common cause of hydrocephalus when that condition is due to congenital malformation (**Fig. 3-38**).

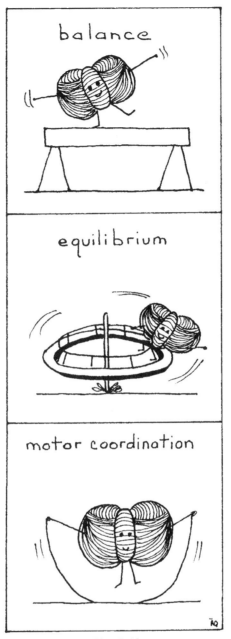

Fig. 5-13
Functions of the Cerebellum:
*It is the cerebellum that is largely
responsible for our ability to balance,
move smoothly, do gymnastics, and not
think about what we are doing.*

The Midbrain

The midbrain, or mesencephalon as it is also called in scientific circles, is a short portion of brain which lies between the pons and the cerebral hemispheres — more specifically, the diencephalic portion of the forebrain portion of the cerebral hemispheres. The midbrain does not divide into two parts during its embryonic development as do the forebrain and the hindbrain. The midbrain structures have strong influence over pleasure sensations, mood, reality contact and motor function. By means of its generous connections with the cortex and the limbic system, the midbrain supplies the dopamine to most of the rest of the brain.

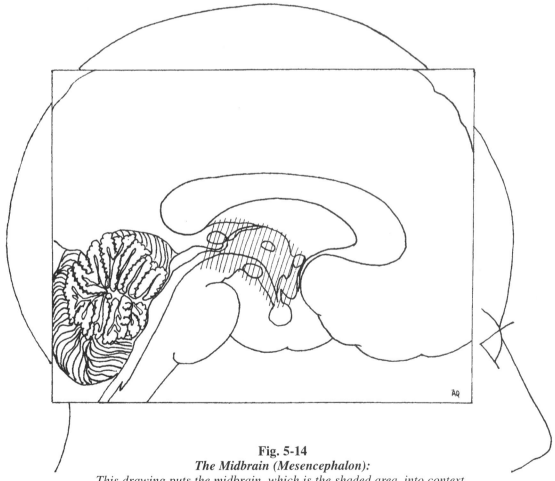

Fig. 5-14
The Midbrain (Mesencephalon):
This drawing puts the midbrain, which is the shaded area, into context.
It is within the midbrain that Parkinson's disease occurs.

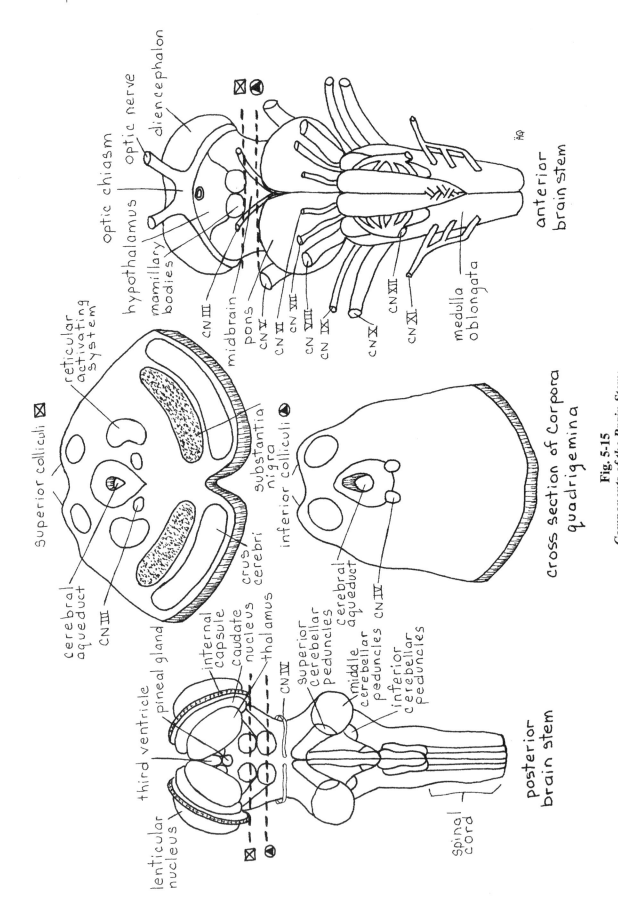

Fig. 5-15
Components of the Brain Stem:
This set of drawings shows many of the components of the brain stem. Front, back and side views are presented. Most of these components are discussed individually in the text.

Components of the midbrain include the tectum, the cerebral peduncles, the tegmentum, the crus cerebri, the substantia nigra, the aqueduct of Sylvius, the nuclei of the IIIrd and IVth cranial nerves, and reticular substance of the brain (**Fig. 5-14**).

The midbrain is the highest level of the brain stem, which includes all of the previously discussed components of the hindbrain as well as the midbrain components listed above (**Fig. 5-15**).

THE TECTUM

The tectum is more or less the roof of the midbrain. The tectum contains the corpora quadrigemina, which are four aggregations of nerve cell bodies with synapses (**Fig. 5-15**). These four aggregations are then subdivided into the two superior colliculi and two inferior colliculi. The two superior colliculi are actually relay stations for our sense of vision or sight. The two inferior colliculi serve as relay stations for our auditory senses, which give us our ability to hear. Therefore, it is clear that problems with the tectum can interfere with our ability to see and/or hear, depending upon which and how many colliculi are involved with the tectum problem.

THE CEREBRAL PEDUNCLES

The cerebral peduncles are two in number. There is one located on each side of the ventral surface (underside) of the midbrain. The peduncle mostly contains connecting fibers that descend from the cerebral cortex down to the midbrain and the spinal cord. The space between the two peduncles is chock-full of blood vessels that penetrate into the depths of the brain and offer blood circulation (**Fig. 5-15**).

THE TEGMENTUM

The tegmentum is the dorsal, or back part of the midbrain. It contains both ascending and descending nerve tracts that connect the brain centers above with the brain stem and spinal cord below. The tegmentum also contains reticular substance of the brain and most of the nuclei for the IIIrd and IVth cranial nerves. Therefore, it is easy to see that problems in the tegmentum can interfere with the communication between the higher brain centers and the peripheral body. These problems involve the ascending and/or descending nerve tracts. When a problem involves the reticular substance as it passes through the tegmentum of the midbrain, there may well be a lack of alertness and/or an inability to respond to or even to notice dangerous or emergency situations. If the tegmentum problems involve the nuclei of the IIIrd and/or IVth cranial nerves, there may be a problem with control of eye movement, since these two cranial nerves (oculomotor and trochlear, respectively) are responsible for the great majority of motor control of the eyes.

THE CRUS CEREBRI

The crus cerebri is made up mostly of nerve fiber tracts that carry messages from the higher brain centers in the cerebrum down to the various nuclei in the brain stem, especially the pons and the spinal cord. The crus cerebri are located in the ventral region of the midbrain. The fiber tracts they contain run longitudinally, for the most part (**Fig. 5-15**).

THE SUBSTANTIA NIGRA

The substantia nigra separates the crus cerebri from the tegmentum of the midbrain. This substance is a part of the system that runs amuck in Parkinson's disease (**Fig. 5-15**). The substantia nigra connects several higher brain centers with the lower centers of the brain stem. It gets its name from its color, which is dark brown to black. The color is due to the presence of cells which contain melanin. Melanin is the pigment that gives skin moles their dark brown, almost black, color. It is also the pigment that gives us a suntan. The substantia nigra is part of the basal ganglia. It secretes lots of dopamine, which is a neurotransmitter related to depression and possibly schizophrenia when it is deficient in quantity. Also, it is the deficiency of dopamine that causes Parkinson's disease. Somehow dopamine seems to facilitate pleasurable experiences.

THE AQUEDUCT OF SYLVIUS

The aqueduct of Sylvius is the "tube" that connects the third and fourth ventricles of the brain (**Fig. 3-38**). It is located in the more dorsal part of the midbrain. It is oriented in a semi-vertical direction between the two ventricles (third and fourth). When the aqueduct of Sylvius, or cerebral aqueduct as it is also known, does not develop or function properly, the result is hydrocephalus (water on the brain). In this case, the cerebrospinal fluid, which is produced within the lateral and third ventricles of the brain, cannot drain into the fourth ventricle for its further distribution into the central canal of the spinal cord and into the subarachnoid space.

NUCLEI OF CRANIAL NERVES III AND IV

The nuclei of cranial nerve III (oculomotor) and cranial nerve IV (trochlear) are located within the tegmentum of the midbrain (**Fig. 5-15**). Problems that contribute to dysfunction of these cranial nerve nuclei result in inability for the eyes to move towards the nose, up and down, and inability to accommodate and focus for distance. The only thing that won't happen is the child won't be cross-eyed. This problem of cross-eyedness relates to cranial nerve VI (abducent), which does not have its nuclei in the midbrain but a little below in the metencephalon.

THE RETICULAR FORMATION

The reticular formation passes through the midbrain in its tegmental region (**Fig. 5-16**). This system of reticular substance communicates particularly with the nuclei of the motor nerves (cranial nerves III and IV) to the eye, and with the substantia nigra. Therefore, the reticular formation (also known as the reticular alarm system and the reticular substance), since it serves as an alerting system, helps the eyes to reflexively track and accommodate in fight-or-flight circumstances. Since the substantia nigra is involved in posturing and smooth coordinated movement, the input from the reticular formation is also very helpful in the production of quick and effective reflex responses when emergency situations arise. Problems that involve the reticular formation as it passes through the midbrain may also interfere with the reflex ability of the child to respond to situations that might require quick eye movements and appropriate posturing and/or smooth coordinated movement in response to alerting or alarm situations.

The reticular formation also plays a major role in emotional responses. Therefore, any problem that compromises its passage through the midbrain region may have an effect on emotional behavior.

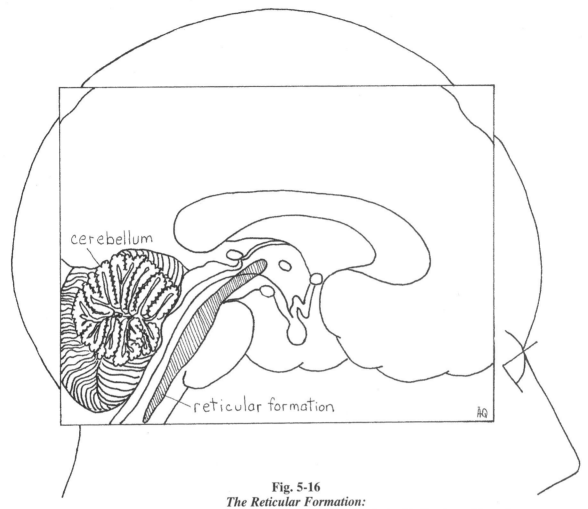

Fig. 5-16
The Reticular Formation:
The reticular formation passes up the spinal cord, through the hindbrain and into the midbrain. It is shown in this drawing as the shaded area.

The Forebrain

The forebrain, or prosencephalon as it is known in scientific circles, divides into two parts during embryonic development. The two parts are named the diencephalon, which is the back/posterior part, and the telencephalon, which is the forward/anterior part. The forebrain itself develops from the forwardmost of the three vesicles that form in the embryonic neural tube **(Fig. 3-12)**. This division into diencephalon and telencephalon occurs during the end of the third week of gestation **(Fig. 5-17)**.

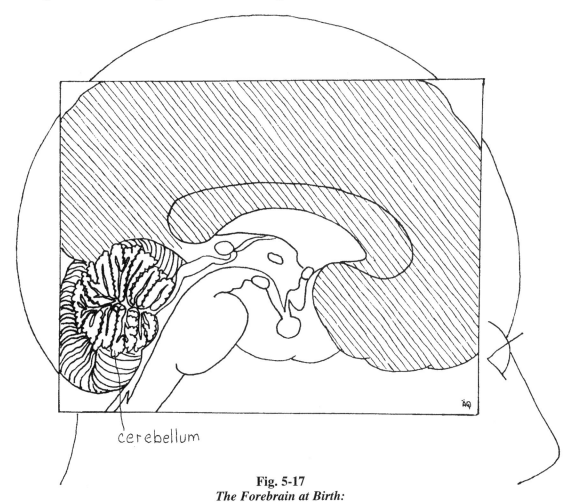

cerebellum

Fig. 5-17
The Forebrain at Birth:
The forebrain is shown as the shaded area. It is divided into telencephalon and diencephalon. The cerebellum is labeled. Do not confuse it as a part of the forebrain because it, too, appears shaded.

THE DIENCEPHALON

The diencephalon develops from the thickened side/lateral walls of the back part of the forebrain. Moving up from the lower brain centers (the medulla oblongata) towards the highest brain centers (the cerebral cortex), the diencephalon is next in line above the midbrain.

The diencephalon encloses the two lateral ventricles and most of the third ventricle of the brain. It also encloses their interconnecting ducts. The list of component parts of the diencephalon also includes the thalamus, the geniculate bodies, the epithalamus, the subthalamus and the hypothalamus.

The diencephalon exercises a great deal of control over the functions of the autonomic nervous system and over the pituitary gland. It also acts as a relay station for sensory messages coming in from lower centers and the periphery of the body.

THE PART OF THE VENTRICULAR SYSTEM IN THE DIENCEPHALON

The lateral ventricles of the brain are connected to the third ventricle of the brain by the interventricular foramina of Monro **(Fig. 3-38)**. These ventricles are part of the brain's ventricular system, which manufactures and distributes cerebrospinal fluid to the spaces that surround and penetrate the central nervous system. All three of the above-named ventricles manufacture cerebrospinal fluid. The lateral ventricles deliver this fluid into the third ventricle, which adds its own production to fluid it has received from the lateral ventricles. From the third ventricle, the cerebrospinal fluid passes through the cerebral aqueduct (of Sylvius) into the fourth ventricle, which delivers the cerebrospinal fluid via its various apertures (foramina of Magendie and Luschka) to the subarachnoid spaces and penetrating canals for interaction with the brain, spinal cord and nerve roots.

THE THALAMUS

The thalamus is paired. That is, each of the two cerebral hemispheres contains a thalamus. The name is somewhat misleading because the singular word thalamus is most often used to signify both the right and the left thalamus. The correct plural name is thalami. The thalami are located one on each side of the third ventricle in the diencephalon. They are connected only by a small band of tissue called the interthalamic adhesion. This small band of tissue is usually, but not always, present. When present it is located just behind the interventricular foramen of Monro **(Fig. 5-18)**.

The thalamus on each side of the third ventricle of the brain is a somewhat oval-shaped mass which is oriented longitudinally. Thus, the thalami run parallel to the third ventricle. In the adult human, each thalamus in its longitudinal dimension is about 1 1/2 to 2 inches long. The thalami extend backwards (caudad) from the third ventricle, and enclose the rather puzzling pineal gland between their caudad parts.

The thalami have a wide variety of nuclei and a myriad of connections with other brain centers and the spinal cord. They function as major relay stations, triage centers, as sensory input enhancers in some instances, and as sensory input screening interceptors in other instances. Actually, all sensations except smell pass through the thalami on their way to the cerebral cortex where they are interpreted and associated. Pain impulses sometimes do not go as far up the

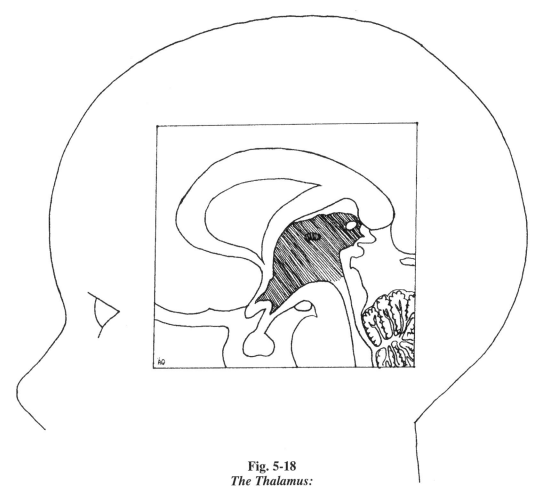

Fig. 5-18
The Thalamus:
The shaded area indicates the general location of the thalamus.
The inset is oriented in the drawing of the head, as shown.

central nervous system as the thalami. About 50 percent of pain sensations do not go above the brain stem. Those sensations of pain that do not reach the thalami for relay to the cerebral cortices (cortices is the plural form of cortex), or which the thalami decide not to relay upward, are probably what we call subliminal pain. This is the kind of pain that we do not feel. Often, we do not feel pain when it goes on and on, or in severe crisis or emergency. At present, this is kind of a gray area, since the blocking of pain perception can also be accomplished by the endorphins. The endorphins function more on a biochemical level. We may discover that the thalamic relays and the endorphins work "en concert," since it appears that the thalamus has many "mu" receptors. These receptors are thought to be the ones that are involved in endorphin reception and in opiate addiction.

Severe alcoholic damage to the brain is often designated as Korsakoff's Syndrome. In this condition there is severe damage to the thalami. Korsakoff's Syndrome shows itself as severe amnesia and dementia, and inability to reason or think rationally. The Korsakoff patient oftimes confabulates incessantly. Infants born of alcoholic mothers often show severe dysfunction of the central nervous system. Most certainly, there is severe thalamic damage in these children with all of the ramifications that occur when the thalamic relay stations are dysfunctional.

More recent research is indicating that the thalamus is also involved in the function of declarative long-term memory, and in conditional fear responses.

THE SUBTHALAMUS

The subthalamus is also paired, so the proper terminology would be the subthalami. The subthalami lie between the thalami and the roof of tegmentum of the midbrain on each side (**Fig 5-19**). The subthalami are oval, gray masses somewhat smaller than the thalami. It is interesting to note that the subthalami are found only in mammals. Problems with subthalamic development result in a condition referred to as hemiballism. Hemiballism is a rather violent form of "jumping restlessness" that involves only one side of the body. Usually, the upper extremity is most severely involved.

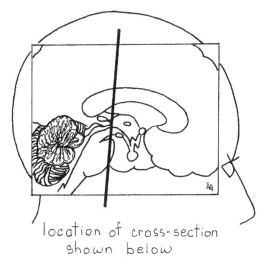

location of cross-section
shown below

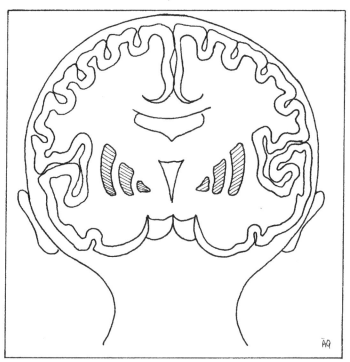

Fig. 5-19
Subthalamus: Globus Pallidus and Subthalamic Nuclei:
The upper drawing is a side view in which the cross-sectional location of
the lower drawing is indicated by the vertical line. The shaded areas in
the lower drawing indicate the locations of the subthalamic structures.

THE EPITHALAMUS

The epithalamus is not paired. It consists of the pineal gland (which we mentioned above as lying between the two thalami), the posterior commissure and the habenular trigone **(Fig. 5-20)**.

The pineal gland is a small mass suspended by a stalk from the crossover (commissural) fibers above it. The pineal gland is thought to have to do with circadian rhythms, directional sense in relationship to the north-south magnetic fields of the poles of the earth, and by some authorities to be related to the immune system. Recent work with rabbits in Europe also suggests that a dysfunctional pineal gland may result in spinal curvature (scoliosis). It is thought that this relationship may be present because the pineal gland urges us to have vertical upright posture. When that urging is not present, the spine begins to collapse to one side or the other. This results in deformity of one or more of the vertebral bodies into a wedge shape. The result is spinal curvature.

The posterior commissure is a region of nerve fibers that connect right and left sides of the brain **(Fig. 3-35)**.

The habenular trigone is a small, depressed triangular area related to the sense of smell. The habenular trigone overlays the habenular nuclei. The habenular structures connect the sense of smell with the limbic system. The result is the memories and emotions stirred by certain odors.

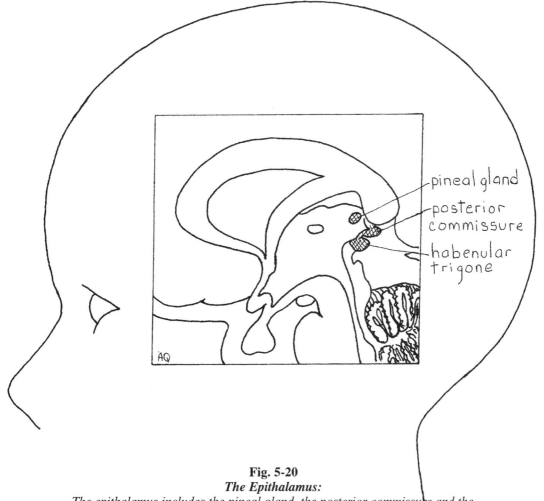

Fig. 5-20
The Epithalamus:
The epithalamus includes the pineal gland, the posterior commissure and the habenular trigone. These structures are shaded and labeled in the drawing.

We don't fully understand how, but the habenular connection is essential to the impact of various smells upon emotion.

Problems with the epithalamus at birth can interfere with natural development of circadian rhythms, sense of direction as it is related to the magnetic fields of the earth, possibly the immune system, the crossover connections between left and right side of the brain mostly involving emotional factors, and the connections between smell and emotion.

THE METATHALAMUS

The metathalamus is in the region of the diencephalon. It is principally made up of the medial and lateral geniculate bodies (**Fig. 5-21**). The metathalamus is the name used for the paired

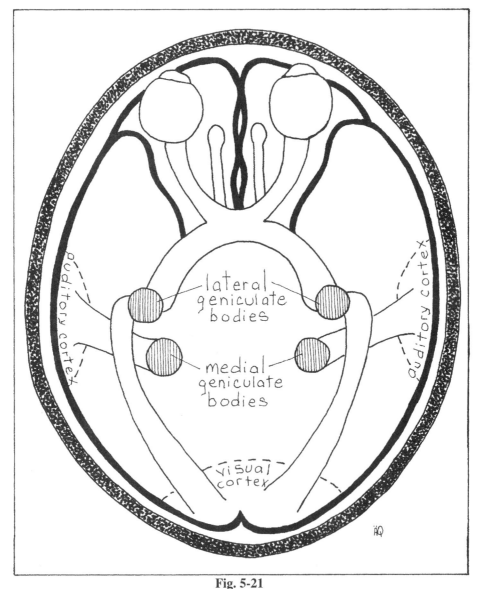

Fig. 5-21
The Metathalamus: Medial and Lateral Geniculate Bodies:
The medial and lateral geniculate bodies, which together are known as the metathalamus, are shown as shaded areas in the drawing. The lateral geniculate bodies relate to our visual sense, and the medial geniculate bodies relate to our sense of hearing.

structures. (There is a metathalamus on the right and left sides of the diencephalon.) Once again, we will use the plural form of the word, metathalami.

The medial geniculate bodies are small, paired and oval-shaped. They serve as relay stations for input coming through our auditory (hearing) sensory system.

The lateral geniculate bodies are small, paired, oval-shaped projections on the rear ends of the metathalami on both sides. They contain nerve cell aggregations which serve to relay visual stimulations to the occipital cortex for organization and interpretation into the visual images that we perceive.

Problems with the metathalamus may interfere with the interpretation and association of sounds and/or visual images, depending upon which of the geniculate bodies are affected.

THE HYPOTHALAMUS

The hypothalamus forms part of the floor and side walls of the third ventricle **(Fig. 5-22)**. It is not paired. It is a singular structure that weighs about 4 grams, which is slightly less than 1/7 of an ounce. A nickel coin weighs more than the hypothalamus. Actually, the hypothalamus weighs less than half of 1 percent of the total weight of the brain. It is located just above the pituitary gland and below the thalami. The pituitary gland is suspended from the hypothalamus by a stalk.

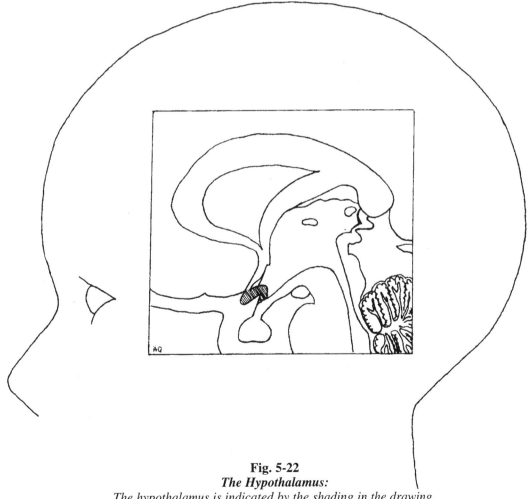

Fig. 5-22
The Hypothalamus:
The hypothalamus is indicated by the shading in the drawing.

It is quite amazing that this tiny structure influences and/or regulates to a great extent the body temperature, hunger, thirst, sexual activity, emotional behavior, ambition (goal seeking), endocrine gland function, and the activity of the autonomic (visceral) nervous system. It is also thought to have influence over sleep and wakefulness. The hypothalamus receives a great deal of nerve impulses and messages from both the cerebral cortex and the limbic system. Both the cortex and the limbic system seem able to override decisions about autonomic nervous system functions made by the hypothalamus. The cerebral cortex apparently has the greatest ability to override the hypothalamus.

This tiny hypothalamus also provides several chemical analyses for the body. For example, it determines the level of salt concentration in your body and sends this information to the appropriate organs, tissues or cells so that proper adjustments can be made. It also monitors sex hormone levels such as testosterone. It then sends messages to the glands that make testosterone in order to regulate the rate of the hormone's production and secretion into the bloodstream. Thus, the hypothalamus can and does influence male libido and sexual potency via its influence on testosterone production. It provides much of the connection between emotion and sexuality.

In addition, the hypothalamus contains several pleasure centers and, in some unknown way, it integrates the pursuit of pleasures with our learned and/or instinctive morals and ethics. Hence, the hypothalamus, at least in part, might be considered a seat of conscience.

The most common neurotransmitters in the hypothalamus are the peptides, which are the most recently discovered neurotransmitters made out of protein. There is a wide variety of peptides thus far discovered, and the list gets larger every month. Among the peptides that are plentiful in the hypothalamus are the endorphins, which are closely related to all the opiates. On this basis it seems reasonable that the hypothalamus may be involved in addictive behaviors.

THE TELENCEPHALON

The telencephalon is the highest division of the central nervous system. It is the forwardmost and uppermost part of the forebrain (of which the other part is the diencephalon).

The telencephalon includes the two paired cerebral hemispheres and the lamina terminalis. The telencephalon is formed in the embryo at about 3 1/2 to 4 weeks of gestation. It develops from the paired embryonic vessels, which were the forwardmost and lateral outpouchings of the forebrain. The cerebral hemispheres are the least fully developed parts of the brain at the time that the newborn infant is delivered from the inside of the uterus to the outside world. However, you may recall that the cerebral cortex, which is a part of the telencephalon, covers most of the brain much as a knitted cap covers your head.

THE CEREBRAL HEMISPHERES

The cerebral hemispheres are the paired structures that form the bulk of the human brain. Together, these hemispheres form the cerebral cortex, the centrum semiovale, the basal ganglia and the rhinencephalon. Some authorities prefer to place the lateral ventricles as components of the telencephalon rather than the diencephalon as we have indicated in the previous section.

Ultimately, the cerebral hemispheres develop into the various lobes of the brain. These lobes are the frontal lobes, the parietal lobes, the temporal lobes, the occipital lobes and the central lobe (also and perhaps more commonly known as the insula) (**Fig. 5-23**).

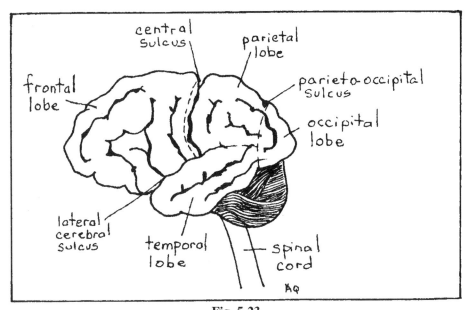

Fig. 5-23
Side View of a Cerebral Hemisphere:
This drawing demonstrates the massive overlay of the underlying (subcortical)
structures of the brain that is provided by the cortical tissue on each hemisphere.

THE CEREBRAL CORTEX

The cerebral cortex is the highly convoluted gray substance that covers each of the cerebral hemispheres. It is about 2 to 4 millimeters thick and is composed of six specific layers of neuronal material. Each layer has its own specific function.

The convolutions allow for a significant increase in the amount of surface area without causing the volume of the skull to enlarge. The grooves or valleys in the surface area are called sulci (singular is sulcus), and the peaks or protruding folds are called gyri (singular is gyrus). There are also deeper grooves in the brain tissue called fissures (**Fig. 3-33 and 5-23**). It is the fissures that separate the various lobes and the right and left hemispheres from one another. It is estimated that about 50 percent of the cortical surface of the brain is located in the sulci and the fissures.

The substance of the cerebral cortex is gray because the neuron cell bodies are gray. The fibers of these cell bodies are white because they are coated with a white substance called myelin. It is part of the function of the myelin to provide an insulating sheathing around the myelinated nerve fibers so that the electrical impulses do not jump from one conducting nerve fiber to another. Nerve "cross talk," as it is called, is much like two electric wires that have defects in their insulation. These wires develop short circuits. Short circuits in either nerve fibers or electric wires cause the end organs, such as muscles in the case of nerve fibers, or toasters and other appliances in the case of electric wires, to dysfunction.

The cerebral cortex has over 10 billion neurons and 100 billion astrocytes within its structure. The structure is organized in six distinct layers. Keep in mind that the neurons perform the actual conduction of messages from the sensory receptors located throughout the body to the brain, between each other, and from the brain to the end organs which carry out the commands. From the time a message enters a neuron through an incoming synapse until the message is delivered to its outgoing synapse, the message delivery is carried out by the conduction of electrical impulses. At the synapse, be it incoming or outgoing, the messages most often cross the synapse by the conversion of the electrical impulse to a chemical process, which involves neurotransmitters. On the far side of the synapse, the chemical process is then reconverted into an electrical impulse, which traverses the next neuron in the chain, or which activates the end organ (a muscle, a gland, etc.). In a minority of cases, a few of the smaller synapses with narrower clefts between the two components may have protein bridges across the synaptic cleft which directly conduct the electrical impulse from the incoming neuron to the outgoing neuron. In these situations the need for conversion to a chemical process is obviated.

The cerebral cortex provides the necessary structures for the highest level of intellectual activities and cognitive functions. It is a key player in perception, in most kinds of memory, in speech and language interpretation, in visual processing, in higher motor function and so on (**Fig. 5-24**).

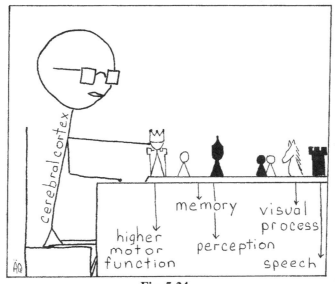

Fig. 5-24
Some Cerebral Cortex Functions:
The cerebral cortex seems to be the home of the intellect.
It also attempts to control our emotions and our instincts.
This control attempt is not always successful. The cortex's
main service to us is problem assessment and solving.

Specific areas of the cerebral cortex have been identified as being related to specific functions, although as research in brain function becomes technically more advanced, it becomes more and more clear that some of our previous "knowledge" about specific cortical areas and specific functions is to be questioned. Be that as it may, there seem to be major areas of cerebral cortex that are quite specific in function. These specific areas are motor cortex, the premotor cortex, the somesthetic cortex, the visual-association cortex, the auditory-association cortex, the planum temporale (word-production) cortex, Wernicke's and Broca's areas (speech motor) of the cortex, and the frontal cortices (**Fig. 5-25**). In general, these areas are surviving the newer research findings but their exclusivity is very much in question. That is, we are seeing that, given the opportunity and encouragement, other brain areas show an ability to take over some of the function of a given area that has been damaged. This ability is referred to as "plasticity." Until recently, brain plasticity was considered impossible in humans.

There were some monkeys in a Silver Spring, Maryland, research laboratory that had demonstrated some very surprising results. These monkeys had the nerves to their arms cut by a neurosurgeon. It was expected that the somesthetic, or sensory cortex areas that had been receiving impulses from the arms with the nerves cut would atrophy and become dysfunctional. This cortex did not atrophy. Instead, the cortex in question began receiving nerve impulses from the monkey's face. This was clearly a "plastic" change in monkey brain function. This raises the question: if monkeys can do it, can humans do it?

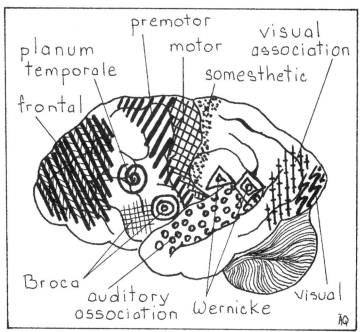

Fig. 5-25
Some Specific Areas of the Cerebral Cortex:
The specific areas of the cerebral cortex shown in this drawing seem to be withstanding the tests of further research. Broca, Wernicke and the planum temporale areas are all involved in language. The somesthetic area is related to sensory perception, and the frontal areas are primarily involved in intellectual activities.

There have also been reports that strongly support the brain's "plastic" abilities in humans. John Lorber, M.D., a neurosurgeon in Sheffield, England, reported an honors math student with a tested I.Q. of 129 had only a 1 millimeter thickness of brain tissue over the surface of the ventricles. By previous standards, this student should have been retarded intellectually. Dr. Lorber states that he has collected over 600 brain scans of hydrocephalic patients with reduced volumes of brain tissue, many of whom were not intellectually impaired as would have been predicted. I have also read an informal report from a research team in California that stated that a significant percentage of the honors students studying science at a university level would be classified as "microcephalic" according to imagery studies of brain size.

These preliminary data do suggest that the old dogma about "the bigger the brain, the smarter the brain's owner" is incorrect. We need to rethink our ideas about mental retardation and perhaps have more hope for normal function in microcephalics and hydrocephalics. Perhaps if we offer more chances for intellectual development we will see some wonderfully surprising results.

Now let's look at some interesting "thought" provokers about brain function. These statements may raise more questions than they provide answers. However, it is time that we questioned and eliminated our dogmatic approach to brain function.

We have seen that the language-related areas of the cerebral cortex seem to atrophy if the infant is not exposed to language. This suggests to me that, when a microcephalic child is born and is expected to be mentally retarded, a few things happen. First, we may not give that child enough external stimulation to cause the "plasticity" of the brain to activate. Second, we may more or less isolate and neglect that child, thus encouraging further brain atrophy. Third, I have this intuitive feeling that people and animals live up to expectations, even when those expectations are not spoken. I'm sure that babies instinctively "feel" what those huge adults expect, and may well nonconsciously begin to fulfill those expectations. So offer a stimulating environment with lots of human interaction, and offer high expectations. It certainly can't hurt anything, and the microcephalic may surprise you.

The hippocampus feeds short-term remembered events into the cerebral cortex for conversion to long-term memories. It was always thought that a memory was stored in one place in your brain. Now we see clearly that the storage of a memory of a single specific event is stored redundantly in several brain areas. Again, the idea that once a brain area is injured the situation for recovery is hopeless is shown to be wrong. If we try we may be very pleasantly surprised.

We were taught in school that specific motor cells or cell groups in the cerebral cortex controlled specific muscles. This is still true, but what we now realize is that the vertical columnar arrangement of neurons in the motor cortex has a very special significance. It seems that a column of neurons in the cerebral motor cortex represents the organized control of all of the muscles that go to a single joint. Therefore, it would seem that the columnar arrangement of neurons in the motor cortex is designed for the purpose of controlling joints, and therefore body positions and postures, rather than focusing their intelligence on single muscle actions.

Speech seems to be a major factor in brain development and function. The cortical areas of the brain normally show a major growth spurt between 6 and 12 months. Then, if a lot of words are given to the infant, these words begin to have meaning and another growth spurt of the language areas of the cortex occurs between 12 and 18 months of age. If there is a lack of language input between 6 and 12 months of age, this second growth spurt will probably not occur. Instead, atrophy may occur and the child will have poor language skills. If there has been a birth trauma to a language area, it seems that language input can activate a compensatory change in brain cell function so that uninjured language-skill areas can develop more than they usually do. Once again, provide input and encourage the brain's "plasticity" to accommodate for problems.

By about 24 months of age, the child begins to lateralize his/her language skills. Usually the left side of the brain becomes dominant in language, and the right side of the brain focuses upon music, singing and creative activities. Damage to one hemisphere before age two years is usually easily compensated by the developing brain so that either the left or the right hemisphere can do it all: language, music, etc.

An interesting observation that is emerging is that females have a larger planum temporale on the right side of the brain, whereas males have a larger planum temporale on the left side of the brain. One of the common problems between the sexes in terms of language communication seems to be that males want the precise facts. Females more often speak intuitively. The planum temporale is the brain area that seems most involved in the selection of the words that we use in order to verbally express an idea. The right hemisphere is more focused on intuition, creative ideas, abstract thoughts and bodily self-image. The left hemisphere is more exacting and objective. It thinks rationally, precisely, and is very focused on logical statements. It won't just "talk." It weighs its words (**Fig. 5-26**).

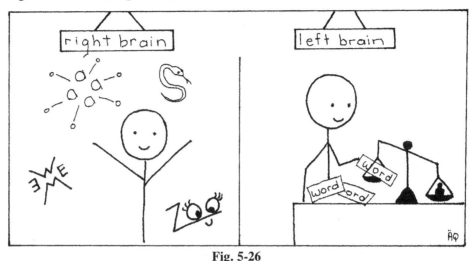

Fig. 5-26
Planum Temporale Functions:
The planum temporale regions of the cerebral cortex have a lot to do with our thoughts and how we express them verbally. The right planum temporale is more spontaneous and less careful about its choice of words. The left planum temporale chooses its words more carefully.

In view of these observations, perhaps there is a sex difference in the use of the language. Perhaps intuitive men and scientific women have made some "plastic changes" in their planum temporale regions.

Statistically, it seems that about 98.9 percent of right-handed adults use the left side of their cerebral cortex to read. About 20 percent of left-handed adults can and do use both left and right sides of their cerebral cortices when they read, and about 10 percent of left-handed adults use only the left cerebral cortex when they read. So, about percent of left-handers still read with the left side of the brain. The answer to this puzzle has not yet been forthcoming.

It does seem to me that an integrated and balanced function of the right and left hemispheres with their individually different focuses, one on intuition and the other on proven fact, gives us a more stereoscopic and balanced view of life, things and the universe. It also seems that when we focus more on one hemisphere than the other, there is an actual inhibition of the hemispheric activity on the side not being used. That is, if you practice hard logic all the time, the left hemisphere gets stronger as if in response to exercise. Concurrently, the right hemisphere weakens as if being neglected. The right hemisphere might be analogous to the "couch potato" and the left analogous to the "body builder" in this case. This hemispheric inhibition leads me to a new concept that has emerged recently as we do more and more PET scan studies of brain function. The new concept is what we might call the "cerebral steal."

Before we describe the "cerebral steal," it is important that you have some idea of what the PET scan is about. PET stands for Positron Emission Tomography. A positron is a positively charged particle in the nucleus of an atom that has about the same mass as an electron. The electron is negatively charged. Positron emission is a process in which an atomic nucleus ejects both a positron and a neutrino at the same time. A neutrino is a particle that has no mass and no electrical charge that we know of. In any case, Positron Emission Tomography is a technique wherein radioactive tracers are given to the subject under study and the emission of positrons is recorded by instrumentation. In the case of using the PET scan to study brain function, a radioactive tracer is administered that attaches to the glucose (sugar) molecule in the blood. Glucose is used by brain cells on a minute-to-minute and second-to-second basis as their principal fuel. The supposition here is that the more active brain areas will use more glucose. Since the glucose has a radioactive tracer attached that emits measurable positrons, it seems reasonable that the more positrons being emitted in a given brain area, the more activity there is in the neurons in that area.

Back to the concept of "cerebral steal." PET scan studies indicate that the brain can only do so much work. That is, it only has a limited amount of energy that must be budgeted throughout all of its structures. For example, the studies suggest that almost one-third of the total cortex is involved in the processing of visual information. So when we are reading, it is hard to listen to music. It is also more difficult to read aloud than to just read or speak singularly. This is because both reading and speaking require a lot of energy. Since there is a cap or an upper limit on the available energy in the brain at any given time, the energy to read and speak (read aloud) must be taken from some other brain area. This "cerebral steal" concept could explain why we get deep in thought or in deep concentration on something and don't notice that our neck is stiff or the house is on fire until our neck is very painful or the smoke from the fire is choking us. Think about this one. It can explain lots of things that we do, and things that escape us.

WHITE MATTER - CENTRUM SEMIOVALE

The white matter which underlies the gray matter of the cerebral cortex is made up of myelinated fibers. The centrum semiovale is simply the name given to the white matter that is seen when you remove the top of the brain (cerebrum) at a given level (the level of the corpus callosum). This white matter is the mass of nerve fibers that interconnect neurons of the cortex between themselves, with sensory input neurons and motor outflow neurons.

Those nerve fibers that interconnect are categorized as: (1) association fibers which interconnect cortical neurons in the same hemisphere; (2) commissural fibers which interconnect neurons located in the two hemispheres, i.e., they cross the midline of the brain and interconnect right and left sides; and (3) projection fibers which connect the neurons of the cerebral cortex with neurons of the numerous subcortical regions such as the thalamus, the internal capsule and so on.

THE BASAL GANGLIA

The basal ganglia are very specific interconnected gray masses located deep in the cerebral hemispheres on both sides (**Fig. 5-27**). These ganglia, which protrude into the brain stem, are involved with the cerebellum in the modulation, control and coordination of all body movements. The interconnections of the basal ganglia include almost everything in the brain and spinal cord.

The structures included in the basal ganglia are the caudate nucleus, the globus pallidus, the putamen, the amygdala, the striatum, the substantia nigra and the subthalamic nuclei.

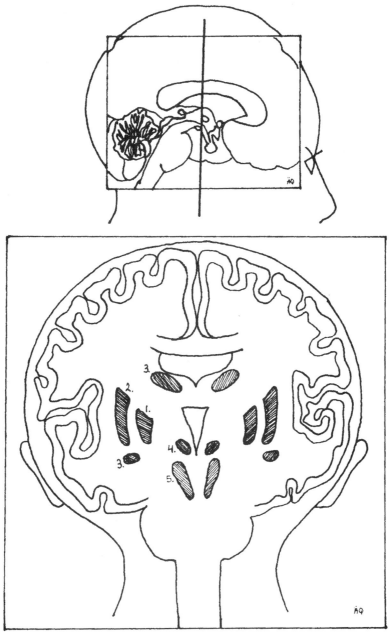

Fig. 5-27
The Basal Ganglia:
The components of the basal ganglia are shaded and numbered as
follows: (1) globus pallidus, (2) putamen, (3) caudate nucleus,
(4) subthalamic nuclei, (5) substantia nigra. The amygdala and the
striatum are not shown on this drawing. See text for further details.

Problems with the basal ganglia manifest as lack of controlled movement. In adults, Parkinson's disease with its difficult movements and tremors is a reflection of basal ganglia problems. In a newborn we typically see abnormal movements, such as the hand going to the side rather than towards an object that the infant is attempting to touch or grasp, when there is a basal ganglia problem.

The basal ganglia are also involved in the integration of sensory input information with motor outflow commands to body parts and internal organs. There is a deep influence of the basal ganglia upon the activities of the internal adaptive responses such as digestion, heart action, breathing, etc., in response to sensory input information.

The basal ganglia are intimately connected with almost all areas of the cerebral cortex, and they receive a large number of nerve impulses from the thalamus. They are involved in planned movements that have multiple components and which require timed sequencing. Examples of this type of activity would be everything you see a gymnast do in a performance, the hop, skip and jumping activities you see in a track and field meet, and so on. Any movement that requires planning and sequencing requires basal ganglia participation, even things that we take for granted, such as walking, eating, swallowing and the like.

THE RHINENCEPHALON

The rhinencephalon deals with our olfactory sense, which is our sense of smell. It has also been called the nose brain. It is one of the oldest parts of the brain phylogenetically. In one sense it is a part of the cerebral hemispheres, and in another sense it is a brain division in its own right. The rhinencephalon includes the smell receptors in the nose. The fibers of these receptors pass up through tiny holes in one of the bones (cribriform plate of the ethmoid bone) into the olfactory bulbs which lie above this bone **(Fig. 5-28)**. From there the stimuli created by the smells are conducted along the underside of the brain through the olfactory tracts to several connections in the brain which coordinate smells with memories, emotions, whetting or diminishing of the appetite, etc. We will

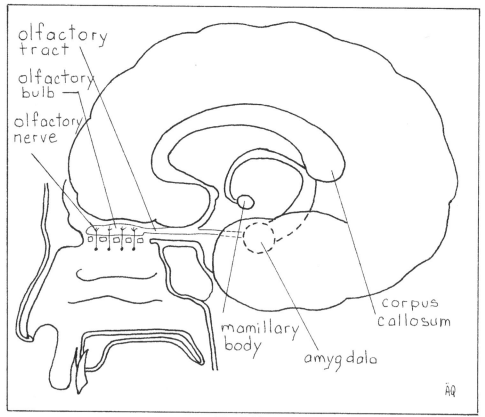

Fig. 5-28
The Rhinencephalon:
The rhinencephalon is the home of the olfactory system. The molecules that stimulate the smell receptors come in through the nose. These stimuli are then sent to the brain via the olfactory nerves, bulb and tracts. This is a very primitive part of us.

talk a lot more about the olfactory system in relationship to the limbic system **(Section V, Topic 20)**, the triune brain model **(Section VIII)** and the reticular system **(Section V, Topic 23)**.

It is of interest to note that more than 8 percent of all head-trauma patients suffer some loss of their sense of smell. However, since the olfactory nerves are capable of regeneration, many of these patients experience some spontaneous recovery of their ability to smell. In fact, it seems that even without an injury to precipitate regeneration of the olfactory nerves, we are always sprouting new olfactory nerves under normal circumstances.

It also seems that the sense of smell is present in the fetus while it is still present in the mother's womb. The olfactory system is one of the first nerve systems to develop completely. Intrauterine injuries may interfere with the development of the olfactory system. When this occurs, the newborn may not be able to smell at birth but will probably develop that ability a little later on in life.

THE LATERAL VENTRICLES

The paired lateral ventricles are located one on each side of the third ventricle. The shapes of these ventricles are illustrated in **Fig. 3-38**. These lateral ventricles are sometimes considered as a part of the diencephalon rather than the telencephalon. I do not wish to become involved in border disputes, so I'll just say that they probably extend into both regions enough to cause a disagreement. The lateral ventricles produce cerebrospinal fluid and pass it on into the third ventricle, which adds some more cerebrospinal fluid to the total volume and passes this fluid on into the fourth ventricle for distribution to the central canal of the spinal cord and the subarachnoid spaces via the foramina of Magendie and Luschka.

Problems with these ventricles may lead to improper quantities of cerebrospinal fluid being formed, which in turn may create a wide variety of brain-function problems, as well as difficulties with the spinal cord.

THE LAMINA TERMINALIS

The lamina terminalis is also considered herein as a part of the telencephalic division of the forebrain, although some authorities consider it a part of the diencephalon. I feel that it is appropriate to consider this structure before we talk about the various lobes of the cerebral hemispheres, no matter where we categorize it. In Latin, lamina means a thin, flat plate or layer. Terminalis means at the end point. The lamina terminalis is a thin plate that originated during the embryonic development from the telencephalon. It was the forwardmost part of the neural tube. Ultimately, it forms the forwardmost (anterior) wall of the third ventricle. At birth it connects the two hemispheres of the brain, and it runs vertically between the roof plate of the diencephalon and the optic chiasm. It separates the telencephalon from the diencephalon **(Fig. 5-29)**. If the final neuropore of the neural tube at the head end fails to close, it seems reasonable that the lamina terminalis would have a defect. To be very honest, I do not know what effect such a defect might have on the newborn. Since this lamina terminalis does form a part of the wall of the third ventricle, it also seems possible that there could be a cerebrospinal fluid leak in the affected wall. This could lead to a type of hydrocephalus. However, please be aware that this is pure conjecture on my part. I choose not to offer further conjecture on the effect of incomplete division between diencephalon and telencephalon. It seems to me that Mother Nature would compensate somehow in both circumstances. What the compensation might cost in terms of functional compromise, I cannot guess.

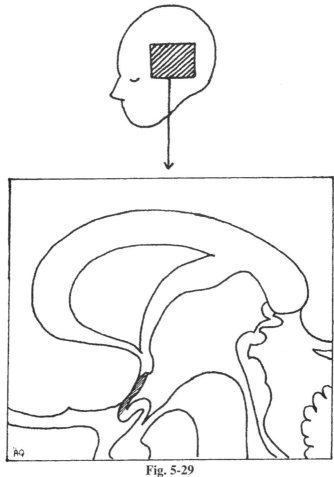

Fig. 5-29
The Lamina Terminalis:
The lamina terminalis is indicated by the shaded areas in the inset drawing. It is the forwardmost part of the neural tube. At birth it connects the two brain hemispheres, and it is part of the wall of the third ventricle of the brain.

THE CORPUS CALLOSUM

We consider the corpus callosum along with the telencephalon at this time, although it, too, crosses boundaries. The corpus callosum is the major crossover connection between the right and left cerebral hemispheres **(Fig. 5-30)**. It contains about 200 million crossover fibers. It is located deep in the brain at the bottom of the very deep sagittal fissure. It is this fissure that divides the brain into its two separate hemispheres. It is larger in women. The presence of the corpus callosum allows integration of the two halves of the brain.

Children are sometimes born without a corpus callosum. This situation interferes with functional coordination of speech, thought and feeling, some motor coordination and the like. My own view is that the deficit, which grows more apparent with the maturation of the child, is the lack of integration between intellect and intuition, and between arts such as music, color, etc., and academic areas such as grammar and arithmetic. They do not have the stereoscopic intellect which I mentioned previously.

THE INTERNAL CAPSULE

The internal capsule is a fanlike mass of white (myelinated) fibers. It connects the cerebral cortex to many subcortical (lower) brain centers. The internal capsule is the most frequent location of adult stroke because its blood supply is extremely vulnerable. It is considered as a component of the basal ganglia system **(Fig. 5-30)**. When it is damaged it causes problems with motor coordination, if not full paralysis. It is also related to sight and hearing, and may be involved in problems of the newborn related to these senses.

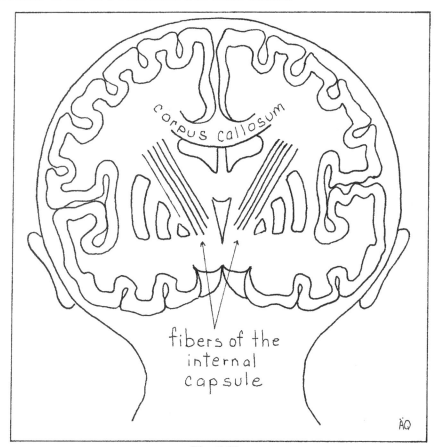

Fig. 5-30
The Internal Capsule:
Internal capsule fibers connect cortical and subcortical brain centers.
This system is considered as a part of the basal ganglia. The corpus
callosum is also labeled.

Topic 19

The Lobes of the Cerebral Hemispheres

There are five pairs of lobes of the cerebral hemispheres. These pairs are the frontal lobes, the parietal lobes, the temporal lobes, the occipital lobes and the central lobes (**Fig. 3-41**). The central lobes are also called the insula or insular lobes. These lobes have been further subdivided repeatedly. The result of all of these subdivisions is a rather complex picture of the brain, the details of which are not necessary for our purposes. Therefore, we will content ourselves with a more generalized overview.

THE MAJOR FISSURES

In general, the major fissures serve to separate some of the lobes from one another, although this is not always the case.

A fissure is defined as any cleft or groove. The major fissures always penetrate or incise the entire 2 to 4 millimeters thickness of the gray matter of the cerebral cortex. The major fissures with which we will concern ourselves are: (1) the longitudinal cerebral (interhemispheric) fissure, (2) the central cerebral (rolandic) fissure and (3) the lateral cerebral (Sylvian) fissure. I have chosen to use the term fissure for these major boundaries between the lobes of the cerebrum. Some authors use the term sulcus for even these major boundaries. Usually a sulcus is more shallow than a fissure. Please don't be confused. You will probably encounter both terms applying to the same structure.

The longitudinal cerebral fissure runs from front to back and is the deep division that separates the brain/cerebrum into right and left halves, or hemispheres. This fissure is occupied by the falx cerebri, which is a membrane structure made of dura mater that divides the skull into right and left compartments. It forms a petition that, among other things, prevents the two cerebral hemispheres from banging into each other. The gray tissue of the cerebral cortex lines the sides of the fissure as the fissure's longitudinal line penetrates the brain substance. At the bottom of our longitudinal cerebral fissure is our old friend the corpus callosum, which connects the two cerebral hemispheres both structurally and functionally across the midline. The longitudinal cerebral fissure divides the frontal region, the parietal region and the occipital region into right and left lobes. Hence, the longitudinal cerebral fissure is the medial boundary for the frontal lobes, the parietal lobes and the occipital lobes of the brain (**Fig. 5-31**).

The central cerebral fissure is also called the fissure of Rolando. This central cerebral fissure is oriented in a side-to-side (transverse) direction (**Fig. 5-31**). It serves to separate the frontal and parietal lobes of the brain. This fissure is also lined with gray matter and it penetrates into the brain at variable depths along its course. These depths usually range between 10 and 20 millimeters. As shown in the illustration, the parietal lobes lie directly behind the frontal lobes (**Fig. 5-31**).

The other major fissure that is important to our general anatomical overview is the lateral cerebral fissure (**Fig. 5-31**). This fissure is located on the side of the brain. Its orientation is almost horizontal. The lateral cerebral fissure separates the lower part of the frontal lobe from the temporal lobe of the brain. It also partially separates the lower forward part of the parietal lobe from the temporal lobe. The back part of the temporal lobe does not have clear separation from the back part of the parietal lobe by means of a fissure. Nor do the back parts of the parietal and temporal lobes enjoy clear fissure boundaries from the occipital lobe on either side of the brain. These latter divisions between the back parts of the temporal and parietal lobes and the occipital lobes are much more man-made and less natural. The conjectured various functions of these brain lobes prompted neuroanatomists to insert arbitrary interlobular dividing lines. Please look at the drawings of these fissures and the cortical lobes. In this case, a picture is definitely worth a thousand words.

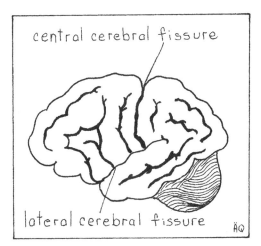

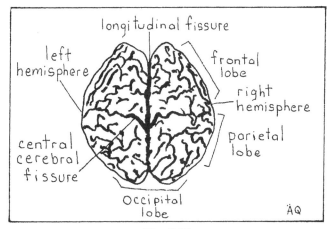

Fig. 5-31
Top and Side Views of the Brain Which Demonstrate the Major Fissures:
In the side view we see the central cerebral fissures, which separate the frontal and the parietal lobes of the brain. We also see the lateral cerebral fissure which partially separates the temporal lobes from the frontal and parietal lobes. In the top view we see the longitudinal fissure separating the two hemispheres, and the central cerebral fissure (of Rolando), which separates the frontal from the parietal lobes.

THE FRONTAL LOBES AND THEIR CORTEX

From a functional point of view, the cerebral cortices of the frontal lobes of the brain are involved in many things. They are involved in movement control of the body. This involvement includes gross and fine motor control of muscles and muscle coordination, as well as involuntary control of postural stance, etc. The cortex of the frontal lobes is also involved in eye movement and focusing. There are a myriad of association areas in the frontal lobes. The cortical interconnections contribute a great deal to thought process, insight, memory, and much of this stuff that we call intelligence, such as decision-making in personal and social matters on a rational or logical level. The cortices of the frontal lobes also moderate and modulate our responses to emotional messages, the majority of which are sent up from the hypothalamus and the limbic system. Also included in frontal lobe cortical functions are attentiveness, ability to categorize and organize information, working memory, and the ability to generalize learned responses from one situation to another. There is also an area of the frontal cortex that relates to our ability to discriminate between various sound pitches.

In general, one might say that the frontal lobe cortex helps us to be rational, to control our temper, to learn the social graces, to solve problems, to be creative, and to move about effectively and appropriately. This seems to be fairly important stuff.

THE PARIETAL LOBES AND THEIR CORTEX

The cortex of the parietal lobes is involved in sensory reception and interpretation as well as in motor speech. The parietal lobes receive information from the world around us as well as from the world within us. Decisions are then made about what should be done, if anything, in response to this input. As you can guess, if we have to move our body, the parietal cortex and the frontal cortex get together and a decision is made as to what action will be taken.

It is also interesting to note that motor speech is shared between the parietal and the temporal lobes. Usually, the left side of the brain controls speech and the right side controls singing. So, it is not uncommon for left-sided problems to prevent speech but allow singing. When the right side of the brain is dominant, the reverse is true. When we are paying attention to velocity of a moving object, it seems that only the left inferior parietal cortex is activated. This observation may change as studies continue.

THE TEMPORAL LOBES AND THEIR CORTEX

The temporal lobe cortices are involved in the auditory senses (hearing) in that they receive and interpret sounds as they are conducted inward to them via the ears. The ears contain the mechanisms for changing sounds into electrical impulses. The temporal lobes are also involved in the interpretation of sight and visual images, as well as visceral function and emotion. The planum temporale is located in the cortex of the temporal lobes on both sides of the brain. It also expands over part of the adjacent parietal lobes. The planum temporale regions are related to our choice of words to express ideas. Usually, women have larger planum temporale regions on the right side of the brain and men have larger ones on the left. This may be why, in general, women speak more on an intuitive level and men are usually more precise in their use of the language.

The temporal cortices also activate when we pay attention to shape. This activation is more pronounced on the right side.

The inferior temporal cortices are involved in visual memory. These areas sort out new experiences and file them away appropriately for future references. Also, the temporal cortices overlay the hippocampus and the amygdala. These parts of the temporal lobes are used by these structures in the transfer of information from short-term memory to long-term memory storage.

THE OCCIPITAL LOBES AND THEIR CORTEX

The occipital lobes of the brain are the posteriormost lobes. Their primary function is in the reception, interpretation and relaying of information brought in via the sense of sight. There has been a lot of work done, and much controversy and resultant confusion about the limits of the occipital lobes and their importance in visual association with memory, emotion and the like. Suffice it to say that we have a distance to travel yet before we fully comprehend the function and importance of the occipital lobes. The same is true of all the cortical lobes, but it would seem that the occipital lobes have gotten somewhat more press than the others. Some of the latest work out of Washington University in St. Louis, Missouri, shows that the right occipital cortex is more active than the left by a ratio of about 2:1 when we pay attention to color.

THE CENTRAL OR INSULAR LOBES AND THEIR CORTEX

The central or insular lobes are buried in the depths of the lateral cerebral fissures. The central lobes are, however, covered with gray matter, which constitutes a cortex or cortical layer which is called the cingulate cortex. By the end of the first year of extrauterine life, the insula is completely buried and attached to the corpus callosum.

The function of these central lobes is still not well-understood. However, it is known that the cortex of the central lobes communicates closely with the amygdala, which are involved in emotional feelings and behaviors, as parts of the limbic system. It is also thought that the cortex of the central lobes has some function in the processing of sensory input as it relates to emotional feelings provoked by these incoming messages. Recent PET scan studies from Washington University in St. Louis suggest that the insula also has a role in attention and listening abilities.

The Limbic System

The limbic system, also known as the mammalian brain, wraps around the brain stem. It is present in all mammals, such as dogs, cows, tigers, dolphins and people. It is the part of the brain that contributes the first altruistic behaviors as we go up the phylogenetic ladder from one-celled animals through all the species to Homo sapiens (humans). There may be some controversy, however, as to just which species occupies the top rung of the ladder. Witness the chaos which surrounds you in our man-made world.

In any case, the limbic system is responsible for the sense of love for your offspring, your sense of family and love of family, your sense of needing to settle into a "home" (be it a cave, a ranch, a mansion or a hut). It is responsible for your sense of loyalty, your feelings of pleasure, sexuality, joy, hatred, anger, rage, fear, panic and so on. It receives communications from the touch, the visual, the auditory, the proprioceptive, the balance and equilibrium, the taste and the olfactory systems. When you are governed by animal instinct in certain situations, your limbic system has a lot to do with it.

The limbic system is a "V-shaped" system that is seated atop the brain stem beneath the diencephalon. It is encircled by the cingulate gyrus rather like a girdle encircles a waist. The apex or point of the "V" points forward, and the "V" itself is oriented more or less on a horizontal plane when the head is in a vertical or standing position. We must be very liberal to use the "V" as a model for the actual shape of the limbic system because, in reality, the structures involved are curved, almost like the horns of a ram **(Fig. 5-32)**.

As in any good functional system, the components of the limbic system are subject to some disagreement amongst brain and nervous system authorities. The list of limbic system components which follows may contradict other lists that you may come across. Please understand that the apparent discrepancies are not necessarily errors, they are more likely evidence of disagreement. Most everyone agrees that the amygdala, the fornix, the hippocampuses, the septal nuclei and the mamillary bodies are parts of the limbic system. Some authorities would include parts of the thalamus, parts of the hypothalamus, parts of the midbrain (mesencephalon) and parts of the olfactory system as components of the limbic system. We will not spend our time entering into the arguments about classification of brain parts.

A great majority of the limbic system is found in the temporal lobes. Seizure problems with the limbic system are called temporal lobe seizures, psychomotor seizures or limbic seizures. The seizures often include hallucinations of the senses, such as smell, taste, touch, vision and hearing. They also often include purposeless movements, such as lip smacking and/or fumbling with

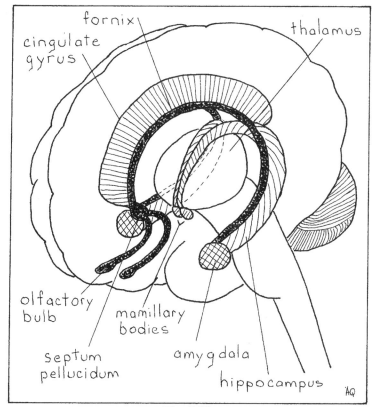

Fig. 5-32
The Limbic System:
The limbic system is a three-dimensional system that is quite difficult to demonstrate on a two-dimensional piece of paper. We hope you get the general idea from this drawing. See text for a more detailed description.

clothing or buttons, much as a very shy person might do. Also, the temporal lobe or limbic seizure often includes marked emotional responses. Patients with this type of problem may experience extreme joy or sadness, or extreme pleasure or pain during a seizure. They may have sexual orgasm or fly into a rage attack or a panic. Any or all of these things can happen.

During the emotionally dominated temporal lobe or limbic seizures, the vital functions of the body respond as though there is an externally induced panic, rage, sexual orgasm, etc. That is, the skin may flush or turn pale, the heart may race to very scary levels, breathing patterns may change, muscle activities will simulate the real thing, and so on. From these observations it is clear that this limbic system has powerful and far-reaching effects.

In an infant, this seizure may be very confusing to observe because it is difficult to separate the seizure from a normal emotional response in the very young child, depending upon the form that the seizure takes.

Many authorities state that the right half of the brain has almost exclusive rights to the creative activities that we pursue. However, there are some very knowledgeable neuroscientists who feel that the limbic system has a lot to do with creativity. At present I prefer to watch this argument from the sidelines and see what happens.

We do know that the limbic system has a great deal to do with our value structures, which involve our morals, ethics, likes, dislikes and our conscience. In conjunction with the midbrain, the limbic system strongly influences our sexual appetites, our consummatory behaviors (gluttony, etc.) and our evolved defensive behaviors.

It would seem that, singularly, the limbic system is responsible for the maternal caring instinct, for the nursing of offspring, warmbloodedness, audiovocal communication between mother and infant in its primary stages, and for the tendency to play.

Now let's consider some of the parts of the limbic system individually.

THE AMYGDALA

The amygdala are walnut-sized masses of gray nerve cells located one on each side of the brain. They are found deep in each side of the lateral part of the forebrain within the temporal lobes **(Fig. 5-32)**.

They are deeply involved in aggressive behavior, in fear reactions and conditioned fear responses. They are in part responsible for self-preservation activities. And they are critical sites for learning.

THE HIPPOCAMPUS

The hippocampus is a major component of the limbic system. It is a curved structure that forms part of the floor of the lateral ventricle in each hemisphere of the brain **(Fig. 5-32)**. So there are two hippocampuses, one on each side of the brain. They can also correctly be called hippocampi. The hippocampus is closely related to the olfactory region of the brain. It is one of the most ancient of brain structures phylogenetically. A hippocampus is completely located within the temporal lobe of the brain on each side. Each hippocampus is about 5 centimeters long, and curves as it extends forward from beneath the corpus callosum. A hippocampus lies adjacent to the amygdala on each side.

The hippocampus is deeply involved in our emotional lives. When your blood sugar is low, your blood level of the amino acid methionine also drops. The hippocampus is heavily and momentarily dependent upon available methionine. It requires large quantities of this amino acid. When methionine falls into short supply, the hippocampus puts out strong emotional responses. This situation is probably responsible, in large part, for the emotional instability that accompanies hypoglycemic episodes.

In addition, the hippocampus is a key player in memory. It retains information for short-term memory, and forwards information for long-term memory on to the various areas of the cerebral cortices for storage. Thus, the hippocampus acts as a triage officer for data to be remembered, and decides whether it can soon be forgotten or whether we will need that information in the distant future. One of the substances that has recently been identified as a neurotransmitter that is necessary for memory to function is nitric oxide. It is abundant in the hippocampus, as is glutamate, which acts as an excitatory neurotransmitter in the hippocampus.

The feeling of anxiety is largely under the influence of the hippocampus. Increased hippocampal activity creates anxiety. Hippocampal activity is quieted by alcohol and opiates. This may be why both of these popular substances quiet fears and make you feel better.

Anxiety may actually be the result of an interpretational conflict between the limbic system, especially the hippocampus and the cerebral cortex. Irrational fears are quieted by reducing hippocampal activity, and many people have learned to use a martini or a fix of heroine to relax. Fear conditioning is also a hippocampal function. That is, if for example a dog bites you, it is your hippocampus that makes you afraid of all dogs in the future.

In conjunction with the midbrain, the hippocampus is largely and deeply involved in hedonistic behaviors and self-awareness. Teamed up with the mamillary bodies, the hippocampus is in charge of penile erections.

The hippocampus is required for higher learning. Without it we cannot add what we are doing today onto what we did yesterday. In fact, if a hippocampus patient takes a coffee break during a task, they have to start all over. But, oddly enough, they know how to do it again. They just can't add on from where they left off.

Also, the hippocampus has a low threshold for seizures. A hippocampal seizure can amount to anything from a panic attack to a sexual fantasy or an out-of-body experience.

THE FORNIX

The fornix offers the connections between the hippocampus and the hypothalamus. The body of the fornix lies above the third ventricle and is attached to the under surface of the corpus callosum. The body of the fornix divides into two columns and connects to the two hippocampuses (**Fig. 5-32**).

Functionally, the fornix seems to be a connector system for the limbic system and for the two hemispheres of the brain. The tissue of the fornix is white, which means that it is made of rapid-conduction myelinated fibers. At this time, there is little known about any specialized fornix function other than as a connector/impulse conductor.

THE SEPTUM PELLUCIDUM

The septum is a part of the limbic system that sends and receives nerve impulses or messages from the hippocampus by way of the fornix. It is a very thin walled structure that is situated between the fornix and the corpus callosum (**Fig. 5-32**).

The neurotransmitter, acetylcholine, is very abundant in the septum. It supplies acetylcholine to the hippocampal tract.

It seems that the septum is significant in mating activities, copulation and procreation.

Topic 21

The Autonomic Nervous System

The autonomic nervous system is believed to be exclusively motor in its function. That is, it sends out impulses to various organs and systems so that the body can function automatically without conscious control by the owner of the body. Until the advent of biofeedback here in the Western world, it was generally agreed that autonomic influences upon organs and organ systems were not to be changed by attempts at conscious control. There were, however, a few radical bioscientists in the last century who used hypnosis and some other offbeat techniques with some success. In the Eastern world, however, yogis and meditators have been influencing autonomic control of organs and organ systems for many decades. Doctors Elmer and Alyce Green were pioneers in the development of biofeedback theory and technique, which they demonstrated as effective in influencing internal organ function. They were in charge of the psychophysiology research laboratories at the Menninger Foundation for many years.

Please do not get the idea that internal organs and organ systems are under exclusive control of the autonomic nervous system. The blood-born molecules that we call hormones, the neurotransmitter molecules, and that whole new class of molecules that we call the peptides, which includes the endorphins and the enkephalins, also exert great influence upon the function of the internal organs and organ systems. However, our focus here will be upon the autonomic nervous system.

Most bioscientists consider the autonomic nervous system as outside of the central nervous system. However, I believe that some acquaintance with the autonomic nervous system is essential for proper evaluation of the newborn as well as the child and the adult. Therefore, we include the autonomic nervous system in our discussion of the central nervous system. It does have its nuclei within the central nervous system.

The autonomic nerve connections, from their central control within the central nervous system to their destination organs or organ systems, all include two nerve cells. The body of the central, or uppermost nerve cell, is in the central nervous system, and the body of the second nerve cell is located in its respective ganglion outside of that system. The central autonomic neuron sends a fiber to the ganglion. This fiber connects via synapse to neurons that have their nerve cell bodies within the ganglion. A ganglion is a collection of nerve cell bodies. Within the ganglion, the nerve fiber that is extended out from the centrally placed autonomic neuron communicates with about 32 autonomic neurons that have their cell bodies within the ganglion. So the central autonomic neuron (often called the first-order neuron) has influence over several ganglionic autonomic neurons (often called second-order neurons). The average ratio has been calculated at about one first-order autonomic neuron to 32 second-order autonomic neurons.

The autonomic nervous system is divided into two parts. They are called the sympathetic nervous system and the parasympathetic nervous system. The sympathetic nervous system ganglia are most often located near the spine. The parasympathetic ganglia are usually located near the end organs that they innervate, send impulses to, and essentially control (**Fig. 5-33**).

The sympathetic nervous system is also called the thoracolumbar division because its roots exit the spinal cord in its thoracic and lumbar regions. The parasympathetic nervous system is also called the craniosacral division because its nerve roots exit the central nervous system from the brain stem, and from the lower or sacral end of the spinal cord (**Fig. 5-3**).

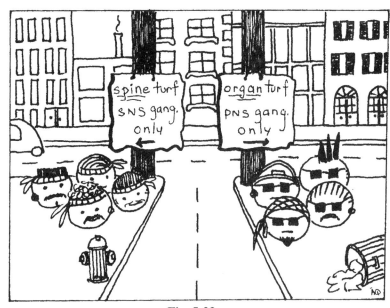

Fig. 5-33
Ganglia Locations:
The parasympathetic ganglia are located near the end organs.
The sympathetic ganglia are located near the spine. PNS=
Parasympathetic Nervous System. SNS= Sympathetic Nervous System.
I do hope that you appreciate our artist's, Ms. Quaid, sense of humor.

The sympathetic division of the autonomic nervous system is the part that takes care of emergency responses. It is the part that helps you perform superhuman tasks when some part of your brain decides that you must do it. The sympathetic division has little or no concern with the long-term effects of its demands, it only wants to get you through the moment. Oftimes the sympathetic division is called into action on a daily basis without being allowed to express the energy that it has procured for the perceived excessive demand. This situation, when repeated over and over, results in an elevated baseline level of activity for the sympathetic nervous system. The result of this sympathetic hyperactivity is chronic stress. This chronic level of increased stress then produces all kinds of stress-related health problems, such as ulcers of stomach and/or bowel, high blood pressure, hardening of the arteries, high cholesterol, coronary artery disease with chest pain (angina pectoris), which may result in heart attack, as well as stroke. So you see, the sympathetic nervous system lacks foresight. It spends your reserves to get you through the day or the specific situation. It seems not to worry about replacement of the energy that it has spent or which it is chronically spending, as happens in the case of chronic increased stress.

On the other side of the coin we have the parasympathetic nervous system, which has the job of restoring the energy reserves to safe levels after the sympathetic nervous system has spent them so freely. Essentially, the parasympathetic division is trying to keep up with these free-spending habits of the sympathetic division. The spending habits of the sympathetic nervous system habits vary with your personality. If you are chronically angry, fearful, guilty, etc., the chances are that your sympathetic nervous system will be chronically in a hyperalert and hyperactive state. If you are complacent and secure, happy and accepting, your sympathetic nervous system's baseline activity level will be lower, and therefore easier for the parasympathetic nervous system to balance. When you consider this state of affairs, it becomes easier to comprehend how techniques that reduce stress, release anger - guilt - fear, and enhance your sense of security and happiness, reduce your sympathetic-division activity and concurrently support your parasympathetic system. These techniques include many forms of mind-body integration work, such as biofeedback and hypnotherapy, as well as CranioSacral Therapy, SomatoEmotional Release℠ and Therapeutic Imagery and Dialogue. In my opinion, the reduction of sympathetic nervous system baseline activity levels coupled with the mobilization of parasympathetic response flexibility constitute the very best preventative-medicine and health-enhancement programs.

Now let's look at some of the specifics of autonomic nervous system influence on the internal organs and organ systems.

The whole body is strongly influenced by both the sympathetic and the parasympathetic divisions of the autonomic nervous system. When stimulated, the sympathetic nerves: (1) increase heart rate, (2) increase blood flow to heart muscle, (3) increase blood flow to skeletal muscle, (4) increase skeletal muscle strength and performance, (5) reduce blood flow to skin, (6) reduce blood flow to all other internal organs, (7) reduce conscious thought processes in the higher brain centers, (8) shut down digestive processes, (9) shut down peristalsis (intestinal activity), (10) shut down kidney function, (11) open the bronchi, (12) raise blood sugar and so on. (You get the idea.) All processes that are not necessary for the immediate activity are inhibited. Even healing that is in process is shut down. For example, experiments have shown that artificial electrical stimulation of the sympathetic nerves to a broken leg will prevent the bone from healing. Once the sympathetic activity is allowed to return to normal, the bone ends heal together. When the sympathetic nerves were cut, the bone healed even faster. Why don't we do that? Because if we did, the healed leg would not be able to muster the necessary strength to do hard tasks.

The parasympathetic division of the autonomic nervous system does almost the opposite of the sympathetic division. The parasympathetic nerves, when active, slow heart rate, lower blood pressure, open the blood vessels to the skin and to the internal organs. The parasympathetics have minimal influence on skeletal muscle but they stimulate the smooth muscles of the gastrointestinal system, thus enhancing peristalsis, digestion and elimination. Most glands secrete when the parasympathetics go into action. The adrenal glands, however, are slowed by the parasympathetic nerves. Adrenals help the sympathetic system. All parasympathetic activities favor anabolic activity. That is, they favor the absorption of nutrients and calories and their conversion to stored energy and/or the formation of protein building blocks. So, you can see that the parasympathetic division is charged with the restoration of the body after the sympathetic division has spent energy and bodily stores as needed in crisis situations.

The sympathetic nervous system has strong allies in the adrenal glands. The medulla of adrenal glands is originally derived during embryonic development from the same neural crest cells that gave origin to the ganglia of the sympathetic nervous system. The medulla of the adrenal glands receive nerve impulses from the first-order (preganglionic) neurons of the sympathetic division of the autonomic nervous system. When stimulated by these sympathetic impulses, the adrenal medullae secrete the hormones commonly known as adrenalin and noradrenalin into the bloodstream. These hormones, also known as epinephrine and norepinephrine, respectively, have very similar effects as the second-order sympathetic neurons have on the body tissues and organs.

You have probably heard a lot about what can be done when you get a "charge of adrenalin." My initial firsthand exposure to the power of adrenalin occurred when I admitted a middle-aged woman to the hospital after she had broken her back. She had fractured several spinal vertebrae when she lifted the rear end of her teenage son's car off of him. He became pinned under the car when the jack slipped while he was working under the car. She heard the noise. She ran outside and saw what had happened. In her words, "Before I knew what I was doing I picked the car up by its rear bumper while my son crawled out. About an hour later I began having these horrible pains in my back." That's adrenalin in action.

The sympathetic nervous system makes use of the adrenalin compounds, both as neurotransmitters and as hormones in times of crisis. The parasympathetic nervous system makes use of acetylcholine as its major neurotransmitter. It is interesting to note that these neurotransmitters are more abundant in the autonomic nervous system than they are in the central nervous system.

The central nervous system's control over the autonomic nervous system is quite loose. That is, the autonomics (as they are often called) enjoy a high degree of autonomy. That control that does come from the central nervous system is largely from the hypothalamus for the sympathetic division. Parasympathetic central control is largely from the brain stem nuclei and from the sacral end of the spinal cord.

Another division of the autonomic nervous system has recently been hypothesized. This is the diffuse enteric nervous system. It is suggested that this is a separate autonomic division, which has some autonomy. This enteric nervous system is largely under the control of the sympathetic and the parasympathetic divisions, and how these two divisions are balanced functionally at any given moment. This newly proposed system exercises control over the gastrointestinal tract if the theory is correct.

Indirectly, the autonomic nervous system divisions (sympathetic and parasympathetic) are very much involved in our responses to emotions such as fear, anger, rage, panic, pleasure, etc. Actually, these emotions are triggered by higher brain centers and the messages are sent to the autonomic control centers, which then dictate many of the bodily responses. These autonomically controlled responses then produce further sensory input, which then contributes to a continuation of the emotional response. The emotional responses may then escalate unless the higher brain centers are able to intervene.

Brain Stem

The brain stem is that portion of the brain that lies between and connects the spinal cord with the cerebral hemispheres. All authorities seem to include the medulla oblongata, the pons and the midbrain as components of the brain stem. Some authorities additionally include the diencephalon (the posterior part of the forebrain) in the brain stem, but this inclusion remains controversial (**Fig. 5-34**).

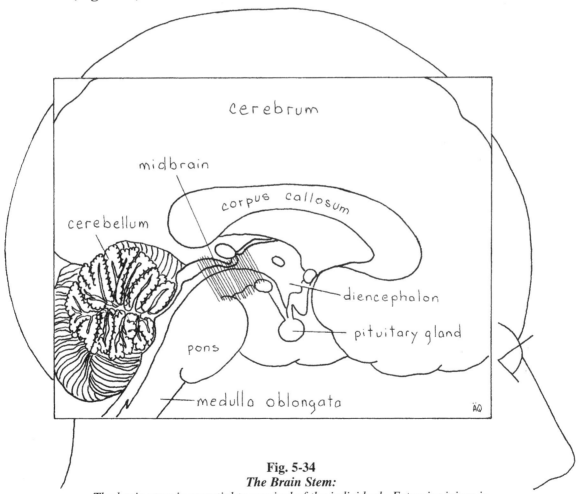

Fig. 5-34
The Brain Stem:
The brain stem is essential to survival of the individual. Extensive injury is deadly. Less-extensive injury almost always results in some degree of disability. The brain stem includes the medulla oblongata, the pons and the midbrain, and some authorities include the diencephalon.

We have listed the brain stem as a separate item in this text because so many parents know only that their child has a "brain stem injury," and that this is very serious. Also, the brain stem deserves special mention because the reticular formation traverses it from its lower end where it connects to the spinal cord, to its upper end where it connects to the cerebral hemispheres **(Fig. 5-16)**.

We have discussed the component parts of the brain stem as we ascended from the spinal cord to the cerebral cortex, and so it should be rather clear just how serious brain stem problems can be. Most of our vital functions, such as breathing, heart rate, etc., have control centers, or at the very least auxiliary control centers in the brain stem. Therefore, a great many brain stem problems require life-support systems in order to sustain life, albeit in a vegetative state.

Less serious injuries to the brain stem may result in dysfunction of cranial nerves III through XII, so you can imagine that less extensive problems within the brain stem can result in a wide array of dysfunctions, depending upon which nuclei and/or fiber tracts leading out from or into these nuclei are affected. Cranial nerves III, IV and VI (oculomotor, trochlear and abducent, respectively) have to do with eye movement, eyelid movement and eye pupil responses to light, distance, and accommodation to that distance and visual focus. Cranial nerve V (trigeminal) is in control of our whole masticatory system, as well as most of the sensory input from the eyeball, the conjunctiva, the eyelids, the nose, the forehead and the lacrimal (tear) glands.

The VIIth cranial nerve (facial) has both sensory and motor functions. Its main function is to provide voluntary control to all of the muscles of the face. Therefore, problems with the VIIth cranial nerve frequently result in some form of paralysis of the face. One side may droop, and so on. It also provides motor control to the salivary glands and the lacrimal glands. So, problems with the brain stem that affect the nucleus of cranial nerve VII may result in inappropriate saliva production and/or tearing from the eyes. Cranial nerve VII also controls the production of mucus from the nose and throat, as well as the perception of taste from the forward part of the tongue, which is mostly sweet and sour. This nerve also carries much of the sensory input from the external ear canal (that part of the ear canal which is outside of the eardrum), and from the soft palate and the nasopharynx. Distortions in any of the sensations and/or motor-control functions mentioned above can result from problems with the VIIth nerve nuclei and/or the related nerve tracts as they traverse the brain stem tissue.

The VIII cranial nerve is variously known as the Vestibulocochlear Nerve, the acoustic nerve and/or the auditory nerve. The latter two titles are older but have not as yet been declared archaic. Therefore, you may encounter these names in some of your travels. At present, it has been declared that vestibulocochlear is the name for the whole nerve, and that the auditory or acoustic nerve shall be called the cochlear branch of the vestibulocochlear nerve. The other branch is known as the vestibular nerve or branch.

Problems with the brain stem, which affect the nuclei of these nerves and/or their related fiber tracts as they pass through the brain stem, can result in difficulty with hearing and/or equilibrium.

We shall consider the IXth, Xth and XIth cranial nerves collectively because they are so inter-related in their nuclei and intertwined in their fiber tracts. These three cranial nerves are also known as the glossopharyngeal (IX), the vagus (X) and the accessory (XI) nerves. Collectively, these nerves influence the production of saliva in the mouth and mucus in the mouth, throat, esophagus, stomach and parts of the large bowel. They monitor blood pressure and blood flow to the brain. In addition, they have a great deal to do with the total digestive and eliminative processes. They strongly influence heart rate by slowing it down, and the respiratory system by reducing the air exchange as they influence bronchial diameter and mucus production. These nerves contribute significantly to the control of neck movement. They also aid the facial nerve in providing taste sensation. And, as if this were not enough diversity, they also provide sensation input from the structures of the ear. You can well imagine from this description how disruptive problems in the brain stem can be with total body function when they affect the nuclei or fiber tracts of these nerves.

Cranial nerve XII is also known as the hypoglossal nerve. It controls the muscles of the tongue. Brain stem problems that affect this nerve will result in an inability to control tongue movement. Often, the tongue deviates to one side when only one hypoglossal nucleus or fiber tract is involved. The deviation will be towards the side of the problem, because it requires tongue-muscle action to protrude the tongue from the mouth. Tongue thrusting can result from excessive activity of the hypoglossal system for a multitude of reasons.

This is a rather straightforward and out-front nerve because, as far as we know at this time, all it does is control tongue movement.

The reticular formation also runs through the brain stem. It is, however, a complete system unto itself. It is therefore considered as a separate subject in the next topic.

The Reticular Formation

The reticular formation is also known as the reticular activating system, and as the reticular alarm system. It occupies the centralmost parts of the brain stem, and it extends downward into the spinal cord to the sacral end **(Fig. 5-16)**. There are several million neurons in the reticular formation, which form a very dense network with their cell bodies and fibers. Although they appear very chaotic and disorganized under the microscope, this system is extremely efficient.

The reticular formation encompasses a wide variety of cell types. Its functional organization is oriented in a longitudinal direction. Tracts of the reticular formation both ascend and descend from the tail end of the spinal cord all the way up to the diencephalon of the forebrain. The afferent, or incoming impulses into the reticular formation, include all of the sensory systems.

The neurons of the reticular formation are very nonspecific. They do it all. The reticular formation receives input from the proprioceptors of all the muscles and tendons, etc., from the censors of balance and equilibrium, from the eyes, the ears, the touch receptors, the hot and cold receptors, the smell receptors, the taste receptors, and any other receptors that exist in the human body.

The intercellular connectors in the reticular formation are incomprehensible in terms of their numbers and complexity. The sorting out and arranging of information that comes in is tremendous. Not only does the reticular formation receive information from all of the sensory systems just mentioned, it also receives partially processed information from the cerebellum, the hypothalamus, the basal ganglia and the cerebral cortex (especially the premotor cortex). It is probably one of the world's best triage officers.

From all of this data, the reticular formation has to decide whether or not the owner of the system should go on "ready alert" or go beyond and be truly alarmed. When incoming data is persistent and/or novel, the reticular formation usually decides to act. In order to execute its decision, that is, in order to set the stage for emergency response action, the reticular formation also has to be able to implement reflex responsive action. In order to do this, the system has fiber tracts that go up to the cortex to let the conscious mind know that there is cause for immediate action. Also, there are long fiber tracts that go down the spinal cord that will initiate the action before the thought processes in the cortex have the necessity of making a decision. It is almost as though the cerebral cortex is awakened in order to observe what the survival system of the body is doing in this emergency.

It should not surprise you, therefore, that any problems with the reticular formation may interfere with the kind of alertness that is necessary for survival. When this activating and/or alerting system has problems, the owner of the system may be approached and attacked totally by surprise. In other words, alertness is reduced.

Also, it should not surprise you that the cranial nerve V (trigeminal) system has copious connections with the reticular formation. Recall that the trigeminal system controls the mouth, biting, chewing, etc. Mammals, of which humans are one species, rely upon their jaws and teeth to a great extent for survival. Thus, the trigeminal system is vital when its owner acts either as predator/hunter or in self-defense. The alarm system must indeed communicate freely with the trigeminal system.

Consider that an overactive reticular formation or alarm system might be the cause of bruxism (teeth grinding) in children and adults. Preventing the teeth from grinding with dental appliances does not reduce the activity level of the reticular formation. One should always treat and correct the cause in preference to the effect. My apologies to those who prescribe dental appliances, but CranioSacral Therapy can and does reduce the level of activity of the reticular formation. This gets closer to the cause. Concurrently, one should focus effort on discovering why the reticular formation is overactive and correct this problem.

The Pituitary Gland

The pituitary gland, also known as the hypophysis, is suspended by a stalk from the hypothalamus. It is divided into two parts, anterior and posterior, which are structurally and functionally different. The anterior pituitary gland does not receive nerve (neural) communications from the hypothalamus, but it has its own private circulatory system with the hypothalamus. Thus, the anterior pituitary receives hormone molecules from the hypothalamus and it responds (appropriately, we hope) to these hormonal messages **(Fig. 5-35)**.

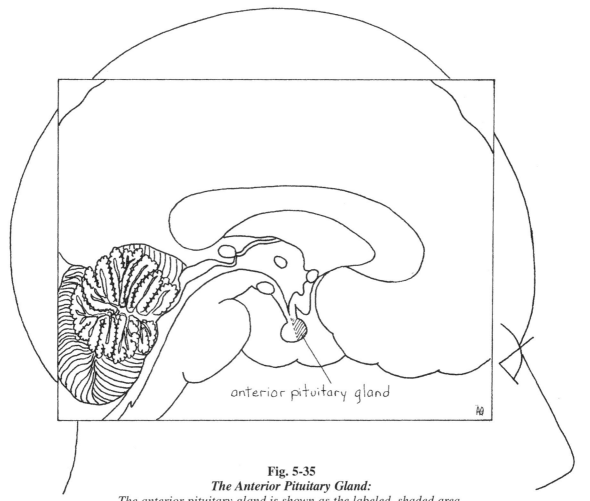

Fig. 5-35
The Anterior Pituitary Gland:
The anterior pituitary gland is shown as the labeled, shaded area.
This is known as the "master gland" of the endocrine system.

The posterior pituitary receives nerve tracts and nerve impulses from the hypothalamus and it also (hopefully) responds appropriately. Both the blood vessel connections between the hypothalamus and the anterior pituitary gland, and the nerve connections between the hypothalamus and the posterior pituitary gland, are two-way streets. That is, both parts of the pituitary gland receive and send messages to the hypothalamus **(Fig. 5-36)**.

The stalk that suspends the pituitary gland from the hypothalamus passes downward through a diaphragm of dura mater membrane which opens wider and closes tighter in response to membrane tensions that are transmitted from distant parts of the dural membrane system (see Topic 26). When the membrane diaphragm tightens a little too much, it interferes with hypothalamic/pituitary gland communication by acting more or less as a tourniquet. Blood flow and nerve impulse flow are both inhibited by pressure.

As we stated earlier, the pituitary gland hangs from a stalk which originates in the hypothalamus. This stalk passes downward through the diaphragma sellae, which is the opening in the dura mater membrane. The pituitary gland per se is then located in the sella turcica. The sella turcica is a protective opening in the sphenoid bone. It is actually a vertically oriented cave. The sphenoid bone forms a part of the floor of the cranial vault of the skull.

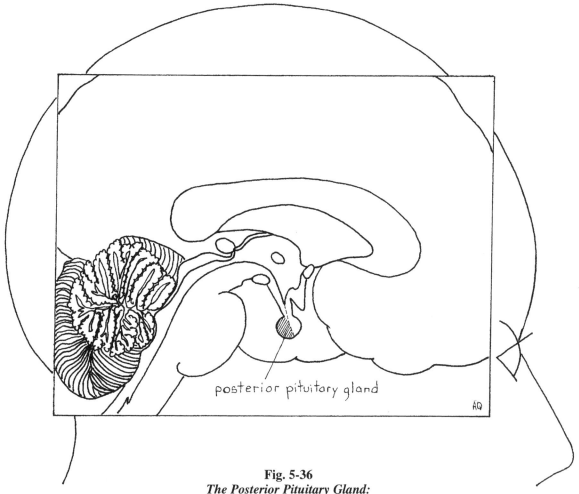

posterior pituitary gland

Fig. 5-36
The Posterior Pituitary Gland:
The posterior pituitary gland is shown as the labeled, shaded area. Although the anterior and posterior pituitary glands are very closely related anatomically, their functions are very different. See text for details.

From this very protected position, the pituitary gland does its work. The hormones secreted into the bloodstream by the anterior pituitary gland regulate thyroid gland function, growth hormone secretion, adrenal cortex hormone secretion, menstrual and pregnancy hormone secretions, and male sex hormones. At the present time this is what we know. There may be much more as yet to be discovered.

The posterior pituitary gland secretes hormones that regulate kidney function and urine output as well as oxytocin, which is involved with memory as well as with the force of contractions during labor. It also secretes hormones that influence blood pressure, and possibly various bodily functions.

We also recognize that the pituitary gland secretes beta endorphins. These newly discovered substances have a great deal to do with pain perception, happiness, euphoria and the like. When you exercise past a certain point of pain and feel great, it is probably the beta endorphins that are responsible for that wonderful feeling which is almost addicting. In fact, the beta endorphins are close chemical kin to morphine and may be just as addicting. The difference is that the beta endorphins are natural substances produced within your body. You can get a "hit" of beta endorphins by self-inducing pain and/or by over-exercising. You may know someone who is hooked on or obsessed with exercise, almost to the point of self-destruction They are probably addicted to their own beta endorphins. The beta endorphins are actually nature's way of giving you mercy when the pain is too much to bear. You become pain-free and euphoric. When the pituitary gland is functionally compromised, a child has tremendous problems with endocrine gland function, fluid balance and pain sensitivity.

Topic 25

The Pineal Gland

In the adult the pineal gland is a small cone-shaped structure about 6-8 millimeters long and about 4 millimeters wide. (1 millimeter is slightly less than 1/16th of an inch.) This gland is situated immediately behind the hypothalamus from which it was derived during embryonic development (**Fig. 5-37**). It draws its blood supply from the enveloping pia mater.

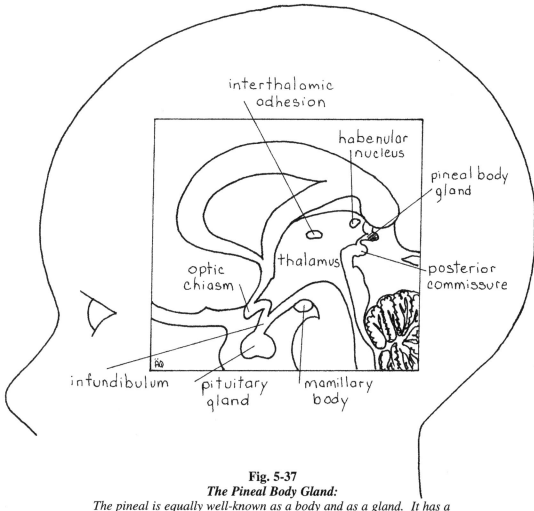

Fig. 5-37
The Pineal Body Gland:
The pineal is equally well-known as a body and as a gland. It has a lot to do with our bodily responses to light and darkness. It also has influences on sexual function and the incidence of cancer. We still have a lot to learn about the pineal. See text for functional details.

A nerve pathway which connects the pineal gland and the visual system travels through the hypothalamus and the brain stem. The relationship between the pineal gland and the visual system seems quite important in that the pineal gland is responsive to light. The light and the darkness seem to influence the pineal gland's level of activity, which in turn influences our levels of hormones and neurotransmitters, and how these levels fluctuate during certain times of the day or night. Circadian rhythm is the term applied to these light/dark-influenced rhythmical physiological fluctuations.

The pineal gland is the richest source of serotonin, which it uses to make its hormone, melatonin. When it is dark the pineal gland makes more melatonin, thus lowering serotonin levels. The increase in melatonin (or the decrease in serotonin) seems to result in: (1) increased incidence of emotional depression, (2) stimulation of brown fat production (brown fat is the hard fat that is used as fuel when we anticipate a period of hibernation during cold weather and food shortage), and (3) inhibition of gonadal hormone production, which results in a reduction of sexual activity.

By a poorly understood process, more noradrenalin is secreted during darkness. This makes us more alert to danger and better ready to respond. This signal for increased noradrenalin production from the sympathetic nervous system and from the medulla of the adrenal glands seems to be coming from the pineal gland. Another interesting relationship is that light decreases noradrenalin and melatonin levels. This may be why we feel safer in the light and more fearful in the darkness. These fears of the dark are instinctive and can be overridden by higher brain centers. It is also true that both noradrenalin and melatonin inhibit sexual activity. Therefore, by this system we are sexier in the light rather than in the dark. Once again, higher brain centers can override these instinctive preferences.

There is yet another very interesting mystery that relates to the pineal gland. The pineal gland contains magnetic crystals which may well be parts of an internal compass that relates to earth's magnetic north. If this is the case, it is possible that all of the magnetic pollution in which we live contributes to a dysfunction of our internal compasses. This, in turn, may be why we get "turned around" so easily in new places until we nonconsciously or consciously become familiar with landmarks and can compensate for our internal compass confusion.

In 1994 on the island of Stromboli (off the coast of Sicily), the third International Seminar on the Pineal Gland was held. There was much research reported that linked pineal atrophy and/or calcification to the incidence of cancer and to the aging of body cells and tissues. The decline of the pineal gland seems to be reversible by the use of supplemental zinc in the diet of the subjects.

There is also some recent work out of Holland that suggests that the pineal gland has something to do with letting our bodies know which way is up. When surgeons removed the pineal glands of monkeys, the monkeys developed scoliosis (spinal curvature). It is as though some intrinsic knowledge in the monkey was lost and the spine no longer knew what the upright posture was. The result was vertebral deformity and spinal curvature.

In summary, although much is still unknown about the pineal gland, it seems to have several important functions within the body system. When I finished osteopathic medical school in 1963, the pineal gland was to be disregarded as unimportant. I was taught that it had a job to do during fetal development and was no longer functional shortly after delivery. The lesson is, don't be afraid to change your mind, and certainly do not cling to dogma just because it feels safe. We are continually discovering different truths about the complex workings of the human body.

The Meningeal Membrane System

The meningeal membrane system is composed of three differently structured layers of membrane. Each layer is separated from the other by fluid. This fluid layer between each of the membranes acts, among other things, as a lubricant which allows for some degree of independent motion between each of the membrane interfaces.

The membrane system envelopes the whole central nervous system, as well as some of its

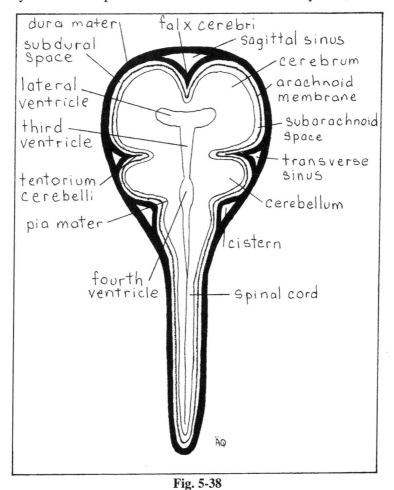

Fig. 5-38
The Three Membrane Layers of the Meninges:
The pia mater, the dura mater and the arachnoid membrane are all shown in this drawing.
The fluid-filled spaces which separate these membranes are also shown. The cisterns and
sinuses are places where the membranes separate and pools of cerebrospinal fluid are found.

roots. More specifically, the brain, the spinal cord, the spinal cord nerve roots and some of the cranial nerves are enveloped by the meningeal membrane system.

The fluid which separates the membrane layers is called cerebrospinal fluid. The make up and characteristics of cerebrospinal fluid is more similar to blood plasma than it is to blood. It normally contains almost no cells and very few protein molecules. Also, the concentrations of glucose and the electrolytes are quite different from blood and blood serum. The details of cerebrospinal fluid constituency will be more fully discussed. (See Topic 30, Section V.)

The three layers of meningeal membrane are, from the inside out: (1) the pia mater, (2) the arachnoid membrane and (3) the dura mater. For our purposes we shall consider the inside as that membrane layer which has direct contact with the tissues of the central nervous system and its major nerve roots **(Fig. 5-38)**.

THE PIA MATER

The pia mater is the innermost of the three meningeal membrane layers. It closely invests the entire central nervous system. That is, the pia mater follows the surface of the entire brain and spinal cord into all the fissures, sulci, cracks and crevices **(Fig. 3-39)**. This layer carries a great number of blood vessels within it which carry nutrients and oxygen to the nervous tissues. They also remove metabolic waste products from the tissues. Considering the moment-to-moment dependence that the brain and spinal cord neurons have upon a plentiful supply of oxygen, glucose and other nutrients, as well as the necessity for quick removal of the byproducts of metabolism, this service provided by the pia mater is of utmost importance to the proper function of the central nervous system.

The pia mater membrane, aside from all of the blood vessels within it, is made up largely of fibers of collagen and elastic, all of which are covered by flattened squamous cells similar to those seen in the skin. The central nervous system tissues also have a great many supporting cells called astrocytes. These cells serve to provide architectural support for the neurons, and they send out projections from the central nervous system tissues into the pia mater membrane. These astrocyte projections serve to attach the pia mater rather closely to the brain, the spinal cord and the enveloped nerve roots. It is not proven as yet, but it is very likely that these astrocyte projections also provide a transportation system for the exchanges of molecules and ions between the pia mater membrane and the tissues of the central nervous system. The pia mater is also very likely involved in the function of the blood-brain barrier which is described under Topic 28 in this section.

Each nerve root that either enters or leaves the spinal cord is ensheathed by a layer of pia mater that extends away from the spinal cord as far as the intervertebral foramen, through which the nerve root passes on its way to the peripheral body. Beyond this intervertebral foramen, the pia mater sheath blends with the sheath called the perineurium that surrounds each bundle of nerve fibers that form the peripheral nerves. Once these bundles pass through their individual intervertebral foramen, they are considered a part of the peripheral nervous system.

The outer surface of the pia mater is intermittently attached to the next (middle) layer of the three meningeal membrane layers, the arachnoid membrane, by very fine fibrous strands called trabeculae. These trabeculae are loose enough to permit independent movement between the pia mater and the arachnoid membrane. The space between these two membrane layers is filled with cerebrospinal fluid. The space is called the subarachnoid space **(Fig. 3-39 and 5-38)**.

THE ARACHNOID MEMBRANE

The arachnoid membrane is the middle layer of the meningeal membrane system. It is very fine and delicate **(Fig. 3-39 and 5-38)**. Under normal circumstances it is as thin and transparent as cellophane. It carries few, if any, blood vessels within it. The arachnoid membrane is somewhat loosely connected to the pia mater membrane which it encloses. The space between the pia mater and the arachnoid membrane is filled with cerebrospinal fluid. It is called the subarachnoid space.

The arachnoid membrane also follows the spinal nerve roots out as far as their respective intervertebral foramen. At these foramen, the arachnoid membrane fuses with the covering of the bone (periosteum). Its fusion also ends the subarachnoid space and hence the circulation of cerebrospinal fluid through this space.

It is interesting to note that the arachnoid membrane seems more vulnerable to swelling due to inflammation than the other two layers of meningeal membrane. I have seen the arachnoid membrane at a time of surgery almost 1/4-inch thick due to swelling. When the arachnoid membrane is swollen and inflamed, it can and usually does become the source of great pain and disability.

The arachnoid membrane is separated from the outermost layer of the meningeal membrane system, the dura mater, by the subdural space. This space also contains a lubricating fluid which allows for relatively friction-free motion between these two outermost layers of the meningeal membrane system. Although the fluid between the arachnoid membrane and the dura mater (the subdural space) is chemically essentially indistinguishable from the fluid in the subarachnoid space, many authorities do not refer to it as cerebrospinal fluid. From a practical point of view and for our purposes herein, we can consider the fluid in both the subarachnoid and the subdural spaces as cerebrospinal fluid.

The arachnoid membrane does not follow the pia mater into all the little sulci and fissures of the central nervous system. It does, however, follow the dura mater as it forms the falx cerebri, the falx cerebelli and the tentorium cerebelli. These three structures form major partitions which separate the right and left hemispheres of the cerebrum, the right and left hemispheres of the cerebellum, and the cerebrum above from the cerebellum below, respectively **(Fig. 5-39)**.

Fiber strands, or trabeculae, connect the arachnoid membrane to the dura mater. The connections between the arachnoid membrane and the dura mater take place only at their common mooring sites onto bone. These mooring sites are located around the entire circumference of the foramen magnum, at the second and third cervical vertebrae, at all of the intervertebral foramen, at the sacrum and at the coccyx. This design allows for a great deal of independent movement between the arachnoid membrane and the dura mater.

The arachnoid membrane is involved structurally in the formation of cisternae, which in some cases are located between the lower surfaces of the brain and the base of the skull. These cisternae may be considered reservoirs for cerebrospinal fluid. Also, the arachnoid membrane forms granulation bodies, which are membranes bunched up into berry-like shapes. These are located particularly in the superior sagittal sinus, and in the forward end of the straight sinus. These arachnoid granulation bodies function as a part of the reabsorption mechanism of the cerebrospinal fluid as it is constantly being taken back into the blood vascular system **(Fig. 3-39)**.

Although it has not to my knowledge been written by authorities, I believe that the arachnoid membrane also serves as a sort of buffer between the pia mater and the dura mater. In this role as buffer, it would allow increased independent motion between the layers of the meningeal membranes.

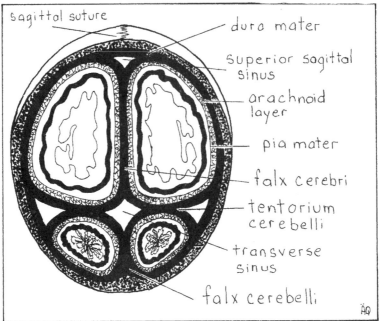

Fig. 5-39
A Coronal Section Through the Brain:
This drawing of a coronal slice which goes vertically through the head right behind the ears shows the formation of the falx cerebri which separates the two cerebral hemispheres, the falx cerebelli which separates the two cerebellar hemispheres and the tentorium cerebelli which is oriented horizontally and separates the cerebral hemispheres from the cerebellum.

THE DURA MATER

The dura mater is the toughest of the three layers of meningeal membranes. It is connected with the arachnoid membrane only at the aforementioned common moorings onto bone. Therefore, the dura mater and the arachnoid membrane are free to move rather independently from each other. When this independent movement is compromised for any reason, severe pain and disability may result.

The space between the dura mater and the arachnoid membrane is called the subdural space **(Fig. 3-39 and 5-38)**. Within that space is a lubricatory fluid that is of very similar if not the same chemical constituency as cerebrospinal fluid. It is not, however, called cerebrospinal fluid by many authorities. Ultimately, I believe we will see that the fluids within the subdural and the subarachnoid spaces are indistinguishable from each other. Then, in another 10 years, the dogma may be overcome and the "two" fluids will both be known as cerebrospinal fluid.

The dura mater is very strong and fibrous. It is waterproof and significantly thicker than either the arachnoid membrane or the pia mater. The dura mater within the skull is in two layers that are closely bound by fibrous strands (trabeculae). When I have dissected both human and baboon skulls, I have noted that the longer the skull has been kept in preservatives after death, the easier these two layers of dura mater separate. The outer layer of the dura mater is actually the inner lining of the skull. It is upon this layer of membrane that the embryo develops the bones of the skull which form the so-called vault. These are the frontal and parietal bones, and the squamous parts of the temporal and occipital bones. Also, within the skull vault the inner layer of dura mater separates from the outer layer at strategic places in order to form the falx cerebri which separates the right and left cerebral hemispheres, the falx cerebelli which separates the right and left cerebellar hemispheres, and the more horizontally oriented tentorium cerebelli which supports the cerebral hemispheres and prevents them from "banging" into the cerebellum.

The cerebral hemispheres are above the tentorium cerebelli, and the cerebellum is below this horizontally oriented dura mater membrane. The tentorium cerebelli is often referred to as the "tent" or the "cerebellar tent." The membrane forms a sort of roof or tent over the cerebellum. The way these membranous partitions are formed creates two layered dividers between brain parts. How it is accomplished is much more clearly seen from the illustrations **(Fig. 5-39)**.

Once the dura mater lines the skull and forms the dividing partitions as described above, both layers of dura mater are very firmly attached at the large opening in the base of the skull through which the spinal cord passes to unite with the medulla oblongata of the brain. Below this large opening, which is known as the foramen magnum, the two layers of dura mater are distinctly separate from each other. The outer layer of dura mater actually becomes the lining of the bones that form the canal of the spinal column through which the spinal cord passes. The inner layer of dura mater is quite separate and free to exercise a great deal of free movement independent from the arachnoid membrane and the outer layer of dura mater. The two layers of dura mater actually only fuse together tightly within the spinal canal at the level of the second and third cervical vertebrae, and at the second segment of the sacrum. And at these levels, the dura mater attachment or fusion is only in the front part of the canal as it passes through the aforementioned levels of the neck and sacrum. Outside of the canal, the two layers of dura mater and the arachnoid membrane all fuse at the intervertebral foramen and at the coccyx. At the coccyx all three of these layers come together to form its outer covering (periosteum). The space between the two layers of dura mater in the spinal region is bounded by these aforementioned areas of fusion.

Nature has engineered this whole meningeal system beautifully so that we can twist and turn and bend our backs forward and backward. Without the ability of the membranes to glide one in relationship to the other, we would lose a lot of our ability to move.

The famous epidural anesthesia is given in the space between the two layers of dura mater in the spinal canal. The fusion at the foramen magnum of the two layers prevents any of the anesthetic from getting up into the head and affecting the brain and/or cranial nerves. Thus, the epidural anesthetic, when properly administered, is limited in its spread of effect to the spinal cord and the spinal nerve roots inside of the intervertebral foramina. This situation makes the epidural approach safer than the spinal anesthetic, which is usually injected into the subarachnoid space.

It is the dura mater that is the cornerstone of CranioSacral Therapy. The approach in CranioSacral Therapy is to use the bones which are attached to the dura mater as "handles" to loosen or correct abnormal membrane tension patterns within the meningeal system. Also, the membranes are used to enhance both blood and cerebrospinal fluid circulation in relation to the central nervous system and its nerve roots, as well as to alleviate any compression of brain, spinal cord and/or spinal nerve roots by abnormally high or distorted meningeal membrane and/or bony tensions and pressures.

Myelin

Myelin is that wonderful white substance that coats, surrounds and insulates many of the fibers of the neurons.

Myelin is about 23 percent protein, which probably doesn't surprise you. What probably will surprise some of you is that the major component of myelin is that "evil" substance, cholesterol. Then there are other fatty substances called cerebrosides, which are major components of myelin. Cerebrosides, if they escape from the myelin and get through the blood-brain barrier, can cause autoimmune diseases. These are the diseases wherein we have an allergic reaction to our own body chemicals. The other important substance in myelin is called sphingomyelin. We can't get allergic to this because it is all through your body, and your immune system knows that it is a part of you. On the other hand, the cerebrosides are not normally anywhere except in the central nervous system, so when they get out into the body by mistake the immune system doesn't recognize them as friends. It attacks in good faith and you get sick.

Myelin serves as an electrical insulator. It keeps the nerve impulse in the nerve fiber. It prevents the nerve impulse from shorting out and not reaching its destination. Remember, the nerve impulse is electrical and behaves as such. Myelin also increases the speed of conduction of the electrical impulse — myelinated nerve fibers have the highest conduction velocity. Also, myelin somehow decreases the metabolic demands of impulse conduction. So, not only do myelinated nerve fibers conduct more rapidly, they have better fuel economy. Myelin is very good stuff, even if it is full of cholesterol.

Myelinated nerve fibers are usually the ones that conduct acute-pain messages. They get the message to the higher centers very quickly so that we can do something about the pain.

Dull aches are usually conducted by unmyelinated nerve fibers. These are the hard-to-localize, nagging types of pains.

The myelinated fibers that conduct acute-pain signals usually go quickly and directly to the thalamus for relay to the cerebral cortex.

The unmyelinated pain fibers usually go to the reticular formation where they can be censored out or passed on to the medulla, the pons, the midbrain, the hypothalamus and, if they haven't been censored out by then, they get to the thalamus for relay to the cerebral cortex.

Please do not get the idea that only sensory pain fibers are myelinated. Many of the motor fibers are myelinated. Myelination occurs wherever speed and efficiency are important.

Myelination is accomplished in the central nervous system by the oligodendrogliocytes and in the peripheral nervous system by the Schwann cells (**Fig. 3-36**).

Problems with myelination are devastating to nervous system function. They are great imitators of other diseases because the type of symptoms that are seen depend upon where the demyelination is occurring. It can be anywhere, so the symptoms can be suggestive of many other problems.

Topic 28

Blood-Brain Barrier

The blood-brain barrier is a system by which substances circulating in capillaries through brain tissue are not allowed to leave the capillaries, and thus cannot enter the substance of the brain. Special cells of brain substance surround the walls of the capillaries and reject entry of large protein molecules from the blood system. Also, certain smaller molecules are selectively rejected from entry into the brain substance. Among these rejected molecules are the neurotransmitters, norepinephrine and serotonin. The brain has to make these substances from their precursor amino acids, lysine and tryptophan, respectively. It would seem that passage through the blood-brain barrier has to do with fat solubility, ionic (electrical) charge and, of course, molecular size (**Fig. 5-40**).

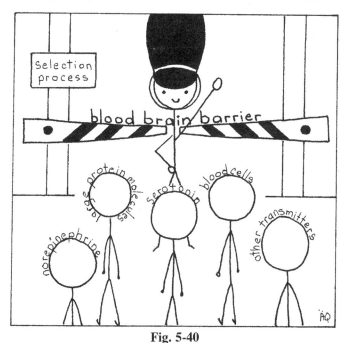

Fig. 5-40
The Blood-Brain Barrier:
Most substances in the blood are denied admission through the barrier into the tissue of the central nervous system. See text for further details.

Nicotine seems to have relatively free passage, which may explain why pregnant women smoking, or second-hand cigarette smoke, affects embryos and infants so powerfully. Also, nicotine has the ability to fool certain synaptic neurotransmitter receptors in the peripheral nervous system. Smokers, be careful of the effect of your habit upon your newborns and nursing infants, to say nothing of the potential effect of second-hand smoke.

Premature babies do not have well-developed blood-brain barriers, and are quite vulnerable to substances taken in by the mother while in utero and after delivery. A faulty blood-brain barrier may be the cause of various brain allergies, which may correlate to bizarre and sometimes psychotic brain function and behavior.

Topic 29

The Choroid Plexus

The choroid plexus is a membrane that lines all of the surfaces of the complete ventricular system of the adult brain. This membrane is actually made up of a series of infoldings of the blood vessels of the pia mater membrane (innermost of the three meningeal membranes), which are then covered by a thin coating of specialized (ependymal) cells. These cells have little hairlike cilia that protrude from their surfaces. The cilia move in such a manner that they facilitate the movement/flow of cerebrospinal fluid **(Fig. 3-31)**.

The infoldings of the pia mater blood vessels into the cavities of the brain ventricles form tufted projections. These tufts actually selectively secrete the constituents of the blood from within the blood vessels of the choroid plexus into the ventricular system as cerebrospinal fluid. In order to make up the cerebrospinal fluid, some of the blood constituents are refused entry into the ventricles while others are allowed to pass through the cellular walls of the choroid plexus and to participate in the manufacture of cerebrospinal fluid **(Fig. 5-40)**. In general, it is fair to say that the fluids pass rather freely through the walls of the choroid plexus. Larger molecules and particles with specific electrical charges do not pass. Blood cells are rejected entry into the ventricular system of the brain. This system is about 90 percent functional at term birth. Most of its function is achieved during the third trimester of the pregnancy.

Cerebrospinal Fluid

Cerebrospinal fluid is extracted from blood by the choroid plexus system, which is located in the walls of the ventricular system of the brain. The cerebrospinal fluid resembles blood plasma more closely than any other body fluid. It has a clear, essentially colorless appearance even though it is extracted from blood. It has almost no cells in it, and protein and sugar content levels are much lower than in blood (**Fig. 3-39**).

The cerebrospinal fluid fills the brain's ventricular system and the subarachnoid space (and I think, in addition, the subdural space). The total volume of cerebrospinal fluid in the adult is about 125 milliliters, or a little over 4 ounces. The rate of formation and therefore reabsorption of cerebrospinal fluid in the adult is about 500 milliliters per day. This amounts to a little over a pint per day. Of course, it is much less in the newborn.

In cases of trauma or sudden jolts, the cerebrospinal fluid serves as a shock absorber for the brain. It also delivers some nutrients and removes some waste products. It helps to maintain the proper water and acid-base balances within the brain and spinal cord. For the craniosacral system, it moves the sutures and membranes via the conduction of hydraulic forces. Also, it is one of the primary tools of treatment for the CranioSacral Therapist.

Recent research by Marshall Rennels, M.D., at the University of Maryland, shows the cerebrospinal fluid also penetrates the brain substance in the spaces between the brain cells. This work was done by adding radioactive tracers to the cerebrospinal fluid. The tracers showed up within five minutes throughout the brain. The implications are that cerebrospinal fluid may be a much more effective delivery system that we previously thought. It may supply nutrients, hormones and neurotransmitters on a minute-to-minute basis throughout the brain. In so doing, it may have a much more powerful influence on brain function than was previously thought. It may influence the metabolic rates of brain neurons, emotional behavior, thought process and so on. This perfusion of cerebrospinal fluid through the brain tissues may also serve as a very efficient waste-removal system for metabolic by-products, as well as for drugs and toxins.

There is no doubt that CranioSacral Therapy enhances this perfusion of cerebrospinal fluid throughout all of the tissues of the brain.

Topic 31

Arachnoid Villi

The arachnoid villi are projections of arachnoid membrane into some of the venous sinuses. These projections serve to increase the surface area between the arachnoid membrane and the venous sinuses. The increased surface area enhances the reabsorption of cerebrospinal fluid back into the venous blood. These projections of arachnoid membrane protrude into the venous sinuses through holes in the dura mater membrane. The majority of the arachnoid villi protrude into the superior sagittal sinus, which is located just under the sagittal suture **(Fig. 3-39)**. The sagittal suture runs front to back on the midline at the top of the skull from behind the frontal to the occipital bone. The superior sagittal sinus also runs in the front-to-back orientation under the frontal bone (forehead). In the newborn the frontal bone is divided into right and left halves by the metopic suture, which is one of the few sutures of the skull that almost totally disappears as we begin to grow up **(Fig. 5-41)**. So, the venous sinus (superior sagittal sinus) that puts most of the cerebrospinal fluid back into the blood supply is located under the top of the skull oriented

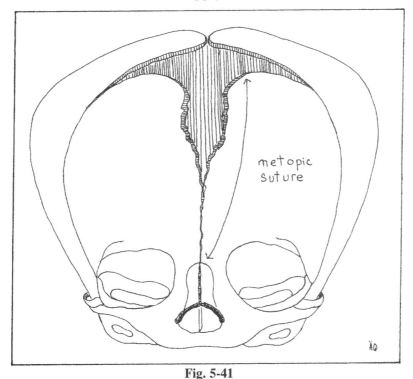

Fig. 5-41
The Metopic Suture:
This is one of the few sutures in the skull that totally disappears as we grow up.

from the forehead to the back of the head in a straight line front to back.

Other venous sinuses have some arachnoid villi and may collect some cerebrospinal fluid for return to general blood circulation, but the distribution of arachnoid villi in other areas is not consistent except for a cluster of arachnoid villi or arachnoid granulation bodies, as they are called, in the forward end of the straight venous sinus. This sinus is located away from the skull bones where the falx cerebri, the tentorium cerebelli and the falx cerebelli all join together. It is thought that, since all membranes that are freestanding partitions (and not skull linings) meet at this juncture, it is very likely that partial control of the reabsorption of cerebrospinal fluid back into venous blood is located in these arachnoid granulation bodies.

Topic 32

The Blood Circulatory System of the Brain and Spinal Cord

The circulation of blood through the central nervous system is most conveniently divided into arterial blood supply, capillary circulation and venous blood return for both the brain and the spinal cord. We will begin with the blood circulation to the brain. The arterial blood delivers higher concentrations of oxygen and nutrients into the capillary system, which offers these supplies of oxygen and nutrients to the cells of the tissues. Coming out of the other side of the capillary system, the oxygen and nutrient-rich blood has been converted to blood that is much poorer in oxygen and nutrients. This venous blood is now more heavily laden with carbon dioxide and other metabolic waste products. This conversion from delivery system to waste-removal system occurs because the walls of the capillaries are semipermeable to the various constituents of the oxygen and nutrient-rich arterial blood. The capillary walls are also semipermeable to the waste products floating around in the (interstitial) fluids. These bathe the tissue cells directly. They are located outside of the blood vascular system. The exchange of usable materials from the blood for the waste materials of the interstitial fluids occurs by the processes of diffusion, osmosis, and by some active conduction.

Diffusion simply means that different concentrations of substances in liquids mix together and reach an equilibrium. The result of this "mixing" is that the different concentrations reach a "happy medium," or equilibrium which is consistent through the mixture of the solutions.

Osmosis refers to the process whereby certain constituents are not allowed to pass through a semipermeable membrane like the capillary wall. However, the liquid solvents in which these rejected substances are suspended or dissolved can pass freely through the membrane. The solvents then tend to pass through the semipermeable (capillary) membrane in an attempt to equalize the pressures on the inside and the outside of the capillary. In our situation, the blood cells and protein molecules are not allowed to leave the blood vessel (capillary) system. This situation creates a higher pressure inside the capillary, which causes the good nutrients to pass through the membranes and leave the capillaries along with some of the fluid, or solvent. This activity occurs in the capillary near its arterial end. As the capillary blood passes along toward the venous end of the capillary, the pressure inside the capillary becomes lower than the interstitial fluid. This difference causes the interstitial fluid to try to equalize the pressures inside and outside the capillary network. In order to do so, this interstitial fluid enters the capillary-network mesh because the capillary walls are permeable to this fluid. Many waste products are dissolved in the interstitial fluid. These waste products are also able to pass through the capillary walls and enter the blood vascular system. They are carried away in the waste-laden blood on the venous side of this ingenious capillary network. As this blood filters through the kidneys, the lungs and the liver, the waste products are removed by these organs and excreted from the body.

Active conduction refers to the mechanism whereby certain substances or molecules are temporarily combined with other substances that actively conduct them through cell membranes. A simple and well-documented example of active conduction is the conduction of a potassium ion attached to a glucose molecule, which is then conducted into the cell (through its membrane) by a molecule of insulin. Thus, an insulin-deficient diabetic has a situation whereby the glucose (sugar) in the blood is high and the potassium in the blood may be high, or at least normal, while inside of the cells (where the metabolic action takes place) there is a deficiency of both sugar and potassium. There are many more examples of active conduction in the nervous system, some of which we will touch upon later.

THE VENOUS BLOOD RETURN SYSTEM

As we said, venous blood is heavy laden with metabolic waste products or, perhaps more politely said, with the by-products of life-giving energy production. The venous blood is collected from the venous end of the capillary network after the usable substance concentrations in the arterial blood have been lowered by the processes of diffusion, osmosis, active conduction and, most likely, some other processes as yet undiscovered. The small veins (venules) become tributaries to larger veins. The waste-laden blood is directed by this system through the lungs where collected carbon dioxide is exchanged in part for oxygen. Neither of these substances goes to zero concentration. The ratio of oxygen to carbon dioxide concentrations is simply reversed in the lungs. The liver and kidney do a large proportion of the waste-removal activity from the venous blood as it circulates through these organs. The liver then puts in a lot of new and good stuff into the blood for use in carrying out necessary body functions. Much of the food we eat after it is digested goes through the liver for processing. This is not true of all the products of digestion, but the liver does an absolutely amazing amount of work.

THE BLOOD CIRCULATION TO THE BRAIN

The arteries deliver between 15 and 20 percent of the heart's pumping output to the brain. The percent varies with changes in demand or request, depending upon how you look at it. As you think harder, your brain metabolism increases and more blood is delivered to that organ, if everything is working correctly. As an aside, the kidneys get about 22 to 25 percent and the liver 27 to 30 percent of blood pumped from the heart. So between brain, kidneys and liver, we can account for as much as 65 percent of the heart's pumping output of blood. These facts may help you to put your body's priorities in perspective. This is also pretty much the normal distribution of heart pumping output for the newborn, except that the brain requirement may be over 20 percent because it is growing and developing so rapidly at the time of birth.

Every good delivery system needs a blueprint or layout. Nature has designed an excellent system for the brain. All of the freshly oxygenated and nutrient-rich blood that gets to the brain is pumped from the left ventricle of the heart into the aorta. The aorta gives off its major branches to the brain early on. These branches are called the common carotid arteries. On the left side the common carotid artery branches directly from the aorta. On the right side the common carotid artery is a major branch from the innominate artery, which comes off the aorta. At the level of, or just a little below the level of your Adam's apple, the common carotid arteries on both sides of your throat/neck divide into the internal and external carotid arteries. The external carotid arteries on both sides deliver arterial blood to the exterior part of the head, the face and the greater part of the neck, so we won't be too concerned about the external carotid artery branches in our discussion of the blood supply to the brain.

The internal carotid arteries are of utmost importance to the brain. In addition to these internal carotid arteries, there are two smaller arterial branches which ascend into the head after they branch from the two subclavian arteries, which lie beneath the collarbones (clavicles) on both sides. These two smaller branches of the subclavian arteries are named the vertebral arteries (**Fig. 5-42**). The vertebral arteries have become famous because, at one point a few years ago, they were implicated as causes of stroke attacks because they, or one of them, got pinched or crimped during forcible neck manipulation. You can make your own judgments as the story of

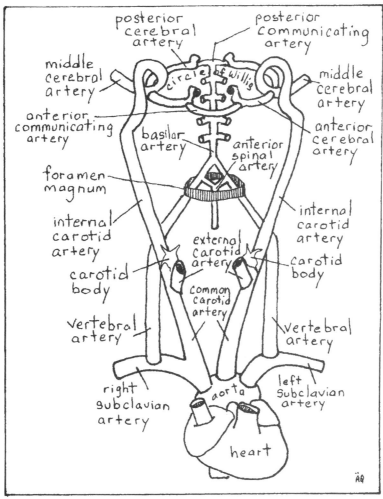

Fig. 5-42
Blood Delivery System to the Brain:
See text for description.

these vertebral arteries unfolds below. Before we get into the details of the internal carotid and the vertebral arteries, we should say a few words about the carotid bodies and the carotid sinuses.

THE CAROTID BODIES

There are two carotid bodies. One is located just behind the bifurcation of each of the two common carotid arteries as they divide into the internal and external carotid arteries on both sides of the neck. The carotid body is a small structure about 1/8 inch to 3/16 inch in diameter (**Fig. 5-42**). It is somewhat of a chemical-analysis station in that it sends information to the autonomic nervous system via the IXth and Xth cranial nerves. This information is reported to the brain on a minute-to-minute basis. It concerns blood levels of oxygen and carbon dioxide, as well as acid and alkaline substances. The carotid bodies are appropriately placed in the neck to monitor blood going to the brain. The brain is sensitive to very delicate and immediate changes in blood chemistry constituency.

THE CAROTID SINUSES

The carotid sinuses are located one on each side of the neck as slight dilations of the terminal parts of the common carotid arteries just before these arteries bifurcate and become the internal and the external carotid arteries. The carotid sinuses may also extend a short distance into the internal carotid arteries as these arteries originate from the bifurcations. The carotid sinuses monitor the blood pressure within the arteries in which they are located. Since the carotids are the principal suppliers of arterial blood to the brain, this information is of utmost importance to brain function. The information is reported to the brain stem via the IXth cranial nerve so that minute-to-minute adjustments in blood supply to the brain can be made in order to insure adequate supply. When you stand up too fast and feel faint, you have probably moved faster than your carotid sinus/brain stem/blood pressure adjustment system was able to work.

THE INTERNAL CAROTID ARTERIES

The internal carotid artery begins at the bifurcation of the common carotid artery in the neck at the upper border of the thyroid cartilage. The internal carotid artery travels almost completely vertically from its origin to the base of the skull. It enters the skull through the carotid canal, which is a hole in the petrous part of the temporal bone. The artery goes through a sharp forward turn within the canal and then enters the skull cavity. Once inside the skull the internal carotid artery runs for a short distance through an area between two layers of dura mater membrane called the cavernous sinus. Within the restricted space of the cavernous sinus, the artery comes in very close contact with the abducent nerve (cranial nerve VI). Excess tension of the dura mater at this location can cause a compression of the abducent nerve and the pulsating internal carotid artery, resulting in loss of nerve function. The presenting symptom will be crossing of the eyes, called convergent strabismus.

After passing through this cavernous sinus, which is really an envelope that is formed by the two layers of dura mater membrane, the internal carotid artery enters the cavity within the skull. Thus, the artery is now fully within the craniosacral system. You will recall that the craniosacral system is a semi-closed hydraulic system that uses the dura mater membrane as its waterproof boundary.

In the neck, the internal carotid artery gives off no branches. As it passes through the carotid canal in the base of the skull, the internal carotid artery gives off a small branch (caroticotympanic artery) that merges with small branches from the external carotid artery and supplies blood to parts of the ear mechanisms. Also, within the carotid canal the internal carotid artery gives off a small branch (pterygoid artery) that joins yet another branch of the external carotid artery and supplies blood to the roof of the pharynx (the throat cavity behind your nasal passages), and to the tube that runs from your middle ear cavity into the pharyngeal cavity (the auditory or eustachian tube). This tube allows an equalization of pressures on the two sides of the ear drum. It is the tube that sometimes requires time to equalize pressures when you get off of an airplane and you can't hear very well. Once the tubes do their job, your ears return to normal unless something more serious is wrong.

As it passes through the cavernous sinus (between the two layers of dura mater membrane), the internal carotid artery gives off some small branches that supply blood to the adjacent bones and sinuses, to the pituitary gland (a very important function), and to the trigeminal ganglion. The trigeminal ganglion is the big ganglionic aggregation of nerve cell bodies related to our masticatory system, as well as to some of the sensation receptors of the eyes and nose. As it passes through the cavernous sinus, the internal carotid artery also gives off branches called the anterior meningeal arteries. The branches provide blood supply to the meningeal membranes of the forward half or third of the intracranial meningeal membrane system.

Once the internal carotid artery penetrates the inner layer of the dura mater membrane, it has entered the domain of the craniosacral system. Inside the dura mater compartment, the internal carotid artery gives branches that supply blood to the eye, the bony orbit within which the eyeball resides, and to the adjacent facial structures. These branches are called the ophthalmic arteries. The internal carotid arteries then contribute to an ingenious design that nature has placed within the skull that insures adequate survival blood to the brain in case one of the carotid arteries becomes obstructed. This is called the circle of Willis. But before we consider the circle of Willis, we will describe the vertebral arteries because they form the basilar artery, which is a big contributor to the circle of Willis.

THE VERTEBRAL ARTERIES AND THE BASILAR ARTERY

The vertebral arteries are paired. One is on each side of the neck. They are usually the first and the largest branches of the two subclavian arteries as they pass under the collar bones (clavicles) on each side of the base of the neck. From their origins behind the clavicles, the vertebral arteries pass backwards to the transverse processes on each side of the sixth cervical vertebra (**Fig. 5-42**). The vertebral arteries enter the foramina of the transverse processes of the sixth cervical vertebra and ascend through the foramina of the transverse processes of the five cervical vertebrae that are located above the sixth to the base of the skull. After exiting the foramina of the first cervical vertebra (the atlas) the two vertebral arteries make sharp turns towards the midline of the body and enter the skull through the foramen magnum. In the neck, the vertebral arteries give off branches that contribute to the blood supply of the spinal cord, the meningeal membranes of the spinal cord, the bony substance of the vertebrae, and some of the deeper muscles of the neck. Much of this blood supply, which the vertebral arteries provide in the neck area, is accomplished in conjunction with other arteries from other sources with which the spinal vertebral arteries conjoin (anastomose). The aforementioned foramina of the transverse processes of the cervical vertebrae through which the vertebral arteries pass are simply holes in these parts of the vertebrae. Some of the branches of the vertebral arteries in the neck also pass through the intervertebral foramen along with the spinal nerve roots. In this way, these arterial branches gain access to the spinal cord and to the layers of the meningeal membranes in the spinal canal.

After passing out of the transverse foramen of the atlas (first cervical vertebra) on each side, the vertebral arteries must pass through a hole in the very tough atlanto-occipital membrane. This membrane binds the atlas to the occiput at the base of the skull. It does have enough slack to allow motion between the atlas and the occiput. However, excessive tension or strain in this membrane can compromise the related vertebral artery's ability to deliver blood into the skull vault on that side. It is at this location that the craniosacral occipital base treatment technique has some of its positive effect upon blood supply to the head. This technique helps to normalize excess and/or abnormal tensions in the atlanto-occipital membranes.

During their passage through the foramen magnum, the vertebral arteries give off small arterial branches to the meningeal membranes in the cerebellar fossa of the skull, including the falx cerebelli. Once inside the cranial vault, the vertebral arteries send out branches that supply blood to the medulla oblongata and the cerebellum. Then, after a very short trip, the two vertebral arteries join to form a single artery, the basilar artery, that courses up the front surface of the pons in a shallow groove. The basilar artery is usually between 1 to 1 1/2 inches long before it joins the circle of Willis. During its short course, the basilar artery, by its branching, offers blood supply to the pons, the internal ear structures, the cerebellum, the posterior part of the cerebrum, and the choroid plexus within the ventricular system of the brain. The basilar artery then loses its singular identity as it joins the circle of Willis.

THE CIRCLE OF WILLIS

All of the arterial blood delivered to the brain comes through a total of four arteries. These arteries are the right and left internal carotid arteries and the right and left vertebral arteries. All of this arterial blood is delivered into a beautifully designed structure called the circle of Willis, which is located at the base (underside) of the brain. Before entering the circle of Willis, the right and left vertebral arteries join on the midline of the body to form the basilar artery. Anatomists call the joining of two or more arteries an anastomosis. The circle of Willis qualifies as such. The incoming blood flow is from the basilar artery and the two internal carotid arteries. The outgoing blood flow is via: (1) the right and left posterior cerebral arteries, which are often considered the terminal branches of the basilar artery, (2) the right and left middle cerebral arteries and (3) the right and left anterior cerebral arteries. The circle itself is formed posteriorly between the basilar artery and the right and left internal carotid arteries by the right and left posterior communicating arteries. The middle cerebral arteries (right and left) depart the circle of Willis opposite the termination points of the two internal carotid arteries into the circle (of Willis). These termination points are about halfway around the circle. The anterior (forwardmost) half of the circle of Willis is formed by the right and left anterior cerebral arteries, which are connected at the very front part of the circle of Willis by the anterior communicating artery. I realize this word picture is complex and perhaps confusing, so please study the illustration of the circle of Willis for clarification (**Fig. 5-43**).

The posterior cerebral arteries, the middle cerebral arteries and the anterior cerebral arteries are the three pairs of blood vessels that offer the great majority of blood supply to the brain. Their names — posterior, middle and anterior — describe which brain regions they supply on each side. The multiple inflow of blood to the circle of Willis gives some insurance that all of these six arteries that go from the circle of Willis to the brain substance can continue to perform adequately for reasonable survival, should there be a blockage/obstruction of the blood flow through one of the vertebral arteries or one of the internal or common carotid arteries. Nature has given us some insurance that our brains can continue to function even if one of the arterial supplies to the circle of Willis is cut off. The other arterial supplies may offer enough blood to the circle of Willis, which then acts as a redistribution center. In this capacity, the circle of Willis equalizes outflow

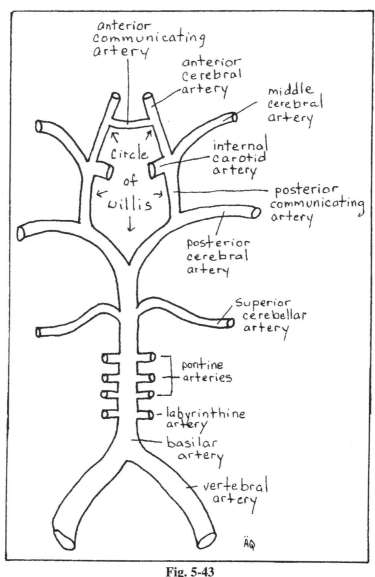

Fig. 5-43
The Circle of Willis:
The Circle of Willis demonstrates one of nature's more
ingenious designs. See text for details.

through the six arteries that supply their respective brain regions. These six arteries enter the brain substance after traveling and branching within the pia mater and into all the sulci and fissures of the brain substance.

The paired posterior cerebral arteries are largely responsible for the blood supply to those parts of the brain that are involved in the visual system. Included in this system are visual perception, eye movement, pupillary reflexes that help us accommodate to light, lens reflexes that help with distance adjustments, and visual memory. Another function is the reception and processing of visual information/data as it comes into the brain and is distributed to other brain areas for responsive action.

The middle cerebral arteries supply large areas of the cerebral cortex of the frontal, parietal and temporal lobes, in addition to the corpus striatum and the internal capsule. This means that interference with the delivery capacities of either of the middle cerebral arteries or their branches can cause problems with sensory perception (more in terms of body awareness), body motor control (paralysis, etc.), personality changes, memory loss, speech problems, and the processing and meaningful interpretation of information. In other words, it may interfere with general intellectual function.

The anterior cerebral arteries duplicate some of the blood supply to the frontal and parietal cerebral cortices, as well as to the corpus striatum and the internal capsule. In addition, they offer blood supply to the corpus callosum, the diencephalon and the choroid plexuses of the lateral ventricles of the brain. Therefore, anterior cerebral arterial problems can result in compromise of information processing ability, intellectual function, right and left brain integration ability, motor control and the production of cerebrospinal fluid.

From these brief descriptions of the major arterial blood supplies to the brain, it can be seen that in several instances the supply to specific brain structures and regions is duplicated so that interference with one part of the arterial blood delivery system can be accommodated by the overlapping of the systems.

As the blood is transported to the interstitial fluids and cellular elements of the brain, it passes through the arterial branching system. The individual arterial branches get smaller and smaller until the smallest arteries (known as arterioles) deliver the blood into the capillaries. It is in the capillary system that most of the action in terms of delivery and pickup of nutrients and metabolic by-products occurs. At the "far end" of the capillary system, speaking from an arterial point of view, the "waste-laden" blood is delivered into small veins (called venules) that are tributaries to larger and larger veins. These veins of the brain empty into venous sinuses, which then empty into the internal jugular veins which return the venous blood into the general blood circulation via the right side of the heart.

The venous sinuses are situated at various strategic locations between the two layers of the dura mater within the skull. It is into these venous sinuses that the arachnoid granulation and the arachnoid granulation bodies protrude. These arachnoid granulation bodies serve to reabsorb cerebrospinal fluid back into the blood system. This reabsorption process seems to be constant and has a great deal to do with cerebrospinal fluid pressure and the function of the craniosacral system.

At birth the newborn blood supply to the brain is pretty much as I have described it. This description has been general, but I believe it serves our purposes at this time. Now let's look at the blood supply to the spinal cord.

BLOOD SUPPLY TO THE SPINAL CORD

The arterial blood supply to the spinal cord comes from three main arteries. These are the anterior spinal artery, and the left and right posterior spinal arteries (**Fig. 5-44**). The anterior spinal artery originates from a union of a branch from both vertebral arteries (left and right) after they have entered the skull through the foramen magnum, but before they join to form the basilar artery. The two vertebral artery branches unite, in most cases, on the anterior or forward side of the medulla oblongata to form the resultant anterior spinal artery. The anterior spinal artery then exits the skull through the foramen magnum and travels down the front (anterior surface) of the

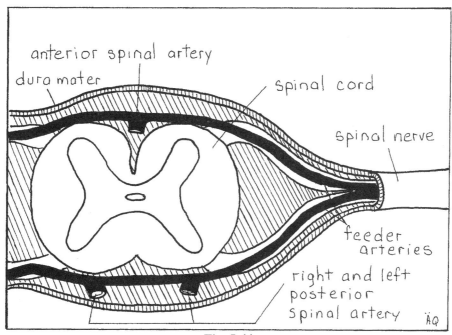

Fig. 5-44
The Spinal Arteries:
This is a cross section of the spinal cord which shows the three spinal arteries and the feeder arteries as they typically enter the vertebral canal with the spinal nerve roots.

spinal cord to its tail end. The anterior spinal artery's ending is quite variable. Sometimes it branches and the branches follow some of the spinal nerve roots out of the spinal canal. Other time it simply terminates within the spinal canal as a group of smaller and smaller branches that penetrate and supply the spinal cord with fresh arterial blood. In this latter case, it terminates into the capillary networks within the spinal cord tissues.

The other main arteries of the spinal cord are the posterior spinal arteries. There is a rather deep sulcus that courses down the length of the spinal cord from its origin at the medulla oblongata to the spinal cord's tail end, the cauda equina. The two right and left posterior spinal arteries originate from the right and left vertebral arteries just before these two (vertebral) arteries enter the foramen magnum and after they have exited the foramina of the first cervical vertebra and passed through the dura mater and arachnoid meningeal membranes. The posterior spinal arteries then accompany the spinal cord throughout its length on both sides of the sulcus. They end similarly to the anterior spinal artery by following nerve roots, or by simply terminating into the capillary networks within the spinal cord.

All three of these spinal cord arteries travel within the pia mater layer of the meningeal membranes and have frequent interconnections (anastomoses) with each other. They receive tributaries from feeder branches from a wide variety of arteries that are located on the outside of the vertebral (spinal) column. These feeder branches from outside of the spinal canal enter with the spinal nerve roots through the intervertebral foramen. Thus, once again Mother Nature has designed a multifaceted arterial blood supply system that gives backup service should one of the arteries become obstructed.

We have previously discussed the delivery of arterial blood into the capillary networks, the exchange of nutrients and oxygen for metabolic by-products and carbon dioxide, and the return of the byproduct-laden blood into the venous side of the circulatory system. This process occurs within the tissues of the brain and the spinal cord as it does in all other tissues throughout the body which are dependent upon an arterial blood supply. Once the smaller veins exit the tissue of the spinal cord they empty into larger veins that pretty much follow the courses of the spinal arteries. Much of the venous blood from these surface veins then exits the spinal canal via the branches that follow the spinal nerve roots through the intervertebral foramina. Once outside of the spinal canal and through the intervertebral foramina, these veins are outside of the dural membrane and, therefore, outside of the craniosacral system. The extradural veins then empty into a wide variety of venous subsystems in the neck, thorax and abdomen for return to the right side of the heart. Then the whole process starts all over again. Remember, the brain and spinal cord are dependent moment to moment upon fresh arterial blood for survival. Nerve cells die very quickly when deprived of nutrients and oxygen. There is good reason for the backup supply systems that deliver arterial blood to the central nervous system.

Inventory of Parts Index

Section VI

The Newborn Evaluation

General Considerations

Within a few minutes of the time of delivery of the newborn infant, a quick evaluation of the child can be done. This offers valuable information about special problems that may require immediate attention and/or the chances of survival for this newborn, as well as some predictors about the probable quality of life.

This initial evaluation should be redone in greater detail at about 12 and 72 hours of post-delivery life, after the effects of maternal anesthesia and/or medications and the shock of delivery have worn off. These follow-up evaluations should be done about one to two hours after a feeding, because a fully satiated infant is less responsive and a hungry infant is more irritable. Either of these circumstances can be quite misleading, and results of examination are therefore easily misinterpreted.

THE APGAR RATING

Usually, an APGAR rating is done within the first few minutes after the delivery of the child, and is repeated within another five minutes.

The APGAR rating system was developed by Dr. Virginia Apgar, and has been used almost everywhere in North America and in parts of Europe ever since. Most parents are familiar with the APGAR rating. In the APGAR system, the newborn is evaluated on five observed parameters and given a rating of 0, 1 or 2 on each of these parameters. A score of 10 is perfect.

Scores of 7 or less suggest depressed function of the nervous system, and a score of 4 or less on the initial rating requires resuscitation of the newborn. Scores below 8 on the second rating suggest a poor or guarded prognosis for the child, and indicate that further examination must be done as soon as feasible.

The APGAR rating system is as follows:

APGAR RATING			
	0	**1**	**2**
Heart Rate	Absent	Less than 100/minute	Over 100/minute
Respiratory Rate	Absent	Slow and irregular	Good respiration Crying with strength
Muscle Tone	Flaccid	Some flexion of the extremities	Making active movements
Reflex Irritability	No Reflexes	Crying weak	Vigorous crying Facial expression
Color	Blue or pale	Body pink Extremities blue	Pink all over

OTHER INITIAL OBSERVATIONS

There are a few other things that give valuable information about the newborn's condition that are usually noted by the healthcare professionals very shortly after the time of delivery. For example, a weight of less than 6 1/2 pounds strongly suggests premature delivery at 37 weeks or less of gestation. Also, the full-term child should be at least 18 inches long. Anything less may suggest prematurity. The newborn head should represent about 25 percent of its total length and, although it usually isn't weighed separately, the weight of the newborn head is approximately one-third of the total body weight under normal circumstances.

Although the APGAR gives 2 points for a newborn heart rate of over 100 beats per minute, it is most often closer to 140 beats per minute. When the heart rate is higher than 140 beats per minute it could signal a problem.

Also, at the time of delivery the chest (thoracic) cage should be about as wide, side to side, as it is deep from front to back. The abdominal movement with breathing represents diaphragm muscle activity. When the diaphragm contracts, it pushes the abdominal cavity down and enlarges the length of the thoracic cage, thus increasing its capacity. The ribs expand the thoracic cage capacity by increasing its side-to-side and front-to-back dimension. Good movements of the diaphragm muscle and of the ribs are a very welcome sight to the folks who are watching this newborn make its transition from inside the uterus, where mother supplies oxygenated blood, to outside the uterus. Once delivery takes place, the child's respiratory system must suddenly take over and inhale air, extract oxygen from that air, attach that oxygen to the hemoglobin in its (the newborn's) red blood cells and deliver it to the tissues. Especially important is the very quick delivery of oxygen to the infant's brain. The human brain requires oxygen on a minute-to-minute basis, more so than any other part of the body. Momentary deprivation of oxygen to the newborn brain can result in injury to brain tissue. Oxygen deprivation is spoken of as hypoxia. This is a word that you will see often in health-related writings.

So, just like in the movies, we want a baby to cry very early on in his/her post-delivery life. For this reason, many of us hold the newborn upside down by the ankles and lightly (very lightly) administer slaps on the butt to get that first cry. We want a loud, vigorous cry to kickstart the respiratory system in a very definite way. We want a good, deep breath to open the lungs and help clear the airway. We will often use suction to remove mucus that could be obstructing the airway because those initial efforts by the infant to activate the breathing mechanisms and the air exchanged via the lungs are so vitally important. Sometimes, in the excitement and concern a newborn can be traumatized in the back of the mouth and/or throat by overzealous use of the suction apparatus. Or, this trauma may be necessary for life and not simply overzealous use of suction. Quick action may be required in order to prevent hypoxia and possible brain injury or death. In any case, time is short and we want to hear a good, healthy cry through an airway that is fairly clear of mucus and other obstructions.

THINGS A CRY CAN TELL YOU

If the cry is high-pitched and shrill it may indicate increased intracranial pressure for any one of a number of reasons. Also, when intracranial pressure is above normal, the fontanelles (soft spots) will often feel as though they are bulging. Normally, the anterior fontanelle is about 1 1/2 to 2 inches in its widest dimension. And the posterior fontanelle is up to about 3/4 of an inch. The anterior fontanelle is normally closed somewhere between six and eighteen months, and the posterior fontanelle closes at about six weeks to two months of age. In severe intracranial pressure elevation related to hydrocephalus, the infant's eyes may deviate in a downwards direction. We will discuss other causes for increased intracranial pressure, such as tumors, in greater detail later.

When the newborn's cry is hoarse, the possibilities of tetany or cretinism must be considered. Tetany is usually due to a low blood calcium level, which results in muscle spasms causing severe flexion of the wrists and ankles, along with muscle twitches, cramps, possible convulsions and sometimes attacks of stridor (difficulty in breathing).

Cretinism is caused by below-normal thyroid function which, when present in utero, results in arrested physical and mental development in the newborn. The newborn cretin shows poorly developed bones and muscles, as well as a reduced or absent nervous system response to various stimuli and tests.

A cat-like cry, which is known as the "cri du chat," is often the harbinger of a genetic syndrome which includes an increased distance between the eyes and facial malformations which are known as hypertelorism. These children also show microcephaly and severe mental deficiency. This problem is of chromosomal origin.

A very weak, feeble, or even absent cry is strongly suggestive of severe illness or a deficit in the development of the nervous system.

MORE INITIAL OBSERVATIONS

Asymmetry of movements from the time of delivery through the neonatal period (first month of life) are strongly suggestive of severe neurological problems, birth injuries and/or congenital anomalies. Even during these first examinations, abnormal movements at right angles to the intent of the movement are suggestive of hypoxia or cerebellar problems. This pendulum-like motor deficit becomes more apparent during the first few days of life if it has serious implications.

This initial examination is also a good time to palpate the neck for deformities, tumors and fistulae. We should include in this evaluation the degree of tightness or looseness of the skull on the neck. If there is tightness, this problem can be taken care of in seconds or minutes right there in the delivery room. If this tightness is not released, it can be the cause of colic. It is always best to deal with this problem as soon as possible in order to avoid the nutritional imbalances that may result as complications of compromised intake of food. Usually, CranioSacral Therapy in the delivery room will solve it on the spot.

Convulsions soon after delivery can be the result of low blood sugar (hypoglycemia), which usually occurs when the mother is diabetic. Postpartum convulsions can also be the result of infection. Even though the newborn infant has some passive immunity protection from the mother for the first four or five months of extrauterine life, infection must be considered. Other causes of newborn convulsions would include delivery trauma to the head with intracranial bleeding, drugs given to the mother during labor, metabolic imbalance, fever, kernicterus, endocrine imbalances and so on.

TIME FOR BONDING

Once the child has been delivered, has started breathing, has been suctioned and wiped off, and the umbilical cord cut, it is time for bonding with mother and father, if he is present. Bonding should be a high and early priority for every infant unless there is some reason of higher priority that precludes this process. By bonding, I simply mean that part of the delivery where, for a few minutes, the newborn is placed upon the recumbent mother's breast and there occurs a sharing of love and energy. The father may join in by simply touching mother and child, or better yet, by joining a sort of group hug that usually occurs quite naturally. We who do CranioSacral Therapy and SomatoEmotional Release^sm work have seen many cases of psychoemotional rejection that has no discoverable basis in reality. These cases of "rejection" are usually in adults suffering a wide variety of etiologically related symptoms. The "rejection" frequently has its roots in a lack of the bonding process soon after their delivery. It has been quite amazing to see how these patients are able to relive the delivery experience, realize that bonding was precluded for some reason, and accept that this absence of bonding was not maternal rejection. Once this realization occurs, we offer the opportunity for the patient to image in his or her mind how it would have been to bond with mother right after delivery. Once this is done, in the great majority of cases the related symptoms, be they physical or psychoemotional, simply disappear.

NEWBORN POSTURE

As soon after bonding as possible, the newborn's posture in the supine (lying on the back) position should be observed. This is important because postural deviations, abnormalities and asymmetries represent an important source of information related to the in utero development of the nervous and musculoskeletal systems. Posture also points to a variety of birth injuries.

The normal newborn posture is called the "flexion posture." In this posture, the upper arms and the thighs are abducted (away from the central line of the body) at the shoulders and at the hips. The elbows, wrists, knees and ankles are all flexed. The fingers are also flexed, and the thumbs are positioned in the palms of the hands. This flexion posture occurs when the newborn is placed upon his/her back in the supine position. After a few weeks of extrauterine life, the limbs begin to extend out of flexion and the thumbs come out of the palms.

Deviations from the normal flexion posture may indicate hypotonia for a number of reasons: excessive sedation of mother during delivery, hypoxia, hypoglycemia, spinal cord dysfunction, neonatal myasthenia gravis, myotonic dystrophy and/or Down's syndrome, amongst other possibilities. A spinal cord problem may look like hypotonia due to other causes, but spinal cord dysfunction is usually accompanied by failure of the urinary bladder to work. Bladder dysfunction is not usually seen in other situations related to hypotonia.

When the newborn's posture is evaluated, the child should be completely naked so that you can evaluate body asymmetries. Observed asymmetries may be due to birth trauma with fractures. These fractures are most commonly of the clavicle and the upper arm, and less commonly of the upper leg. Lack of symmetry in the pelvis and hips should also be noted. When present, it may suggest congenital hip dislocation. This problem is easily confirmed or denied by feeling the hips, and the relations and movements of the femoral heads to the hip sockets (acetabula), which are located in the pelvic bones.

THE SKIN COLOR

While viewing the naked newborn, skin color is another important factor to observe. A yellowish color indicates a neonatal jaundice (icterus). The less serious type of jaundice, known as physiological jaundice, does not usually show itself until day two or three of extrauterine life. It usually goes away by itself by day 20. The "bili" light is often used to reduce the jaundice. It is not quite known how shining a blue light on a jaundiced newborn solves the problem, but most often it does. This type of jaundice is due to an excessive, or perhaps even normal breakdown of red blood cells. It is the liver that excretes the metabolic by-products of disintegrating red blood cells. Excessive red blood cell destruction could be the result of delivery trauma which produces more by-products than a normal liver can manage. On the other hand, a liver that is not yet functioning at a normal newborn level may not be able to handle a reasonably normal metabolism of red blood cells.

More serious causes of neonatal jaundice include erythroblastosis fetalis, which is the scientific name for the Rh-incompatibility problem between mother and fetus. It means that maternal antibodies from an Rh (-) mother have gotten across the placental barrier into the fetus. These maternal antibodies have attacked and destroyed many Rh (+) fetal blood cells. The Rh (+) factor in the infant must have been donated by the father.

Other more serious causes of jaundice in the newborn include serious infection, failure of development of the bile duct and other congenital problems. Icterus, or jaundice, are the names which mean that there is an elevation of bilirubin, or bile, in the blood. Very high levels are called kernicterus. The high blood levels of bilirubin can cause convulsions, spasticity and brain damage.

There are times when an exchange blood transfusion is life-saving for the infant.

Blueness of skin, lips and nail beds is called cyanosis. Cyanosis usually indicates that, for some reason, the blood is not getting enough oxygen, and/or that the heart is not effectively pumping the blood through the vascular system to the body parts and regions that reflect the blueish (cyanotic) color.

Both jaundice and cyanosis require investigation for cause and proper treatment in order to prevent brain injury and dysfunction, and/or death.

EDEMA

Another sign that is easily observed at this time is edema. Edema is an excess of fluid accumulation under the skin. It shows itself as a swelling under the skin. Edema may be due to heart dysfunction, kidney dysfunction, low blood proteins, endocrine problems and/or mineral imbalance. There are also other, less common reasons for edema. The cause must be identified.

EARLY MOVEMENTS

The newborn infant should be observed for concurrent chest and abdominal movements related to breathing. Also, the chest wall may move with the heartbeats. The abdominal movements related to breathing represent the action of the diaphragm muscle. The diaphragm enlarges the thoracic cage by increasing its vertical dimension. The rib cage movements represent front-to-back and side-to-side dimension changes of the rib cage. Both diaphragmatic and rib cage movements should be apparent.

It is a simple task at this time to observe general alertness and responsiveness to stimuli, as well as spontaneous movements. It is also quite easy at this time to evaluate the strength of the sucking reflex, as well as many other reflexes that we will discuss in greater detail.

Topic 34

Head, Skull and Craniosacral System

Following the general assessment of the newborn infant, sometime within the first 72 hours of life a more in-depth evaluation should be carried out. This evaluation should include the head (the skull in particular), the craniosacral system, and a look at the brain for more obvious problems. It is true that the craniosacral system does not as yet have its proper place in traditional medicine. However, the positive results of quality craniosacral work with newborns and children are amassing and the benefits are beginning to look irrefutable. In any case, the craniosacral evaluation and treatment of newborns is included in this description.

During fetal life, the brain as it is forming is initially covered by the previously described three layers of meningeal membrane. These three layers from the inside (next to the brain substance) out are: (1) The pia mater, which covers the brain quite intimately. It follows the brain tissue into all the crevices and sulci that characterize its surface. (2) The middle of the three layers of meningeal membrane is called the arachnoid because it somewhat resembles a spider web in the way in which its fine fibrous strands are woven through its fabric and connect it to the pia mater. The arachnoid membrane does not follow the brain surface into all of the crevices and sulci as does the pia mater. The subarachnoid space between these two innermost meningeal membranes is filled with cerebrospinal fluid. (3) The outermost layer of meningeal membrane, the dura mater, is tough by comparison to the delicacy of the arachnoid and pia mater membranes. The dura mater membrane is actually double-layered in the skull. But, the two layers are rather closely adhered together by connecting fibers. The outermost of the two layers of dura mater within the skull doubles in later life as the inner lining of the skull bones. However, during fetal life this dura mater membrane actually calcifies in specific patterns. It is this calcification of the dura mater layer of the meninges that becomes the bones of the outer skull. That is the part of the skull that is accessible to us as we feel through the scalp to evaluate the bones. On the inside of the skull, the bones of the floor of the skull cavity are formed from cartilage rather than from dura mater membrane.

This "hardening" of the dura mater membrane begins during the fourth month of gestation within the mother's womb. You should also know that the dura mater is not tightly adhered to the arachnoid meningeal membrane layer. There is a subdural space which allows for some independent movement between dura mater and arachnoid meningeal membranes. This space is filled with a fluid that greatly resembles cerebrospinal fluid in its composition/consistency. However, it is not known as cerebrospinal fluid as yet. Perhaps one day it will be so designated.

At the time of obstetrical delivery, the skull bones are largely developed. However, the interfaces between the bones are not yet clearly formed. These interfaces are known as sutures after they are formed. Sutural formation at the time of delivery would interfere with overriding of skull edges. This overriding, which is known as head-molding, allows the fetal head, which when it is expanded would be too large to pass through the mother's birth canal, to collapse as it passes through this birth canal. The fetal head can thus gain access to the outside world without too much damage to either mother or newborn child.

THE HEAD AND SKULL

Now let's consider what an average newborn head feels like within the first day or two after its delivery. First of all, within a few hours the shape of the newborn head should be almost symmetrical. Any overriding of bone edges that persists after 24 hours can usually be corrected by the proper application of CranioSacral Therapy. The sooner the treatment is applied, the better it is for the child.

There are two soft places in the normal newborn head. One is toward the front just behind the frontal bone which forms the forehead. The other is farther back by a couple of inches. Both soft places are on the front-to-back midline of the skull. These soft places are officially called fontanelles. The front one is the anterior fontanelle and the back one is called the posterior fontanelle. The anterior fontanelle is about an inch to an inch and a half at its widest diameter at birth. It normally closes between a year and a year and a half after obstetrical delivery. The posterior fontanelle is usually about the size of a fingertip and it closes about six to eight weeks after delivery. The fontanelles are key areas that allow fetal head molding during passage of the "too large head" through the "too small birth canal" (**Fig. 3-40**).

Most parents get almost "spooked" when they feel their newborn infant's soft spots (fontanelles). It is kind of eerie when you realize that, if you press on the soft spot of your child's head with your finger, you are only separated from the child's brain by some skin, membranes, a little connective tissue and some fluid. Your child is extremely vulnerable to pressure through his/her "soft spots."

So, during the initial evaluation, we are interested in the "feel" of the fontanelles and the sutures. Fontanelles that are bulging are strongly suggestive of increased intracranial pressure. When this bulging is coupled with vomiting, you must be very concerned about the newborn's chances of survival without specific and definitive treatment. Causes of increased intracranial pressure would include tumors, intracranial hemorrhages, hydrocephalus, rickets, even neonatal syphilis. A sign that increased intracranial pressure has been going on for a while within the uterus is palpable and visible dilation of the veins of the scalp. If left unattended, increased intracranial pressure for any reason will cause a belated closure of the fontanelles. Another cause of late fontanelle closure that is unrelated to intracranial pressure is achondroplasia with dwarfism. In this case, the problem interferes with normal skull-bone development.

The sutures should feel essentially undeveloped in the newborn skull. That is, the bone edges should move rather independently from one another. Premature closure of the skull sutures is called cranial synostosis. This premature closure prevents the skull from growing in volume in accordance and compliance with the requirements of the expanding brain. This may be a genetic problem but the cause remains unknown at present.

If the fontanelles feel excessively soft and are easily depressed or are actually indented, it signifies that the intracranial pressure is too low. This happens most often in cases of dehydration for any reason. Those reasons include maternal dehydration and illness just before delivery, newborn vomiting, inability to absorb fluid and so on. When the fontanelles are depressed, the bone edges are more tightly abutted than usual and there is a greater propensity for persistent overriding of bone edges after the molding that has occurred during delivery.

If fontanelles actually close prematurely as opposed to being in a soft and depressed condition, it may indicate microcephaly, oxycephaly, or scaphocephalous **(Fig. 6-1)**. All three of these conditions are accompanied by brain-function deficits. Microcephalus is a condition in which the size of the head is abnormally small. Oxycephalus is a condition in which the top of the skull is pointed, owing to premature closure of the coronal and lambdoid sutures. Scaphocephalous is an abnormal length and narrowness of the skull as a result of premature closure of the sagittal suture.

During this general evaluation of the head, in addition to evaluating the general symmetry of the shape of the head, the fontanelles and the sutures, we should feel for irregularities of bone hardness or density, especially in the frontal and parietal regions. The frontal region is from the brow back to the anterior fontanelle. The parietals are the bones that meet at the front-to-back midline of the skull between the two fontanelles, and extend down over the sides of the skull to their sutural junction with the temporal bones. These temporal/parietal junctions are slightly above the ears on each side. Craniotabes is one condition that can be found with your fingers by

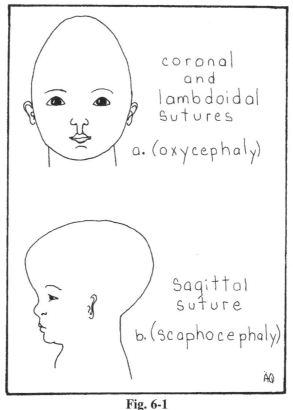

Fig. 6-1
Head Shapes Related to Premature Sutural Closure:
The pointed head in drawing (a) is due to premature closure of
the coronal and lambdoidal sutures. This is called oxycephaly.
In drawing (b) the sagittal suture closed prematurely resulting
in a long, narrow head called scaphocephaly.

feeling the skull vault. In craniotabes, the bone is soft and demineralized. This condition can signal the presence of rickets, which is a deficiency of vitamin D and/or neonatal syphilis.

There is another less severe problem that results in a softened area in the newborn skull bone. This problem is named cephalhematoma (**Fig. 6-2**). In this case there has been trauma to the head during the delivery process, often caused by forceps. The trauma has caused bleeding within the bone just underneath the outer surface (periosteum). This bleeding separates the outer layer of the bone from the rest of it. Since the separation is caused by a fluid, namely blood, the bone surface that your fingers feel is soft. After a few days the outer circumference of the cephalhematoma becomes hard through calcification. When this occurs it can be mistaken for a depressed fracture of the involved skull bone. However, when the infant cries the increased intracranial pressure does not transmit to the cephalhematoma. Therefore, there is no palpable change as there would be in other conditions such as depressed skull fracture, or a formation defect with protrusion of the meningeal membrane and perhaps part of the brain through the bone defect. There is also a condition called the lacunar bone deformity in which the cells that produce bone (osteoblasts) convert to, or become outnumbered by, cells that absorb bone (osteoclasts), and the bone begins to reabsorb. The result is a defect in the bone.

Other conditions that can be discovered simply by feeling the newborn head include swollen areas in the scalp due to bleeding, which is usually due to birth trauma. We should also feel for nodules in the skin of the scalp, abnormal connections between arteries and veins which present as swollen areas, and caput succedaneum, which is just a swelling of the scalp due to the force of

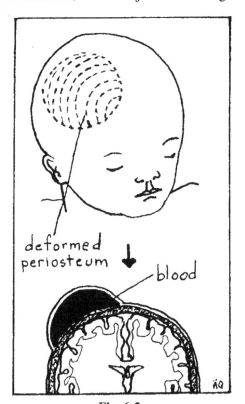

Fig. 6-2
Cephalhematoma:
Note that the blood has accumulated beneath the
outer surface of the skull bone causing a
deformity of that layer (periosteum) of the bone.

the head pushing against the resistance of the birth canal. Dilated or prominent scalp veins may suggest rickets, neonatal syphilis and/or internal hydrocephalus.

The circumference of the newborn head should be measured at its largest transverse area. The normal measurement is between 34 and 36 centimeters. Large heads occur in cases of hydrocephalus with or without abnormality of brain size, and in megacephalus wherein the brain is grossly enlarged. Small heads occur in microcephalus, certain genetic defects, and in a variety of congenital infections.

The stethoscope should be used to listen for abnormal sounds (bruits) in the newborn head. Usually, these bruits are insignificant, but they should arouse suspicion of the possibility of increased intracranial pressure and/or abnormal connections between the arterial and venous systems in the head.

CRANIOSACRAL SYSTEM: EVALUATION AND TREATMENT

It is at the time of the more in-depth evaluation of the newborn that the first craniosacral evaluation and treatment may be most efficiently carried out. Since I am firmly convinced of the value of this craniosacral work in the newborn, I shall describe in detail the methods I use at this early time in the infant's life.

The treatment is immediately begun as it is indicated by the evaluation. The whole procedure usually takes about five minutes and, even in complicated situations, it seldom requires longer than ten minutes. More often than not, one or two treatments are all that are needed to correct the craniosacral problem in the newborn, unless there is some congenital defect that is resultant to either intrauterine problems or genetic abnormalities. In these cases, ongoing CranioSacral Therapy may be indicated to reach the maximum potential, even though that level of function may not reach the average. Good examples wherein CranioSacral Therapy is helpful in congenital problems would be in Down's syndrome and in spina bifida. There may always be a deficit, but ongoing CranioSacral Therapy seems to increase the maximum level of function. In these cases we have no desire to create dependency. Therefore, we are most happy to train willing parents to do CranioSacral Therapy with their children.

My own approach to the craniosacral evaluation begins by placing one hand on the newborn cranial vault. I'm feeling for symmetry or lack of same, for the overriding of bone edges, and for the vitality of the craniosacral rhythm. Craniosacral rhythm is felt as a gentle widening of the skull as it shortens slightly from front to back. This change in skull shape alternates about eight to ten times a minute with a subtle narrowing and lengthening of the skull. If this motion is not symmetrical on both sides of the head, I will, with my hand, very gently inhibit the side that moves the most. Since this movement is caused by a rhythmical fluctuation of hydraulic force within the dura mater membrane, when the movement of one side of the head is inhibited, the other side experiences a small increase in fluid pressure. This increase is frequently enough to liberate any restriction to movement on the side that was moving the least. Frequently, at this early age this is all the treatment that is required.

Next, I place one finger in the newborn's mouth while I hold my other hand on the skull vault. I want the newborn to suck on my finger as hard as he or she will do it. As the sucking occurs, I place just a little pressure in coordination with the sucking rhythm on the midline of the roof of the mouth. Between the sucking action and my adjunctive pressure, the tendency for the natural widening of the cranial vault (skull) is increased. If the infant does not suck on my finger, I will apply my finger pressure to the roof of the mouth in a rhythmical fashion. If I can feel the craniosacral rhythm with my other hand, I will coordinate my roof-of-the-mouth pressure with this inherent craniosacral rhythm. If there is no perceptible cranial rhythm, I will simulate what I think is normal in the roof of the mouth. This simulation will quite often sort of "jump start" a craniosacral rhythm that, for one reason or another, has been inhibited and has failed to start.

I find this time (with one finger in the mouth enhancing the amplitude of the craniosacral system's activity and the sucking action of the infant) to be the best time to correct the problem of one skull bone overriding another. Sometimes, the internal fluid force enhanced by the sucking and your finger are enough to make the corrections. If this is not the case, I often place one finger (of the hand which is on the skull vault) on each of the involved overriding skull bones and spread them away from each other. This technique is almost always successful, but in that rare exception you may have to go back and try again later. I believe that the sooner the symmetry and balance of movement in the skull are achieved and the overriding is corrected, the better it is for the newborn. Therefore, I might go back and try again two or three times in one day.

The next thing I do in the newborn craniosacral evaluation and treatment is what we call releasing the occipital cranial base and condyles. This technique is designed to release any jamming or residual compression of the occiput that might continue to exist subsequent to the obstetrical delivery.

When the newborn is presenting its head through the birth canal in a face-down position, it is quite easy for the head to become bent backwards excessively into the upper neck. The joint surfaces of the occipital bone and of the top (first) cervical vertebra form an incomplete "V" with the projected apex pointing forward. When the back of the head/neck juncture passes under the mother's pubic bone, it is not uncommon for the head to excessively bend backward on the neck. Sometimes, this forces the occipital joint surfaces forward into the "V" shaped joints of the first cervical vertebra (also called the atlas), and they get stuck. The jamming, or compression of the head on the neck is then maintained by the ongoing contraction of the soft tissues (muscles, etc.) in the area. These soft tissues remain in a contracted state in order to offer protective splinting against further injury. It is as though they just don't know enough to relax when the danger is past.

The technique that I use is simply to hold the skull vault in one hand with my third and fourth fingertips, straddling the vertical midline of the newborn's head. On this same hand, my thumb is reaching towards the forehead as near to the vertical midline as I can get it.

I place my index finger of the other hand horizontally across the top of the neck very near the base of the skull so that I am supporting the first cervical vertebra in a forward position. Next, I move the baby's head around an imaginary transverse axis that would pass horizontally through the ears on both sides. The force I use is very gentle but persistent. This gentle force is applied in a circular direction around the aforementioned transverse axis. The direction of the force is such that it moves the newborn's head backwards, off of the neck, the back of the head is urged to move upwards, and the top of the head would move forward. All of these aforementioned force directions are actually arcs rather than straight lines.

This application of force is comparable to the amount of force that it takes to pick up a nickel. It is indeed a small force that will cause no trauma to the infant. But when the small force is applied for a prolonged time, perhaps one or two minutes, it will cause the soft tissues to relax and alleviate the jamming or compression of joints of the skull and the top of the neck.

In our experience, this jamming between head and neck is frequently and markedly present in children who suffer from the hyperactivity syndrome which is more recently becoming better known as Attention Deficit Disorder. When this craniosacral problem is present in the hyperactive child and it is corrected by treatment, we have seen marked improvement, if not complete alleviation of the problem in over 50 percent of our patients. The relief comes very quickly when it comes, so you know by the rapid and dramatic response whether or not CranioSacral Therapy will be the answer for any given child. The therapist simply works until the correction is made. When the correction of the jamming is complete, if this is the cause, the child is better within minutes. The correction may have to be repeated three or four times over a period of a month or so. I believe that recurrence of the jamming happens because the soft tissues have become habituated to over-contraction and the habit must be broken. We have also witnessed rapid relief in colicky babies when this head/neck jamming is alleviated. Anatomically, this seems related to the alleviation of excessive pressure on the vagus nerve as it passes out of the skull and into the neck. We will discuss the vagus nerve and its workings in Topic 36, which gives a detailed discussion of all of the cranial nerves.

The next part of the craniosacral evaluation and treatment involves the spinal column, the spinal canal and the meningeal membranes, especially the dura mater and that part of it which forms a tube around the spinal cord and the two inner membrane layers. This dura mater tube also forms sleeves for all of the spinal cord nerve roots. These sleeves offer protection to these delicate nerve roots until they exit the spinal column. It is at the transverse foramina where these sleeves attach and end.

The technique is carried out as follows. Continue to hold the newborn head with one hand as you have for the previous techniques. Remove your other hand from the neck and move it down to the pelvis so that your fingers are under the child's sacrum. (The sacrum is the larger bone at the tail end of the spine.) Now apply a small stretching force or traction upon the spinal column by pulling your two hands away from each other very gently. Continue this stretching for a few minutes. The newborn may cry but your force is very small. You are not causing pain. You may, however, be causing pain from the recent delivery to be remembered and re-experienced as you allow release of the kinks and twists that were put in during the passage through the birth canal. If during this process the head or the pelvis show any tendency to twist or turn, you follow these intended movements as you continue the gentle traction.

It is my own belief that well-intentioned obstetrical delivery persons sometimes become overzealous and pull the newborn out of the mother too rapidly. This overzealous pulling may cause defensive tissue contraction or guarding in the infant that may persist after the danger has passed. The treatment that I have just described is designed to release residual soft tissue guarding, splinting and contraction. You can feel the releases when they occur, and when the technique is complete there is a marked sense of relaxation in the newborn's body.

Personally, I believe that unless there is necessity to pull the infant out of the mother, we should passively catch the child. We may gently assist in rotations and so on, but we should intrude as little as possible. I envision the passage through the birth canal as carefully designed by Mother Nature to offer skull and spinal mobilization treatment, a soft tissue (perhaps neuromuscular) massage, and a stimulating skin rub that helps to activate the sensory nervous system. In my opinion, Mother Nature has good reasons for everything she does. She also does it best.

This completes the routine initial craniosacral evaluation and treatment. Obstinate problems may require more work, but an amazing amount can be accomplished in this first session. In addition to the craniosacral work done, I also like to mobilize and balance the rib cage and the pelvis at this time. It only takes a few more minutes to do these things, and the assistance that can be offered the infant by helping to organize and make the breathing easier, as well as helping the bowel and bladder function better, makes it well worth the effort.

Topic 35

The Brain

GENERAL CONSIDERATIONS

In general, it is fair to say that a functional evaluation of the total brain of the newborn above the level of the brain stem is unreliable. This is the case because so much functional brain development occurs after delivery. Newborn reflexes are essentially primitive and rarely go above the level of the midbrain (mesencephalon). Actually, an evaluation of complete cerebral cortex function cannot be reliably carried out until the child is about seven years of age, when cortical development is complete. Therefore, the presence of a brain dysfunction may not be detectable until the child matures to that level of neurological development when a specific functional landmark should normally appear and it fails to do so. For example, after about two or three weeks of extrauterine life, the normal flexion posture as previously described begins to disappear. The limbs begin to extend, the palms of the hands open up and the thumbs come out and begin to assume the normal position, which allows them to grasp objects more effectively between the fingers and the opposing thumb. The oppositional use of the thumb depends on functional development and dendritic (interneuronal) connections in the "hand" region of the motor cortex in the cerebral hemispheres. These functional connections are not usually present at birth.

It isn't until age three that a preference towards right- or left-handedness occurs. It seems that the handedness correlates to the development of speech, which is dependent upon temporal lobe development.

The startle or Moro reflex, when it persists after four to six months of age, is indicative of slow development of the cerebral cortex.

There are many more examples of these developmental landmarks. We will encounter a large number of them as we discuss the specific evaluation of the motor division of the nervous system.

BRAIN SIZE

The physical examination for the presence of the brain and its form in the newborn is carried out largely by head measurements. A circumference of between 34 and 36 centimeters is considered within normal limits.

Transillumination is another screening test of brain size and symmetry that seems quite reliable. During transillumination, you shine a flashlight through the newborn's head from the back to the front. The amount of light coming through the orbits of both eyes should be equal. The orbit is the skull's accommodation for the eyeball. If the brightness of light is greater in one eye than the other, there may be a discrepancy in the size of the two hemispheres (halves) of the brain. This is a very straightforward test. Brain mass obstructs the passage of light. Brain mass should be equal on both sides. If it isn't, there may be a lesser amount or an absence of brain mass on one side; or there may be a brain cyst on one side filled with a fluid which conducts light more efficiently than normal brain tissue.

NO-NEW-NEURONS DOGMA

It has long been thought that the infant develops no new neurons after delivery. Functional developmental progress is supposed to be totally dependent upon the formation of neuronal dendritic connections or synapses that develop in response to stimuli coming into the brain via the sensory division of the nervous system. I'm still not quite convinced that no new neurons can develop after being born. I have had a few patient experiences that cast doubt upon the "no-new-neuron" theory. For example, I worked with a young lady who lost a significant portion of her cerebral motor cortex along with a generous portion of her skull to a motorboat propeller. She was in a coma for several weeks. Her neurosurgeon predicted that she would never be able to voluntarily move anything below her neck again. Today, she has good use of her arms, hands and most of her trunk. She still requires braces and a little assistance to walk. This progress has been made over a period of approximately five years. I'm very suspicious that she grew some new neurons.

SLEEP

On a different subject, it is of interest to note that researchers are beginning to see that the newborn infant spends about 50 percent of its time in a special kind of sleep called REM sleep (Rapid Eye Movement). Premature infants spend about 75 percent of their time in REM sleep. It is presently believed that during REM sleep the brain is aroused and the body is essentially paralyzed. This may have something to do with conservation of energy and the facilitation of brain development when that energy is available.

CLASSIFICATION OF NEUROLOGICAL PROBLEMS

Neurological problems are usually classified as either static or degenerative. The static problem does not progress. The disability stays the same but it may seem to be increasing because, as the child should develop more skills, he/she doesn't. It simply means that whatever is wrong remains static, but it prevents development of brain regions or circuitry. Examples of static neurological problems would be cerebral palsy, Down's syndrome, meningocele and so on.

Degenerative neurological diseases progress. That is, the disease or problem spreads and will take away neurological function that has been present. Tumor growth, multiple sclerosis, amyotrophic lateral sclerosis, other demyelinating diseases are examples of degenerative neurological problems. It is important to know which classification of problem you are dealing with. It is also sometimes quite difficult to make the classification in the newborn simply because so many nervous system functions are not yet present.

Probably the most reliable observation in the newborn is the symmetry or lack thereof of movements from the time of birth. Another fairly reliable sign is the ability of the eyes to fix on a light or bright colored object, and then to follow this object to one side or the other. The eyes cannot move right away, but the newborn does follow by moving the head. These signs can tell you when something is wrong but they don't tell you what it is.

When the fontanelles are bulging and the pressure in the newborn head is elevated, the eyeballs are harder to press inwardly. In order to know the normal eyeball resistance to pressure, you should have pressed many newborn eyeballs so that you have a subjective baseline for comparison.

Tumor is one cause for increased intracranial pressure. It is interesting to note that the majority of newborn and, indeed, childhood tumors are found in male children. This could be related to the dominance of testosterone in males. Some studies show that testosterone stimulates neuronal cell multiplication and growth. The possibility of a tumor-formation/testosterone relationship does therefore exist.

It is also of interest to note that the majority of childhood brain tumors occur below the tentorium cerebelli. This means most childhood tumors are of the cerebellum, the pons and/or the medulla. In adults the majority of brain tumors occur above the tentorium cerebelli. I haven't a clue as to why this would be the case except that most cortical growth occurs after delivery. The cerebellum, pons and medulla develop before the upper brain structures.

Another observation that you might find of interest are that newborns have strokes. These strokes, when they occur, are identifiable because the onset of the problem is very sudden. Coma produces a group of specific reflex abnormalities that relate to depressed function of the brain stem. At the onset of coma, spinal cord reflexes may be depressed, but they may return even though the coma persists. In coma, the newborn posture is called a decerebrate posture. This posture is rigid. Muscles are tight and do not allow extreme ranges of motion. Turning the head right causes increased muscle contraction on the left side, and vice versa.

Grand mal seizures, when they occur, are of two types: tonic and clonic. The tonic seizure means that muscles contract and continuously maintain their contraction. During a clonic seizure, the muscles alternately contract and relax. The clonic seizure is less dangerous to the infant than the tonic seizure. Both types require diagnostic tests to discover the cause.

During the initial evaluation of the brain, it is also helpful to discover at what level of the brain the problem exists. A problem with the medulla oblongata may produce dysfunction of the trigeminal nerve. This nerve is generally in control of mouth movements like chewing, opening and closing the jaw and so on. The abducent nerve controls the muscles of the eye that prevent cross-eyedness. However, eye movement control is not present in the newborn, so it is a few weeks before this sign of medulla problem shows up.

The glossopharyngeal, vagus and accessory cranial nerves are also affected by problems in the medulla. Dysfunction of these nerves will show up as difficulty in swallowing, frequent regurgitation, colic, and difficulty in breathing. The child may also have difficulty making sounds, and poor control of neck posture and movement. Also dysfunctional in medulla oblongata problems is the hypoglossal nerve, which controls tongue movements. When my finger is in the mouth during the craniosacral evaluation, it is very convenient to evaluate tongue movement and strength, and thus to evaluate hypoglossal nerve function.

Medulla oblongata problems may also show up as nystagmus, which is a rhythmical movement of the eye without ability to focus or track. This movement can be either vertical or horizontal. Paralysis may be variable in problems with the medulla oblongata. Depending on what part or parts of the medulla oblongata are affected, the child can be paralyzed or weak (paretic) on one whole side of the body (hemiplegia), on all four limbs of the body (quadriplegia), or only of the lower parts of the body (paraplegia). Usually the medulla oblongata will not cause bladder control problems. When bladder control is impaired, it more strongly suggests spinal cord problems. Usually, a child will fall chronically and consistently to one side or the other in problems of the medulla oblongata.

Pons problems involve almost the same cranial nerves as the medulla oblongata problems, but there is less effect on the sound-making apparatus on the ear and on swallowing. The differential factor is that there is often a facial paralysis with pons problems. One side of the face may be expressionless while the other side may be essentially normal. Body paralysis may be of the same types as produced by the medulla oblongata. Eye movement may be increased and purposeless, and look like a very exaggerated form of nystagmus.

Midbrain (mesencephalon) problems produce more severe eye movement dysfunctions in all directions except cross-eyedness. The midbrain problem does not cause the eyes to cross — they will diverge, they won't be able to look up and down, but the child will not be cross-eyed. Paralysis can be of any of the types described above. The posture will be tilted and there will usually be an intention tremor so that, when the infant reaches for something, the arm and hand that are reaching will tend to shake or tremor. When the reaching extremity goes markedly side to side, much like a pendulum, it is often the cerebellum that is the problem.

The newborn has no signs that are specific above the midbrain. Therefore, it is almost impossible to diagnose problems above this level until a little later in life.

If there is a problem below the foramen magnum in the spinal cord, there will be no cranial nerve problems, no nystagmus, no seizures and no mental changes. There may well be dysfunction of the urinary bladder manifest as an inability to urinate with any force.

The Cranial Nerves

GENERAL INFORMATION

In an effort to keep some semblance of order and organization, we shall now discuss the cranial nerves. These nerves are the pairs of nerves that either exit or enter the brain rather than the spinal cord. Therefore, it seems more rational from an anatomical perspective to look at these nerves before moving to the spinal cord, which is considered the lower part of the central nervous system.

There are 12 pairs of cranial nerves. They are interchangeably identified by Roman numerals I through XII, and given names which bear some relationship to their function and/or anatomical location. For a change, there are no anatomist's or neurologist's names attached to these nerves.

To be absolutely correct, the first two pairs of cranial nerves, namely the olfactory (I) and the optic (II) are not nerves at all. They are actually extensions of brain tissue into the nose and the eyes, respectively. The criteria used to designate a peripheral nerve as compared to the brain (or spinal cord) extension include the requirement that there must be a synaptic connection between that nerve and the brain. For the olfactory nerves (I) and the optic nerves (II), these synaptic connections do not exist. Therefore, there are two brain tracts which are misnamed cranial nerves I and II. This leaves us with only 10 pairs of true cranial nerves. The names of the cranial nerve pairs are as follows:

I	Olfactory nerves (brain tracts)
II	Optic nerves (brain tracts)
III	Oculomotor nerves (true peripheral nerves)
IV	Trochlear nerves (true peripheral nerves)
V	Trigeminal nerves (true peripheral nerves)
VI	Abducent nerves (true peripheral nerves)
VII	Facial nerves (true peripheral nerves)
VIII	Auditory or vestibular or vestibulocochlear or auditory/vestibular nerves (true peripheral nerves)
IX	Glossopharyngeal nerves (true peripheral nerves)
X	Vagus nerves (true peripheral nerves)
XI	Accessory nerves (true peripheral nerves)
XII	Hypoglossal nerves (true peripheral nerves)

Of all the nerves in the body, the nerves that enter or exit the brain between the areas bounded by and including the midbrain (mesencephalon) above and the medulla oblongata (myelencephalon) below are the first to myelinate during the gestation period of the embryo. This myelination process of the cranial nerves (and some others nearby) occurs during the third month of intrauterine life. This myelination is carried out by the Schwann cells for the IIIrd through the XIIth nerves, and by the oligodendroglia cells for the olfactory and optic nerves. Oligodendroglia cells myelinate the brain nerve cells. Schwann cells myelinate peripheral nerve cells.

THE OLFACTORY NERVE - CRANIAL NERVE I

During the newborn evaluation, the olfactory nerve is not usually examined. This omission is based upon the theory that there is no way to test for smell in the newborn, and that probably the sense of smell is not operational in the newborn infant. It is difficult to argue one way or the other, but I have some bias that a one-day-old newborn has some primitive sense of smell. I have seen them grimace and recoil in a rather primitive way from rubbing alcohol when it is held near their nose **(Fig. 5-28)**.

THE OPTIC NERVE - CRANIAL NERVE II

The optic nerve (brain fiber tract) is also known as cranial nerve II **(Fig. 6-3)**. This is the "nerve" that perceives the light waves that go through the pupil of the eye and strike the retina of the eyeball. Vision is quite primitive at birth, as is eye motor control, but simple testing of optic nerve function can be carried out. The newborn is rather nearsighted (myopic), so it is optimal to use a light stimulus about 10 to 12 inches away from and in front of the newborn's eyes. Close observation must be made to see whether or not the infant's eyes fix on the light. A bright colored object may also be used. If the infant's eyes are seen to fix on the visual stimulus, the stimulus should be moved slowly first in one direction about 60 degrees, then in the opposite direction about the same distance. A normal infant will retain fixation on the visual stimulus by moving its head. The newborn's eyes do not have good movement control, and so the whole head is rotated in order to enable the eyes to follow the stimulus. If the newborn does not fix his or her gaze upon the visual stimulus and follow it as you move it, the possibility of blindness must be considered. Within a few weeks of delivery, a blind infant will usually develop what is called "wandering nystagmus." This is often called a "blindism." It means that the eyes keep moving rhythmically because the infant can't see and therefore the eyes do not "fix" on anything. This eyeball movement is also seen in adults who are blind. It makes most people rather uneasy to see it, but it only means that there is nothing to look at. It would seem that without something to look at our eyes keep wandering about.

The use of the ophthalmoscope to look into the newborn's eye is difficult, but sometimes it can be accomplished. There is an area in the retina called the optic disc. This is where the optic nerve enters the retina. This area should be gray or white. The rest of the retina should have a bright red coloration. When there appears to be an atrophy or shriveling-up of the optic nerve as it enters the eyeball, this suggests some type of serious problem inside the skull. Further investigation is mandatory. There are other signs within the eyeball that may suggest congenital infection of various types, or a maternal infection such as German measles during the pregnancy.

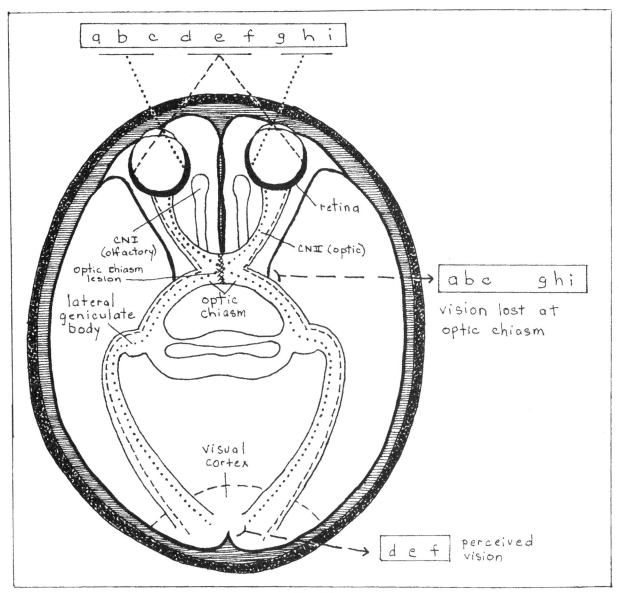

Fig. 6-3
The Visual Nerve Conduction System with Tunnel Vision:
The visual stimuli come into the retina and follow the optic nerve back to the optic chiasm where the stimuli from the nasal retinal fields cross over to the opposite side. Those stimuli from the temporal visual fields do not cross over. After passing through the optic chiasm, the nerve signals follow the optic tracts to the visual cortex. There is communication with the lateral geniculate bodies en route. An obstructive lesion in the optic chiasm as indicated in the drawing will result in "tunnel vision" because the stimuli from the nasal retina do not reach the visual cortex. Therefore, the areas labeled (a) (b) (c) and (g) (h) (i), whose images would stimulate these nasal retina, are not perceived. The external images cross over to the opposite side of the retina as they enter the eyeball.

EYE-MOVEMENT CONTROL

The movements of the eye are under the control of the oculomotor (III), the trochlear (IV), and the abducent (VI) cranial nerves. Although controlled eye movement does not usually occur in the newborn until about 10 days after delivery, it is somewhat inconsistent, so we will discuss the details of eye movement at this time.

OCULOMOTOR NERVE - CRANIAL NERVE III

The oculomotor nerve (III) supplies several muscles of the eyeballs. They are the superior rectus muscles, the inferior rectus muscles, the medial rectus muscles, the inferior oblique muscles and the levator palpebrae muscles. In addition to these muscles, the oculomotor nerves also control constriction of the pupils of the eyes through the circular muscles in the irises, and accommodation of the lenses. Accommodation has to do with the thickening and thinning of the lens so that focus can be made on objects near or far.

Paralysis of the oculomotor nerve results in an eyeball that can only move laterally (sideways) and down. The result is a divergent kind of strabismus. In addition, the eyelid may droop on the affected side, the pupil will not constrict on that side, and the lens will not accommodate to distance focus. A problem with the oculomotor nerve on one side will affect mostly the eye on the same side. However, if the problem is in the brain near the central connections of this nerve, it may affect both eyes to some extent, because a minority of fiber tracts within the brain do cross over to the oculomotor nerve on the opposite side. The most apparent clue that relates to oculomotor nerve problems for any reason is that the pupil of the eye, which is innervated by the affected nerve, will not constrict when you shine a bright light into it. The presence of the pupillary light reflex usually appears in the newborn infant before controlled eyeball movements are present.

TROCHLEAR NERVE - CRANIAL NERVE IV

The trochlear nerve (IV) only innervates one muscle of the eyeball. This is the superior oblique muscle. All of the fibers of the trochlear nerve cross to the opposite side, and so the situation is greatly simplified (**Fig. 6-4**). When the trochlear nerve on one side is not working correctly for any reason, the eyeball on the other side cannot look down and to the side (laterally). The affected eyeball may actually drift so that it is looking up and towards the center (medially).

THE ABDUCENT NERVE - CRANIAL NERVE VI

It is just as easy to evaluate the abducent nerve (VI) as the trochlear nerve. The abducent nerve does not cross to the opposite side at all, and it only innervates one muscle of the eyeball. This is the lateral rectus muscle (**Fig. 6-4**). When this muscle doesn't work right, the affected eyeball crosses. If both eyes are affected, we get a totally cross-eyed child. More commonly, only one abducent nerve is in difficulty, and therefore only one eye, the eye on the same side as the affected nerve, crosses abnormally.

EYE MOTOR CONTROL - "EN CONCERT"

The nuclei of all three nerves that control eyeball movement are very closely related in the brain tissue just in front of (anterior to) the aqueduct of Sylvius. As you may recall, this aqueduct connects the third and fourth ventricles of the brain, so that cerebrospinal fluid can flow out into the subarachnoid spaces and down the central canal of the spinal cord.

All three of the motor nerves to the eyeball exit the brain from the area of the diencephalon in

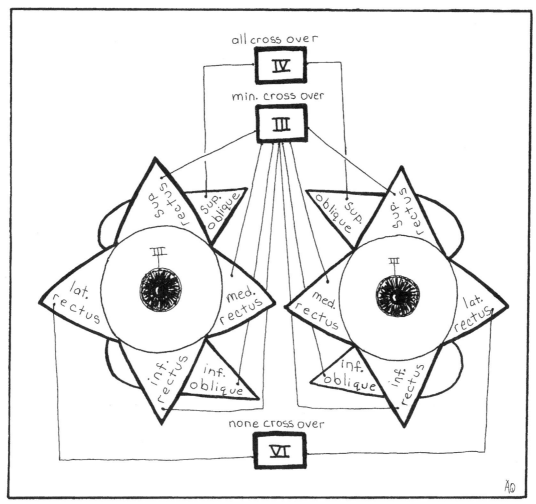

Fig. 6-4
Control of Eye Movement:
The drawing illustrates which cranial nerves control the eyes on the same sides and on opposite sides.
It also shows which eye muscles are controlled by which nerves. See text for further explanation.

the posterior cranial fossa. They then travel in close proximity to each other in the space between the arachnoid membrane and the pia mater (subarachnoid space) towards the orbits of the eyes. As they go forward they pass between two layers of the dura mater membrane that forms the horizontal support system for the cerebral hemispheres and separates these hemispheres from the cerebellum. This horizontal support system is called the tentorium cerebelli. There are several conditions that can make this tentorium cerebelli abnormally tight or tense. Among these causes of excess tentorium cerebelli tension are distortions in skull bone relations secondary to delivery trauma. These excessive tensions often cause abnormal pressure on one, two, or all of the three motor nerves to the eyeball. This pressure, in turn, may compromise nerve function and result in paralysis of the related eyeball muscles. The result may be lack of control of eyeball movements.

When this abnormal tension occurs, more often than not it can be corrected in one or two treatments by a skilled practitioner of CranioSacral Therapy. I strongly suggest that, before a surgical correction is considered for improper motor control of the eyeball, a conservative approach should be tried. That conservative approach is often quite successful when it is CranioSacral Therapy. If correction does not occur, there has been no risk involved. It won't take long to find out, because results are very quick in coming.

During the newborn evaluation, a dilated pupil on one side may be due to eyedrops which have been recently put in the infant's eyes. Or it may be due to trauma, seizure activity, excessive tension in the tentorium cerebelli, or even a blood aggregation (hematoma) in the tentorium cerebelli. Hematoma that involves both sides of the tentorium cerebelli may be due to hypoxia, infection, abnormal fluid retention (edema), and/or intracranial hemorrhage (bleeding inside the skull).

When the child cannot look upwards, it suggests the possibility of a problem in the upper brain stem. Problems in the cerebral cortex usually affect only the voluntary eye movements. In cerebral cortex problems, reflex eye movements may be left intact even though voluntary eye-movement control is impaired.

Nystagmus (a constant purposeless rhythmical eye movement) in the absence of blindness suggests the possibility of cerebellar or vestibular (equilibrium) problems. Absence of a "blink" reflex suggests blindness.

THE TRIGEMINAL NERVE - CRANIAL NERVE V

Now let's go back and look at the Vth cranial nerve, which is called the trigeminal. It is called trigeminal because it has three major branches. These three branches are the ophthalmic, the maxillary and the mandibular nerves (**Fig. 6-5**). The trigeminal nerve, before it divides, has the largest trunk diameter of any of the cranial nerves. It is responsible for sensation from the eye, for sensation from the teeth and gums (yes, it's the one that lets you know you have a toothache), and it is the one that gives you the ability to bite and chew, as it has motor control over the

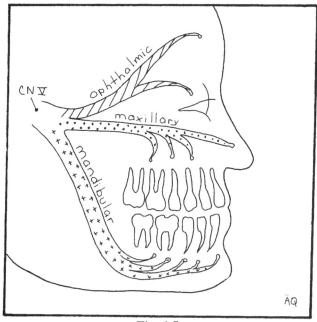

Fig. 6-5
The Trigeminal Nerve Divisions:
After passing through its ganglion, which is located on the temporal bone's contribution to the floor of the skull cavity, the Vth cranial nerve (trigeminal) gives off three major divisions: (1) the ophthalmic nerve, (2) the maxillary nerve and (3) the mandibular nerve. See text.

muscles related to the jaws.

Testing the function of the trigeminal nerve in the newborn is done simply by judging the strength of mouth closure during sucking and or (toothless) biting on your finger. Also, you should observe whether or not the infant's mouth opens symmetrically, or whether the lower jaw deviates to one side when it opens.

Problems with trigeminal nerve function in the newborn can be due to abnormal tensions in the dura mater membrane of the meninges. These abnormal tension patterns in the membrane are usually corrected with relative ease by the use of CranioSacral Therapy. The earlier the correction is attempted, the easier it is to do, and it is "the sooner the better" for the newborn. That newborn has enough to cope with as its adaptation to the outside world is carried out. Working against excessive intracranial membrane tensions is a needless expenditure of adaptive energy, because these problems are most often easily correctable early on, even in the delivery room.

THE FACIAL NERVE - CRANIAL NERVE VII

The facial nerve is the VIIth cranial nerve (**Fig. 6-6**). A quick evaluation of facial nerve function can be done by simply observing the newborn's facial symmetry or lack thereof. This observation should be done both when the infant is at rest and when he or she is moving.

When the whole nerve or its nucleus is dysfunctional, the forehead doesn't wrinkle and the eye will not close effectively on the involved side. The mouth will be drawn over towards the side that has normal facial nerve function. Excessive drooling can also be a sign of facial nerve problems, because the mouth cannot close effectively and the salivary glands are controlled by the facial nerve. So too much saliva may be produced, and the child does not have the ability to close its mouth and swallow the saliva rather than drool.

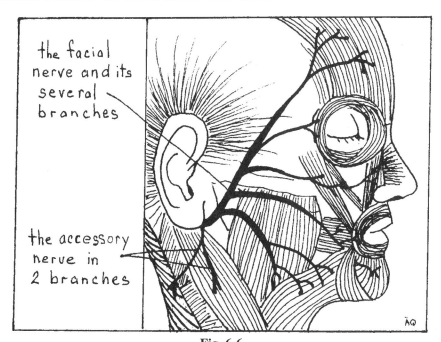

Fig. 6-6
The Facial Nerve (VII) and the Accessory Nerve (XI):
Because of their anatomical proximity, the facial and the accessory nerves
are both shown in this drawing. See text for details.

The facial nerve is rather vulnerable during obstetrical delivery, because it passes out of the skull through the stylomastoid foramen, a little canal that is located below and behind the ear. As the infant ages, this nerve is protected by the mastoid process of the temporal bone of the skull. The mastoid process has not yet formed by the time of delivery, and so the facial nerve sits out there exposed and unprotected from various external forces and pressures. It can receive injury in the birth canal as the newborn head passes over some bony prominences projecting from the mother's sacrum or the pelvic bones. It is also subject to injury by the blade of a forceps during a forceps-assisted delivery.

THE AUDITORY/VESTIBULAR NERVE - CRANIAL NERVE VIII

The VIIIth cranial nerve has a name that has been in transition. It used to be called the auditory nerve; some folks call it the acoustic nerve, and others call it the vestibular nerve. Quite often, it is also called the vestibulocochlear, or the auditory vestibular nerve (**Fig. 6-7**). In order to avoid confusion, I'll just call it the VIIIth nerve.

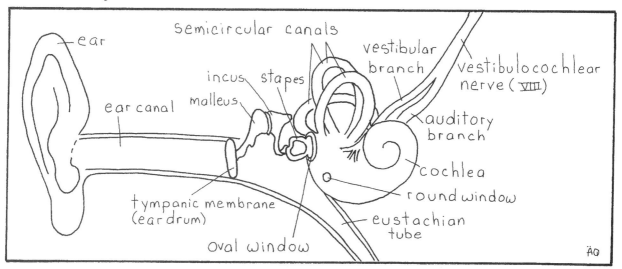

Fig. 6-7
The VIIIth Cranial Nerve:
The VIIIth cranial nerve has several names. (See text.) It services the senses of hearing and equilibrium. Thus, it has two major branches. The drawing gives a general idea of the structures of the hearing/auditory system, which are all those shown except the semi-circular canals, which relate to equilibrium and balance.

In order to test this VIIIth nerve, we have two major components to consider. From the mixed nomenclature, you can probably guess that cranial nerve VIII has to do with both hearing and equilibrium. In order to test hearing, you need only clap your hands sharply near the newborn's ear. The sharp noise should produce an eye blink and a startle reflex. This clapping should be done on both sides. If you don't get a blink or a startle response, you must suspect deafness. When you look in the ears with the otoscope (the hand-held instrument with the light and the funnel-like attachment), you can only tell if the ear canal is open and reasonably properly formed. You cannot see the ear drum (tympanum) because it is covered with vernix caseosa (the substance we described earlier that covers the newborn at the time of delivery).

In order to test the newborn's equilibrium, you need simply hold the infant out at arm's length facing you. Then spin around three or four times while holding the infant. When you stop spinning, the infant's eyes should deviate in a direction opposite to your spin. This spinning, or rotation test, is also a good way to elicit nystagmus if that problem is present.

THE GLOSSOPHARYNGEAL NERVE - CRANIAL NERVE IX
THE VAGUS NERVE - CRANIAL NERVE X

The IXth (glossopharyngeal) and Xth (vagus) cranial nerves can be evaluated at the same time in the newborn by testing the gag reflex. This is done by touching the back part of the mouth/tongue with your finger or a tongue blade. Normally the infant will gag rather easily. You should also look inside the mouth to see if the uvula is hanging in the midline. If there is deviation of the uvula from the midline, it will deviate towards the side of the normal innervation. The strength of the muscles of the soft palate also give information as to the function of the IXth and Xth cranial nerves. You can feel if these muscles are soft and flaccid on one side as compared to the opposite side with your fingertip. If so, there may be a problem with one or the other of these two cranial nerves.

The glossopharyngeal nerve does most of its work in the mouth and throat. The vagus also works in the mouth and throat, but it extends farther down. In fact, it is one of the longest nerves in the body. It offers nerve supply to the esophagus, trachea and bronchi, and to the sinus node of the heart, which has great influence over the heart rate and rhythmicity. The vagus nerves then continue down through the chest and offer innervation to the stomach and the large bowel (**Fig. 6-8**). We find that colicky and constipated babies often have irritation or pressure on the vagus nerve.

Before we discuss these nerves in detail, let's look at cranial nerve XI, the accessory nerve. We sometimes think of the glossopharyngeal nerve as a branch of the vagus nerve because they are so closely interrelated, both anatomically and functionally.

THE ACCESSORY NERVE - CRANIAL NERVE XI

The accessory cranial nerves give motor supply to the sternocleidomastoideus muscles of the neck (**Fig. 6-6**). These are rather large muscles that run from the skull behind the ear diagonally downward, and attach to the top of your breast bone (sternum) and the middle part of your collar bone (clavicle). The tone and/or strength of the sternocleidomastoideus muscles can be judged by feeling their firmness or flaccidity with your fingers, and by getting the newborn to rotate his or her head one way and then the other. The action of the muscles is to tighten on the side opposite to the direction of rotation.

The accessory nerve also offers innervation to the upper part of the trapezius muscle, which is found in the back of the neck on both sides. The trapezius muscle, when it contracts, causes the head to bend backwards. If the head is fixed in one position it causes the shoulder to go up towards the head. The back bending of the head is not a good test because other muscles besides the trapezius can also produce this motion. Testing this muscle singularly in the newborn is not easy, because you have to get the infant to raise (shrug) his or her shoulders against your resistance. The trapezius also receives innervation from some of the cervical nerves, as well as from the accessory cranial nerves, so it is difficult to draw conclusions from the action of the trapezius muscles.

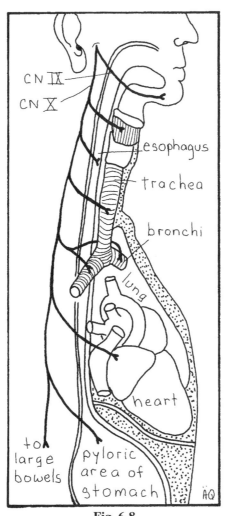

Fig. 6-8
The Glossopharyngeal Nerve (IX) and
The Vagus Nerve (X):
The IXth and Xth cranial nerves are
very closely interrelated, both
anatomically and functionally. This
drawing shows diagrammatically the
major innervations of these two nerves.

CRANIAL NERVES IX, X AND XI - "EN CONCERT"

When there is a problem with the IXth, Xth and/or XIth cranial nerves, it is often easily corrected by the use of CranioSacral Therapy techniques to release the head at the base of the skull (occipital base) from the top of the neck (atlas bone). This treatment technique has been described previously in detail in Topic 34 on craniosacral evaluation and treatment. All three of these paired nerves pass through an opening on each side of the base of the skull called the jugular foramen. When the skull is jammed forward excessively onto the neck of the newborn (most often during the delivery), the soft tissues (muscles, etc.) become contracted in order to prevent further injury. Due to proximity of the jugular foramina to the skull/neck joints, the contraction of these muscles and other connective tissues often exerts undue pressure upon the IXth, Xth and XIth cranial nerves as they exit the skull through these jugular foramina **(Fig. 6-9)**. This pressure

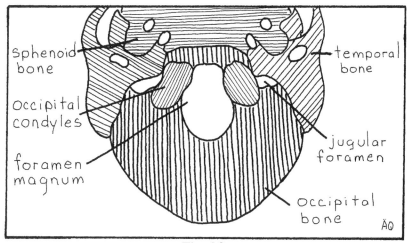

Fig. 6-9
The Jugular Foramina:
This is a view of the underside of the base of the back part of the skull.
The IXth, Xth and XIth cranial nerves exit through the jugular foramina.
Problems with the occipital condyles can cause soft tissue tension, which
may compress these nerves at their exit points from the skull.
The clinical effects are discussed in the text. This excessive tension of
the soft tissues may also partially compress the jugular veins which
carry blood out of the skull. This partial compression may cause an
excess of fluid accumulation in the skull vault with secondary headaches,
poor concentration/mentation and, in children, it may contribute to
attention deficit disorder.

can then interfere with nerve conduction/function. The results may include difficulty in swallowing, bronchial congestion, heart rhythm problems, colic, pyloric spasm of the stomach and/or poor bowel function. A myriad of colicky babies have been helped by craniosacral release of the base of the skull from the neck.

Another problem that can have the same cause is torticollis, because the accessory nerve may be pinched at the jugular foramen. Once again, CranioSacral Therapy may correct the torticollis problem quickly and easily.

THE HYPOGLOSSAL NERVE - CRANIAL NERVE XII

The XIIth cranial nerve is the hypoglossal nerve **(Fig. 6-10)**. This is the nerve that controls the muscles of the tongue. The tongue should be observed for narrowness and furrows. If you gently pinch the nose so that the newborn cannot breathe through its nose properly, the mouth will open and the tongue will go to the roof of the mouth. If the tip of the tongue does not remain on the midline, the side to which it deviates will be the side that has a dysfunction of the hypoglossal nerve.

Before we decide that this is a congenital or hereditary neurological disease, we should once again release the base of the skull from the neck by the use of CranioSacral Therapy. The XIIth cranial nerves pass right through the occipital condyles to the skull/neck joints on both sides. Jamming of these joints can interfere with hypoglossal nerve function, which presents itself as lack of control of the muscles of the tongue on one side or the other.

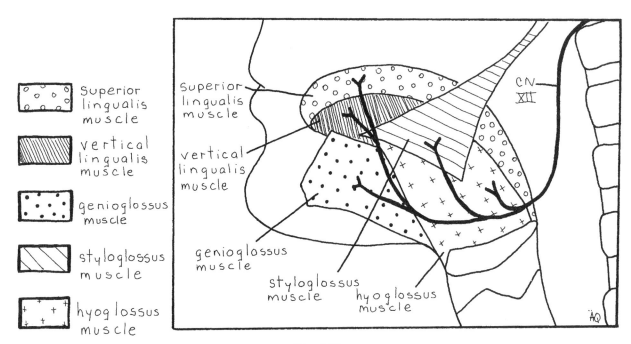

Superior
lingualis
muscle

vertical
lingualis
muscle

genioglossus
muscle

styloglossus
muscle

hyoglossus
muscle

Fig. 6-10
The Hypoglossal Nerve (XII):
The hypoglossal nerve services the muscles of the tongue as indicated in the drawing.
It controls all of the gross and subtle movements of the tongue.

Topic 37

Evaluation of the Vertebral/Spinal Column and the Spinal Cord

THE EVALUATION OF THE VERTEBRAL COLUMN FOR MOTION

A general evaluation of the vertebral column and the spinal cord can be done quite easily at the time of this initial evaluation. Personally, I like to do this examination at the same time that I do the craniosacral system evaluation. In my evaluation of the bony vertebral column, I rely largely upon my sense of touch and my palpatory skills. You can begin at either the head end or the tail end of the vertebral column, as long as you feel and move each vertebra in the column. The soft tissues that relate to the vertebrae must also be evaluated for tightness (tonus), tenderness to the touch, increased warmth or coolness as compared to surrounding areas, and skin texture. Watch the infant's reaction to your touch in one place as compared to another. A grimace, a cry, a pulling away and so on can be interpreted as signs of increased tenderness.

When I speak of feeling and moving each vertebra in the whole column, I mean that you should be able to identify with your fingers the spine (spinous process) of each vertebra as it protrudes slightly backwards from the vertebral column. This palpation of spinous processes is quite difficult at the base of the skull because spinous processes of the first cervical vertebra (atlas) and the second cervical vertebra (axis) are both very tiny. They are very hard to find if you are not experienced. The rest of the spinous processes (the third through the seventh cervical vertebrae, the 12 thoracic vertebrae and the five lumbar vertebrae) are much more readily accessible and prominent to the searching finger.

As each vertebra is located, it should be gently moved side to side and up and down in relation to the adjacent vertebra above and below it. If there is an increased resistance to these movements, which you are gently inducing with your fingers, it indicates that something about that immobile vertebra is not working right. Stabilize the vertically adjacent vertebra with your other fingers; retest. The resistance to motion may be caused by muscle contraction in that area of the spine. This muscle contraction will be signaled by the increased tissue tonus, increased tenderness, temperature changes and skin texture differences which I mentioned above. The skin surface will usually be drier and rougher over the area of the immobile vertebra. Keep in mind that the part of the vertebra that you feel is just a small percentage of the total bone of that vertebra. It spreads out sideways so that the vertebra's transverse processes extend perhaps an inch laterally from the midline in both directions.

The vertebral movement of which I speak is very small and subtle. Use a gentle pressure in the direction that you are testing. Continue your gentle pressure until you get a response in the form of a "floating" type movement in that direction. The "prolonged push" is often enough to correct non-serious vertebral immobility. The longer it takes the vertebra to respond, the greater is the resistance. If the soft tissue changes remain present after the vertebra in question moves, gently touching the involved area for a few minutes may be enough to normalize the soft tissue tightness. This work, in conjunction with craniosacral treatment of the dural tube (dura mater layer of the meninges within the spinal canal), is usually enough to correct any problem that does not have basis in structural deformity of the vertebrae.

The type of problem we have just discussed is usually resultant to undue strain and/or trauma during the delivery process, or perhaps a difficult position into which the fetus was locked and maintained during the later part of the pregnancy. The maintenance of the problem after delivery is usually due to intervertebral joints originally jammed together, then sticking together one joint surface to another, or being held by abnormal adjacent soft tissue contraction. This abnormal contraction can be maintained for a long time by the nervous system. It may actually result in vertebral bone deformity as the bone tries to grow against increased resistance. It is much better to deal with this type of problem in the beginning and perhaps avert a spinal curvature or dysfunction later.

SPINA BIFIDA

Spina bifida is a congenital deformity in which the back (posterior) parts of the vertebrae do not fuse together at the proper time during the pregnancy. This leaves a bony defect in the posterior part of the spinal canal which may offer opportunity for the protrusion of meningeal membrane, cerebrospinal fluid and, in extreme cases, even the spinal cord out of the spinal canal (**Fig. 6-11**). The results of this defect in the spinal canal can range from minimal to very severe. When the spinous processes of the vertebrae are evaluated one by one manually for both presence and movement, such a deficit can usually be discovered. Other signs of spina bifida may present as a tuft of hair growing from the skin in the area of the defect. Also, you may see a red discoloration (flame nevus) over the area.

PILONIDAL CYST

One of the more common defects is located in the lower spinal (sacral) region, and often presents as a "dimple." This may be the clue that a pilonidal cyst is present. It may travel under the skin and open through at the lower end of the tailbone (coccyx). The pilonidal cyst may contain hair. It is simply a question of some cells not doing what they are supposed to. Perhaps they got the wrong orders from genes, or they interpreted these orders incorrectly.

ERB'S AND KLUMPKE'S PALSIES

Paralysis of the arm of the newborn may result from problems with: (1) the vertebral column, (2) the spinal cord and/or its nerve roots, (3) the nerve (brachial) plexus that goes to the arm,

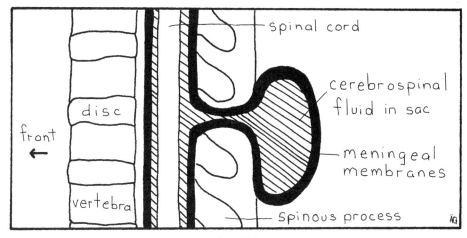

Fig. 6-11
Spina Bifida:
In this drawing the meningeal membranes protrude abnormally to form the sac which is filled with cerebrospinal fluid. This deficit may be corrected successfully by surgery.

(4) the soft tissues through which these nerves pass, and (5) the dural tube and/or the fascias (connective tissues) that relate to the arm and shoulder. This paralysis may be called Erb's Palsy if it involves the nerves from the neck (cervical) region of the spinal cord exclusively. If it involves the lower cervical and upper thoracic nerves to the arm, it is called Klumpke's Palsy. If it involves both areas from mid-cervical to upper-thoracic region, it is called a "mixed" palsy. What this looks like is the newborn's arm pulled in towards the body and rotated inwardly. The child can't use the arm.

In Erb's Palsy, the child may be able to use the fingers but not the arm. In Klumpke's Palsy, the child cannot grasp with the fingers. A fractured clavicle may mimic any of the above palsies. When the problem involves both arms and/or hands, the spinal cord may have been injured during the delivery.

SPINAL CORD INJURIES

Spinal cord injuries may occur during breech delivery. This is because the smaller pelvis is pulled out of the birth canal first, and the larger head follows. Therefore, the birth canal is not ready for the delivery of the largest part. The traction on the pelvis necessary to pull the trailing head through the unprepared birth canal is sometimes enough to injure or even tear the spinal cord near the area of the juncture between the lower neck and the thorax.

It is not always easy to differentiate spinal cord problems from less serious problems involving bony vertebrae, nerve roots, nerve trunks, dura mater and/or other soft tissues. Two reasonably reliable and quick methods involve bladder function and anal reflexes. Normal bladder function is signified by a healthy stream of urine being produced with some force behind it. This tells you that the spinal cord is intact because it is getting the nerve impulses to the bladder. The anal reflex is elicited by scratching the area around the anus *lightly* with a pin or other sharp object. The normal response is a tightening of the anal sphincter. This tightening reflex is visible to the naked eye. If this reflex is absent it suggests the possibility of spinal cord dysfunction.

It is important to observe bladder and anus function, because problems involving the lumbosacral plexus in a way similar to those described above for Erb's and Klumpke's Palsy can cause pelvic and lower-extremity dysfunction. It can look like spinal cord injury. But when bladder function and anal reflexes are intact, the spinal cord is okay.

As a point of interest, at birth the spinal cord extends down to the level of the fifth lumbar vertebrae within the spinal canal. Since the vertebral column grows more than the spinal cord, the cord only reaches the first or second lumbar vertebrae in the adult **(Fig. 3-18)**. Also, it is of interest to note that complete myelination of the spinal cord does not occur until one or two years of age. The last tracts within the spinal cord to myelinate are those originating in the brain and serving as motor tracts to the body. They are called the corticospinal and the tectospinal tracts. In the brain, myelination is carried out by specialized cells called oligodendroglia. In the body, the Schwann cells do the myelination of the peripheral nerves.

Miscellaneous Extras

THE AUTONOMIC NERVOUS SYSTEM

Evaluation of the autonomic nervous system of the newborn must rely on observation of function. The autonomic nervous system regulates bodily functions which are not ordinarily under voluntary/conscious control. Therefore, the newborn autonomic function is estimated based on blood pressure, temperature control, perspiration, bladder and bowel function, and eye-pupil responses to light.

THE NEWBORN SENSORY SYSTEM

The evaluation of the sensory system is indirect, because it must rely upon observed responses to stimuli. In the newborn these responses to touch, temperature and pain are slow and rather insensitive. Therefore, the stimulus must be applied for several seconds in order to elicit a response. Those responses upon which we rely to indicate that the newborn has received the stimulus are changes in heart rate, breathing rate, skin color, alertness, withdrawal from the stimulus and the like. These are all indirect responses which we suppose indicate that the infant felt the touch, the heat/cold or the pain. Infants do not complain of sensory deficits. You must find them.

Topic 39

Screening Tests

GENERAL CONSIDERATIONS

Reflexes

In general, the evaluation of the newborn's reflexes is fairly reliable if these reflexes are mediated by the spinal cord and the brain stem, because these structures are fairly well-developed at birth. Since the higher brain regions develop subsequent to birth, many of the birth reflexes disappear because the cerebral cortex begins to exercise control over the lower regions of the central nervous system, namely the brain stem and the spinal cord. Therefore, it is normal for the Moro (startle) reflex, the rooting-response reflex, the sucking reflex, the palmar grasp reflex, the Babinski reflex and others to disappear as the cerebral cortex develops during the first year or two of postpartum life. On the other hand, absence of these reflexes at birth strongly suggests problems with the central nervous system beneath the cortical level.

Deep tendon reflexes are not very reliable indicators of the condition of the newborn's nervous system. These deep tendon reflexes are only valuable when the same reflex is present on one side of the body and entirely absent, or responds differently, on the other side. These are the reflexes that you see elicited by the famous "rubber hammer" which is used to tap various points on the body. Incidentally, any observed reflex may be considered as the summation of automatic body responses to a stimulus. Those responses are mediated only by the nervous system. The deep tendon reflexes are a special category of reflexes that are elicited by hitting tendons with the rubber hammers and watching the related muscles jump (contract).

Posture

The first screening test of the nervous system that is carried out is usually a simple observation of the newborn's resting posture, and the quality and symmetry of the voluntary motions. The normal newborn resting posture is called flexion posture. The presence of this posture persists in a full-term infant for about the first two or three weeks of post-partum life. It persists even while the infant is sleeping.

In the flexion posture, the newborn's arms and legs will be slightly flexed at the elbows and the knees. The upper arms and legs will be aimed away from the body's vertical midline at the shoulder and hip joints, respectively. There will also be some periodic rhythmical movement of the arms and legs wherein the elbows and knees will straighten for short periods of time. These movements should be symmetrical, but they will alternate chronologically between the arms and the legs. That is, when the arms straighten at the elbows, the legs will remain flexed, and vice versa. This spontaneous motor activity is normal. If it is not present, you must be suspicious of nervous system problems. Also, the fingers will usually be flexed into tight fists, often with the thumbs inside against the palms. Periodically, the fists will relax and the fingers will straighten. The newborn infant may put his/her hands up to the face periodically. All of these movements should be relatively smooth and well-coordinated. If the movements are jerky, there may be a central nervous system problem.

The flexion posture is symmetrical except for the head-neck complex, which may be turned slightly to one side or perhaps flexed forward on the midline. In the latter case, the posture will be totally symmetrical if all is well. When there is persistent asymmetry of posture, predominant extension of the arms and/or the legs, and/or constant turning of the head from one side to the other, it suggests a problem inside of the cranium. If that problem involves an active infection, a hemorrhage of the brain stem or an irritation of the meninges, the neck will be stiff and hyperextended, in addition to the aforementioned signs.

Crying and Sucking

In addition to the observation of the newborn's resting posture and voluntary movements, we gain a great deal of information from the strength of the cry and the strength of the sucking response. Weakness of cry and/or sucking is strongly suggestive of a significant problem in the central nervous system, and demands further investigation. The range of problems that manifest as weakness of cry and sucking can be metabolic or biochemical, as well as a primary nervous system dysfunction.

Motor Control and Strength

At the same time that we are observing posture, we can observe the ability of the newborn to work against gravity. Poor muscle strength, as demonstrated by the infant's inability to hold body parts like the arms, legs and head up from the bed, indicates a dysfunction of some part of the motor system. That is, it could be upper motor neuron, anterior horn cell, lower motor neuron (peripheral nerve) or effector (muscle). It could also be that there is damage to soft tissue or bone as a result of delivery.

Voluntary movements by the newborn rely upon the intactness of function of the whole motor system. A voluntary movement, such as putting the hand to the face, originates in one side of the motor cortex of the brain. This cortex, as we said previously, is not fully developed at the time of delivery, but there is enough of it present to initiate the movement of the hand to the face. From the motor cortex the signal must go through the internal capsule, then into the brain stem where, in the medulla oblongata, the impulses cross over to the other side of the body. The medulla oblongata is the lowest part of the brain that connects with the spinal cord. From the crossover in the medulla oblongata, the impulses go into the spinal cord. It is lower in the spinal cord where the upper motor neuron ends by synapsing with the anterior horn cell. The anterior horn cell that receives the nerve impulse is usually at that level of the spinal cord where its nerve fiber exits the spinal cord and goes out into the periphery of the body to one of the muscles that enable the hand to move to the face. The nerve fiber from the anterior horn cell (including its cell body) is spoken of as the lower motor neuron. At the muscle, the lower motor neuron forms a myoneural junction, which is the synapse between the nerve and the muscle. Once the nerve impulse crosses the myoneural junction, the muscle is ordered to contract **(Fig. 6-12)**.

There are a few complicating factors in the motor nerve unit. Its function is also influenced by the extrapyramidal system, which does not cross over in the medulla oblongata, and includes the basal ganglia of Parkinson's-disease fame. The extrapyramidal system, in concert with the cerebellum, serves to coordinate and smooth out the voluntary and involuntary movements. Together, they offer some control over repetitive movements. So, keep in mind that the jerkiness of movements that you may see in newborn movement relates to lack of mature and coordinated influence by the extrapyramidal tracts and the cerebellum. The development of these brain parts may not be complete at birth, but excessive jerkiness suggests less than normal development.

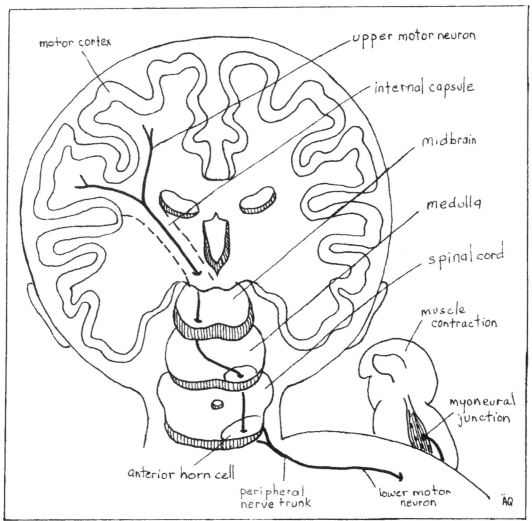

Fig. 6-12
Voluntary Movement Pathway:
The cerebral cortex of the motor area orders a movement. The order, in the form of electrical impulses, is sent via the upper motor neuron through the internal capsule and the midbrain, then it crosses over in the medulla oblongata and descends in the spinal cord to the level of the anterior horn cell. It synapses with this cell, which is the lower motor neuron. The impulse then goes out the axon of the lower motor neuron via the peripheral nerves to the significant muscle which it will cause to respond.

In summary, when there is an upper motor neuron problem in the brain or spinal cord above the synapses with the anterior horn cell, there is a lack of voluntary movement, but spinal cord reflexes remain intact. These spinal cord reflexes are the involuntary movements. When there is a problem with the anterior horn cells in the spinal cord, fasciculations occur. Fasciculations are small, localized, involuntary muscle contractions that occur spontaneously and rhythmically under the skin. These contractions are the muscle's response to the spontaneous discharges of nerve fibers related to single myoneural junction units. When the lower motor neuron is dysfunctional, there is a loss of both voluntary and involuntary muscle activities. The muscle is essentially cut off from its nerve supply. It therefore begins to autonomously fibrillate. Ultimately, the denervated muscle will atrophy or shrink up and, for all practical purposes, become irreversibly nonfunctional, or so they say. There are also occasional exceptions to this rule.

Remember, the voluntary movement control on one side of the body comes from the brain's motor cortex on the opposite side.

Specific Reflexes

THE MORO REFLEX/RESPONSE

Moro response is also called the startle response and/or the Moro, or startle reflex. It is a very frequently (almost universally) used test. In order to perform the test, the infant is placed lying on his/her back. The examiner places his/her hands under the thorax and shoulders. The upper torso, head and neck are then lifted about 30 degrees from the horizontal plane. The infant is then suddenly dropped onto the crib mattress. Alternatively, the infant can be held up in the supine position and then suddenly lowered about two feet. Either of these techniques will elicit the Moro, or startle response. The desired (hoped for) response is a straightening of the elbows and fingers, and an initial pulling away from the body's vertical midline of the arms so that arms are pointing outward. Then, rather quickly, the arms are pulled inward towards the midline of the body, the elbows bend, and the fingers flex into fists. There is also a response in the legs. The knees bend and the thighs flex onto the body at the hips. The infant will also usually cry.

Under normal circumstances, the Moro response is gone within the first four months of postpartum life. If it persists beyond four months, it is suggestive of a neurological problem. If it persists after six months, there is a definite neurological problem.

If the Moro response is not present in a newborn and the Perez reflex, which I will describe next, is also absent, there is definitely a severe problem either in the cerebrum, the spinal cord in the upper neck area, or a severe generalized myopathy (muscle disease). An asymmetric response in the extremities suggests the possibility of brain injury on one side. This is called hemiparesis. An absence of response in both legs, called a paraparesis, suggests a low spinal cord problem or a congenital hip dislocation. If one arm fails to respond, it could be due to a fractured clavicle or humerus, or an injury to the brachial nerve plexus, which supplies innervation to the arm. A problem with the craniosacral system at the lower neck or upper thoracic level will also cause asymmetry of arm response.

THE PEREZ REFLEX

The Perez reflex, if absent in conjunction with absence of the Moro response, suggests serious problems. It is evaluated as follows. The newborn child is held suspended face down (prone) over the examiner's hand and arm. Beginning at the sacrum, the examiner's other thumb is moved up the spine, exerting a firm pressure on each spinous process as it moves. A positive response is considered to be a backward bending of the head and the spine, a flexion of the knees towards the chest, a cry, and an emptying of the bladder.

Both the Perez and the Moro reflexes are summation responses that show normal development and control by subcortical brain. The cortex, as it develops, will normally obliterate these reflexes within three or four months. If the reflexes persist after four months, something is probably wrong with cortex development. If these reflexes persist after six months, this probability is very high.

THE ROOTING REFLEX

Another very popular reflex is the rooting reflex. To elicit this reflex, you simply touch the newborn infant's cheek with your finger. The normal infant response is to turn the head towards the side of the touch and open the mouth as though to capture the touching finger in the mouth. Absence of this reflex suggests a decreased level of awareness. This condition of decreased awareness often occurs in serious generalized problems of the central nervous system, or in more localized problems involving the medulla oblongata. Medullary (medulla oblongata) problems are often referred to as "bulbar disease," because the medulla oblongata is often spoken or thought of as a bulb. On occasion, the rooting reflex will be suppressed by sedation given to the mother during the delivery. It may also be suppressed by a recent feeding, which causes an increased blood flow to the digestive organs and a proportional reduction of blood flow to the brain.

Variations or extensions of the rooting reflex may include a touch on the upper lip which causes a backward flexion of the head, and/or a touch on the lower lip which causes a dropping of the lower jaw. The rooting reflex and its variations are gone at about three to four months when the higher brain centers are more fully developed.

TETANY

While looking at the face it is well to test for Chvostek's sign. This is done by simply tapping the infant's face just above the cheek bone (zygomatic arch) about a half to a full inch in front of the ear. Normally, the facial muscles give one or two short contractions in response. A prolonged contraction is suggestive of calcium deficiency or tetany due to other causes, such as vitamin D deficiency, acid-base imbalance and/or parathyroid deficiency.

HAND REFLEXES

The hand can also give reliable information about the normalcy of nervous system development. Assuming that there is no Erb's, Klumpke's or mixed palsy as previously described, the palmar grasp and digital response reflexes will tell you about the intactness of the central nervous system.

THE PALMAR GRASP REFLEX

The palmar grasp reflex is elicited by simply pressing your finger against the palm of the newborn's hand. The newborn's fingers should flex in order to try to grasp the object that is pressing on the palm. In this case, that object is your finger. Compare both sides for symmetry and strength of response. A weakness of bilateral response suggests central nervous system dysfunction. Response strength can usually be increased by getting the infant to suck. Asymmetry of response or strength can be due to the same more-localized causes as Erb's, Klumpke's and mixed palsies. Persistence of the palmar grasp reflex after four months of age suggests cerebral dysfunction.

THE DIGITAL RESPONSE REFLEX

The digital response reflex is elicited by doing a light stroking of the ulnar side of the hand and the little finger. The response that is considered normal is an extension, or spreading out of the thumb and other fingers. Absence or asymmetry of response have similar implications as do abnormal responses to the palmar grasp reflex.

FOOT REFLEXES

Similar reflex tests are also done on the infant's feet. The plantar grasp reflex is elicited by pressing on the ball of the foot. A normal response is seen as the toes attempt to flex around the pressure stimulus.

Pressure on the heel of the infant's foot should produce a plantar flexion of the big toe. An extension of the big toe usually relates to a spinal cord problem.

Exaggeration of all of the palmar and plantar reflex responses in the newborn child usually means that there is some dysfunction involving the central nervous system. A common cause of central nervous system dysfunction is hypoxia at birth. Hypoxia, which refers to an inadequate supply of oxygen to the newborn brain and/or spinal cord, when prolonged, may cause "permanent" damage to the central nervous system. Sometimes "permanent" damage is reversible. You never know unless you try. Acceptance of a level of disability more or less cements that level of disability into place.

THE PLACING RESPONSE

Another good general screening test for function and normalcy of the central nervous system is the "placing response." This test may not be totally reliable until about three to four days after delivery, but it is certainly worth doing and re-doing a few days later if there are confirming results that make you suspicious of problems. The placing response is elicited by holding the newborn infant in an upright position and then allowing the upper surface (dorsum) of one foot to touch an object, such as the under surface of the examining tabletop. The infant should flex the hip and the knee in response to the touch, and place the stimulated foot on top of the table. A normal response signifies good function of the peripheral nerves to the leg and foot, as well as intact function of the spinal cord and lower brain centers. Absence of response means that you have to start looking for a problem.

THE SPINAL CORD REFLEXES

Now let's look at some tests that are more specifically aimed at giving information about spinal cord function.

First, please recall that intactness of urinary bladder function and the anal reflex are good indicators that the spinal cord is in reasonably good working order. Urinary bladder function is indicated by the force of the stream of urine which flows. Poor bladder function produces a dribble. The anal reflex is a tightening of the anal sphincter when a light scratching is done with a pin point next to the anus.

When the infant is held upright with your hands as support under the armpits (axillae), the head should be maintained on the midline and the legs should be flexed at the hips and the knees. When this is not the case, the spinal cord needs further investigation. A spastic paraplegia is indicated by a scissoring of the legs when held in this position.

GALANT'S REFLEX

Galant's reflex is a reasonably good indicator of spinal cord function. In this reflex test the infant is held horizontally in the prone (face down) position. The examiner uses the thumb or a finger to press on one side in the midback (thoracolumbar) region about one half an inch lateral to the vertical midline of the infant's back as signified by the palpable spines. The shoulders and pelvis should flex towards the side of the pressure making a "C-curve" of the torso. Repeat with the pressure on the opposite side of the spine, and the shoulders and pelvis should move towards the side of the pressure. The examiner may get a similar response by simply running a finger in the paravertebral region from the infant's buttock up to the base of the neck to stimulate the paravertebral muscles on one side and then the other. If there is no response to the pressure or touch stimulation, there may be a complete transverse lesion of the spinal cord. If the response is not symmetrical, the search is on for a possible sensory or motor deficit involving the spinal cord. Cranial nerve functions are not affected by spinal cord injury.

Topic 41

Muscle Tone and Motor Function

Muscle tonus can be normal, hypotonic or hypertonic. This sounds easy, but because the nervous system is so complex, we often get contradictory results when looking for tests that should confirm each other.

Initially, it is well to test for motor function by putting each joint through its range of motion and evaluating the muscle tone for excessive spasticity or flaccidity. It is difficult to perform this range-of-motion testing on the individual joints of the vertebral column. But the spine's range of motion can be tested more generally by simply bending and rotating to test for symmetry of compliance and/or resistance to your testing movements. Asymmetry implies a hypertonic condition (tightness) of the muscles on the opposite side of the direction into which the motion is restricted.

It is much easier to test the joints of the extremities and simply feel the muscles related to these joints for excessive tightness or flaccidity.

THE HYPOTONIC NEWBORN

When motor function is subnormal, the infant is spoken of as hypotonic. The hypotonic newborn shows a different resting posture, which is often referred to as "frog-leg posture." The upper arms and the thighs are markedly abducted from the torso. They often approximate a 90-degree angle (right angle) from the vertical midline of the body. This abduction is much greater than the normal resting postural position, which is usually not more than 45 degrees from the vertical body midline. The hypotonic child will also show a marked exaggeration of flexion of the elbows and knees. The angles at these joints may be 90 degrees or less. The hands will be open and the palms will be up as compared to the finger-flexed fists that are present in the normal resting posture. The hypotonic infant's feet will be flopping downward at the ankles. The proper term for this is "plantar flexed." The hypotonic infant's chest diameter is reduced in the forward/backward (anterior/posterior) dimension. This gives the child a flat-chested look. I'm referring to the appearance of the thoracic cage as a whole. It looks as though it has been pressed with an iron. The respiratory movement is largely from the diaphragm. That means that you see the child breathing from its belly and very little from his/her chest. There is very little rib cage motion.

If the cause of the hypotonia involves a generalized metabolic or brain problem, the face muscles will also be lax. If the problem involves only the spinal cord, facial expression and mouth movement will be intact.

Generalized problems that cause hypotonia include hypoxia (not enough oxygen), hypoglycemia (low blood sugar), hypothyroidism (low thyroid function), elevated blood magnesium levels, Down's syndrome, and other congenital diseases such as neonatal myasthenia gravis, myotonic dystrophy, cerebrohepatorenal syndrome, Werdnig-Hoffman syndrome, and a variety of congenital brain anomalies.

Causes of hypotonia can be localized to some extent by certain characteristics. When the problem lies in the anterior horn cells (you may recall that these are the cell bodies of the lower motor neurons, which receive impulses from the upper motor neurons located in the brain), you will see reduced muscle mass, muscle weakness, fine tremors of the fingers and toes, and singular muscle fasciculations. Abnormal movements which are at 90-degree right angles to the intended direction of the movement signal that a problem such as hypoxia has involved the cerebellum. These movements go back and forth like a pendulum, side to side, as the infant tries to move a body part (hand, foot, etc.) forward.

THE STEPPING REFLEX

There is a reflex called the stepping reflex, which is absent in hypotonic newborn infants. It normally disappears at about four months of age. It simply means that, when held upright, the infant will normally bear some weight with the feet and legs. The hypotonic child will not do this. Also, the normal infant will rather awkwardly try to place one foot forward, and if you move his/her body forward, he/she will step forward with the other foot.

THE HYPERTONIC NEWBORN

The spastic or hypertonic response is best demonstrated in the newborn in the thenar muscles, the mentalis muscle and the tongue. The thenar muscles are located in the palm of the hand near the thumb. They cause the thumb to be pulled into the palm. When they are spastic, the thumb cannot easily be extended away from the palm. The mentalis muscle pulls the corner of the mouth down towards the chin so that the child looks perpetually sad. The spasticity of the tongue muscles causes immobility and protrusion of the tongue.

Hypertonus is also suggested by movements of the upper or lower extremities as a "block" when you shake the hand or the foot. The flexibility is minimal at the elbow, wrist, knee and ankle.

Other signs of hypertonus or spasticity are clonus when crying. Clonus is an involuntary and rapid alternating contraction and relaxation of muscles. Do not confuse clonus with normal tremors, which occur during vigorous crying. The stepping reflex, described above, is abnormal in hypertonus in that, when the infant is held upright, both legs extend forward and are held in that position.

Signs of more serious hypertonus include scissoring of the legs and rigidity of the neck in a backward bent (hyperextended) position. This latter condition is spoken of as opisthotonos. Nuchal rigidity is severe tightness of the ligament which connects the back parts of the cervical vertebrae. These are the spinous processes of the vertebrae. Nuchal rigidity suggests a severe hypertonus problem, which could be due to spinal meningitis.

Hypertonus can be caused by some of the same problems that cause hypotonus if the severity is not too great. Examples of problems that could go either way would include hypoxia and hypoglycemia. When hypertonus is more severe, it may be due to intracranial hemorrhage. Severe hypertonus suggests an upper motor neuron problem or a severe metabolic problem. A prolonged or maintained opisthotonos is suggestive of drug toxicity, kernicterus (very high bile salts in the blood), congenital infection such as toxoplasmosis, or a congenital defect such as maple sugar disease. Prolonged severe nuchal rigidity, as stated above, strongly suggests spinal meningitis.

Topic 42

Breech Delivery and Caesarean Section

BREECH DELIVERY

Breech delivery presents some unique problems. In simple language, the part of the fetus that is coming through the birth canal first is the rump **(Fig. 6-13)**. This complicates matters significantly because, left to its own devices, if the breech infant could get through rump first, he/she would be coming through with knees against the chest and in a complete position of flexion of the pelvis on the lumbar spine. This rump and pelvic-spine flexion posture would then be trailed by the chest, the shoulders, and finally by the head. The stresses that are placed upon the newborn's body by such a delivery are quite immense. The rump is smaller than the legs bent on the torso, smaller than the shoulders and smaller than the head. Therefore, there is increased circumferential pressure on the trailing parts of the infant for which his/her body is not well

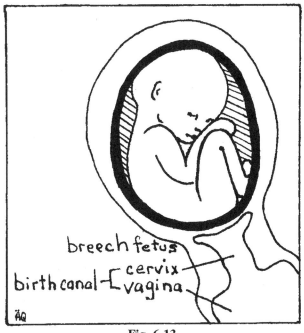

Fig. 6-13
Breech Position in Utero:
In a breech delivery the part of the fetus that presents
to the inner opening of the birth canal is the rump.
Successful vaginal breech delivery requires
considerable obstetrical skill. See text for description.

equipped. From a craniosacral point of view, the fluids of the body are forced up into the head, thus increasing fluid pressure inside the skull. This abnormally increased intracranial pressure is prolonged, because the passage of a breech newborn through the birth canal is difficult and almost always takes more time.

This situation of prolonged increased fluid pressure can be damaging to the intracranial membrane system. Breech delivery can also result in aberrations of normal skull bone positions and functional mobilities. Under normal head-first delivery conditions, the newborn head is usually large enough to dilate the birth canal so that the trailing body parts can slip through without difficulty, except for perhaps an arm or shoulder that may require a little further stretching of the birth canal's circumference. Also, the fluids are forced from the head into the body during normal head-first delivery, thus alleviating excess fluid pressure and volume within the vault of the skull (cranial vault) early on. This squeezing of fluids out of the head into the body during the passage through the birth canal (which may be thought of as a passage through a tourniquet or a wringer) greatly reduces the likelihood of intracranial membrane damage or skull bone problems.

If the breech delivery is carried to completion with the assistance of a qualified and/or knowledgeable person, that person may use his/her fingers to reach into the birth canal and to gently stretch and dilate it. This will enlarge the opening through which the rump-first newborn must pass. As an alternative, the delivery person may try to push the fetal rump out of the birth canal. If the fetus is not too far engaged, and if the mother's uterus is relaxed enough to allow it, a rotation of the fetal body might be possible. The breech delivery might then be converted to a normal head-first delivery. If this rotation cannot be accomplished, the next best thing is for the delivery person to engage a leg of the fetus and get that leg into the birth canal so that it precedes the rump in the delivery. Hopefully, if one leg can be brought through, so can the other. Now you have the feet coming out first followed by the legs, the torso, the shoulders and the head. With some assistance by the dilating fingers of the delivery person, the squeezing of fluid into the head can be minimized. However, the probability of hip dislocation and/or pelvic injury during the process of bringing down the legs is significant. Less probable, but not to be overlooked, is the possibility of fracture of the femur (thigh bone). Also, as the shoulders are delivered in the reverse order to that intended by nature, a fracture of the clavicle (collar bone) is not uncommon. Less common is a fracture of the humerus (upper-arm bone).

We must also consider that a rather small but significant amount of overzealous pulling by the delivery person on the feet and legs can traumatize the spinal cord and/or the neck as the large trailing head is pulled through. Therefore, it is common for reflexes that test the integrity of the spinal cord in the breech-delivered newborn to be abnormal. Also, it is not uncommon for the breech-delivered newborn to suffer Erb's palsy, Klumpke's palsy, mixed palsy and/or a torticollis of the neck. The torticollis of the neck is often due to an excessive stretching force being placed upon some of the neck muscles. This force may result in a strain or even an intramuscular bleed, which may cause abnormal contracture of the involved muscle or muscles. Most commonly the sternocleidomastoidus muscle is involved in torticollis. Torticollis is a condition wherein the muscle or muscles of the neck on one side contract, and either stay contracted or they episodically release and contract, causing the head to be abnormally side-bent and rotated in conjunction with the contractions. This abnormal position is usually accompanied by a significant amount of pain.

CAESAREAN SECTION

It is with all of the aforementioned breech-delivery information in mind that the majority of breech-presenting fetuses are taken from the mother's uterus by Caesarean section. Caesarean section, however, presents its own problems for the newborn. But most of these complications can be more easily dealt with than those that might occur in breech delivery.

I have three major concerns with Caesarean section that could be eliminated if a few treatment techniques were to be carried out routinely. The first concern involves a simple precaution during the operation itself. The second is a treatment of the newborn that would be done either immediately after delivery or within the first few days of life. The third can be done almost any time, but ideally it would be done sooner rather than later.

First, the technique which involves the operation per se is to reduce intrauterine pressure more slowly. When you consider that there is often a significant pressure differential between the inside and the outside of the uterus, it cannot be good for the fetus to make this change too rapidly without time for the fetal body to adapt. I have seen the intrauterine fluid spout out of the uterus three or four inches into the air when a quick incision is made in the uterus during Caesarean section. This quick and dramatic pressure change subjects the fetus to a very rapid decompression, which in turn induces a very rapid abnormal expansion of the fetal head within the decompressing uterus. This rapid increase in head volume can suddenly stretch the intracranial membranes. The result may be tissue strains, tiny hemorrhages within the membranes and/or actual membranous tears. These problems can wreak havoc with the craniosacral system and its function. They could be essentially eliminated by gently and slowly reducing intrauterine fluid pressure over a period of a minute or two, thus allowing the fetal body time to adapt.

This situation may be considered as analogous to the decompression precautions that divers take in order to avoid the problem caused by rising too quickly to the surface of the water. I believe that a very small incision in the uterus, which only allows a small stream of intrauterine (amniotic) fluid to escape over a prolonged period of time (two to three minutes), would eliminate a majority of these decompression problems. In 1976-78, while doing clinical research at Michigan State University, I saw a significant increase in craniosacral system problems related to Caesarean section deliveries as compared to vaginal deliveries.

My second concern that accompanies Caesarean section delivery is one of deprivation. By this, I mean that the newborn is deprived of its trip through the birth canal. This passage through the birth canal, I believe, is tantamount to its first spinal adjustment and mobilization treatment, its first skin-stimulation treatment and its first craniosacral treatment. When Caesarean section is performed, these treatments could be carried out by a well-trained professional very soon after delivery. I believe that the newborn would benefit a great deal from the replacement of the lost natural treatment which normally occurs through the birth canal, by treatment from a skilled pair of caring hands.

My third concern has to do with the completion of a natural birth process. This birth process has been interrupted for both the newborn and the mother by the Caesarean section procedure. It is my opinion that natural processes are programmed within the body sequentially by some mechanism or system. Quite possibly, this program is imprinted in our genetic structure. My observations have led me to conjecture that when a woman becomes pregnant, or perhaps when uterine implantation occurs, there is an inner intelligence that says that the process is not completed until vaginal delivery (with all of its therapeutic benefits) and bonding with the mother have occurred. These processes are interrupted for both mother and child by the Caesarean section delivery. We have found that, by the use of Therapeutic Imagery and Dialogue and/or SomatoEmotional Release[sm] techniques, these processes can be effectively completed, and certain frustrations that relate to lack of vaginal delivery and bonding can be effectively resolved.

Topic 43

The Premature Infant

About 10 to 15 percent of infants are born prematurely. In general, it is agreed that an infant with a gestation period of less than 38 weeks is considered premature. The premature infant is usually less than 5 pounds. 8 ounces at birth, with a crown-rump length of less than 18 1/2 inches.

As the problems of our society change in relationship to drug usage, the malnutrition of poverty, etc., we are finding exceptions to the generally accepted criteria of prematurity, especially in the newborn weight. Smaller babies are more often born even though the gestation period may be more than 38 weeks. Aside from these new "societal epidemics," some of the more "traditional" causes for premature delivery of newborn infants include the following: hypertensive toxemia of pregnancy; intercurrent acute infection; chronic infection of the mother such as syphilis; constitutional non-infectious illness of the mother such as diabetes, heart disease, kidney disease and the like; hydramnios, which is excessive amniotic fluid; abnormalities of the placenta, such as placenta previa (abnormal attachment); multiple pregnancies; severe emotional upsets, fatigue, overwork, etc., of the mother; maternal malnutrition; and maternal age over 40. In addition, deformity of the fetus often results in either early miscarriage, stillborn delivery, or premature delivery of a live fetus.

There are many clinical signs of prematurity in a newborn. The newborn will, of course, be small. He/she has a soft, delicate, almost transparent skin that is covered with a delicate hair called lanugo. This hair has a peach-fuzz quality. The premature newborn's fingernails and toenails do not extend past the tips of the fingers and toes as they do in the full-term infant. Also, there is minimal fat under the skin (subcutaneous fat), so that the premature child looks drawn, malnourished, and perhaps appears dehydrated. The full-term baby usually has a subcutaneous fat layer that offers the appearance of healthy plumpness. This fat content offers caloric nourishment to the full-term child during the period of time when the abilities to absorb and digest food are getting into effective working order. A blueness of the lips, finger and toenail beds and, in more severe cases, of larger skin areas of the body, is frequently present in the premature newborn. The extent of this blueness, called cyanosis, is dependent upon the level of effective development and function of the cardiovascular and pulmonary systems of the premature child. Most often the premature infant will demonstrate a lack of alertness or awareness of his/her environment. His/her body will be floppy and limp. The muscle strength is poor as demonstrated by lack of voluntary movement of extremities and torso. The sucking and swallowing abilities will probably be poorly functioning, if at all, and the newborn child's body temperature is often subnormal.

The handicaps of prematurity include an inability to properly regulate body temperature. The skin often radiates excessive heat. The child may not as yet have developed the ability to sweat. Sweating or perspiring is one of the ways that mature infants have of getting rid of excess heat, and lack of sweating is a way of conserving internal heat. Control of internal body temperature is very important as it affects metabolic efficiency, as well as the vitality and function of internal organs. Excessive internal body heat can cause damage to vital organs such as the brain. On the other hand, consider that hypothermia is a method which is currently under investigation. It allows the preservation of living tissues by reducing the need for nutrients and oxygen, and perhaps by other factors as yet unknown. This works because the activity of the hypothermic tissues is significantly reduced. The newborn needs all of his/her tissues to be working. The premature newborn's existence is in a very precarious balance as it tries to complete its development without the assistance of the uterus and the placenta.

The respiratory system of the premature child is underdeveloped, and therefore the child lacks good oxygenation. We hope as we see the cyanosis of the premature infant that the reason for the blue coloration is related exclusively to the pulmonary system, and that it does not involve the cardiovascular system. The pulmonary system and the brain are two of the last systems to develop, so pulmonary cyanosis in the premature infant is essentially normal, and chances are good that the efficiency of oxygenation by the pulmonary system will naturally improve as the days pass into weeks.

The same is true of the absorption of nutrients by the digestive system. Nutritional absorption will improve as we buy time for the prematurely delivered newborn. Therefore, a very high caloric food intake is provided during these early days and weeks of premature extrauterine life. The percentage of caloric waste for food taken by mouth is higher because the digestive system is not yet functioning efficiently. In order to compensate, nutrition may have to be provided intravenously. The same is true of the premature infant's immune system. Therefore, extra precautions are taken to prevent exposure to infections until the premature immune system has achieved a higher level of efficiency.

The Far-Reaching Effects of Traumatic Experiences of the Newborn Infants

Until recently it has been believed by the traditional medical community that newborn babies and infants were not capable of experiencing remembered pain and/or emotional trauma. On this basis, many invasive and painful diagnostic and treatment procedures have been and still are (although it is improving) being carried out on newborn babies and infants without regard for the child's experience of pain or discomfort. Perhaps even more significant has been the almost total disregard for emotional scars that could be and definitely have been imposed upon many of these babies by the attitudes and handling techniques of the healthcare professionals carrying out these procedures. We know now that both physical and emotional traumatic experiences are recorded in the memory banks of the newborn baby and infant. These experiences are there but are suppressed. They are also exacting a cost to the adult patient in order to keep them out of the conscious awareness. These costs take the form of many aberrant behaviors, such as unreasonable fears and phobias, unwarranted guilt problems, and a variety of other neuroses and obsessive and/or compulsive behaviors.

I believe that you shouldn't judge another until you have worn his/her shoes for awhile. In fact, I have worn these shoes and I share some of this guilt because I recall doing procedures such as circumcisions, spinal taps, venipunctures and the like on newborn and two- or three-day-old infants without regard to the piteous cries and screams that were elicited by my actions. I did these things because, as an intern, I was ordered to do them. I was taught that a child this small did not as yet have the brain development to truly perceive and remember pain. We were instructed not to worry about it, just get the job done. I was also advised that there was no such thing as an emotionally traumatic incident to a newborn or infant. So most certainly there would be no long-lasting effects or psychoemotional scars from these experiences.

As I have worked with and taught the therapeutic and facilitative techniques of SomatoEmotional Release℠ and Therapeutic Imagery and Dialogue over the past 15+ years, I have come to know by hundreds of observations and patient experiences that the fetus in the uterus, the fetus going through the delivery process, the newborn child and the infant in the nursery are all capable of and do, in fact, experience and record in their memory banks both the physical and emotional trauma to which they are exposed. Some of these traumas are imposed by nature, some by ordinary people and parents, some are the result of accidents and/or physical conditions, and some are imposed by well-meaning healthcare professionals.

All of us who do CranioSacral Therapy, SomatoEmotional Release℠ and Therapeutic Imagery and Dialogue have seen many cases of adults suffering from low self-esteem, lack of self-worth, guilt about being alive and the like. A significant percentage of these problems have been traced back to conversations between the pregnant mother and the father as she informed him of her condition for the first time. Typically, in these cases the father becomes angry because he doesn't want the child. The pregnant mother becomes emotionally distraught. Abortion is often discussed. The details can take a myriad of turns. The bottom line is that a fetus in the uterus somehow senses the problem between the expectant mother and the father. The result is that, at a repressed, non-conscious level, the child grows to adulthood living with serious doubts about his/her self-worth, and/or whether or not he/she deserves to be alive. Often when we get deeply into these problems with patients, they feel as though they should not have been born. This feeling often seems to spring from that first emotional conversation between expectant mother and father, during which the patient somehow perceives, while still a developing fetus in the mother's womb, that he/she was not wanted. This is a very common scenario in my experience. The details vary but the central theme remains the same.

Another typical scenario that I have encountered on several occasions with male patients who were suffering from sexual dysfunction is the interpretation that the matter-of-fact or impatient or hurried attitude of the doctor doing a painful circumcision somehow means that the penis is bad. This interpretation of this early and painful experience is recorded in the infant's memory bank. It then surrounds the penis with guilt. Confusion occurs when the normal libido begins to develop and confronts the guilt about normal reproductive penis function and so on. In my experience the details must be cleared and resolved in order to normalize sexual function. In order to resolve the details, we have to unearth the incident and re-experience the feelings that went along with it originally. It is amazing how much experience the newborn child and nursery infant perceive, store in memory banks and suppress.

I recall one circumcision-related problem that threw me for a complete loop. It was a great affirmation to our rule that we don't lead the patient. By this I mean that I make the patient move, but he/she decides in which direction to travel. This was a 34-year-old Jewish male who was suffering from increasing fear that "people" were out to kill him. The surfacing of this fear was not yet a year old. He was not psychotic (as yet), but he was quite distressed about this irrational fear of being killed. He recognized the fear as irrational. Further, when the fear gripped him he had great difficulty speaking about it. More often it was quite impossible for him to say anything at all.

Our SomatoEmotional Release℠ process took us back to his Bris. I conjectured that this might become an interpretation of the circumcision as an attack upon him with murder as its intent. Not so. It was the gauze soaked in kosher wine that was put into his mouth that he interpreted as the attempt to kill him through suffocation. That wine-soaked gauze was put into his mouth in the hopes that the wine, as it is absorbed in the mouth and throat, might offer some anesthetic or calming effect before circumcision. In this case the child interpreted the gauze in his mouth with the wine and its repugnant taste and aroma as an attempt by the Rabbi, in conjunction with his father and several other strange men, to kill him. Apparently, his repressive mechanism wanted to let go, so it started to release the feelings related to the incident into his conscious awareness.

So much for the idea that newborn babies and nursery infants and even fetuses in the uterus don't feel pain or emotion. Just think about all the invasive attacks, pains and suffering that we have undergone before the doctors thought we could perceive and record. It is a miracle that most of us do as well as we do.

Section VII

Congenital Malformations

Congenital means present at birth. It does not tell you whether the malformation is due to a genetic problem which is inherited, a gene defect that has been created by some external agent such as radiation, or whether the malformation is due to something that happened during the pregnancy that interfered with the normal development of the child inside of the uterus.

In 1994, there were over 4,000 known genetically induced and inherited diseases that initially present as congenital malformations. These problems show up in over 250,000 newborn infants in the United States each year. As research into genetic diseases continues at a very rapid rate, the number of known genetic problems will continue to rise.

Some of the genetically induced problems are such things as Down's syndrome, cystic fibrosis, muscular dystrophy, sickle cell anemia, Klinefelter's syndrome, Turner's syndrome and so on. It would require an encyclopedia to list them all. And the way things are going, that encyclopedia would need to be rewritten each year.

It must be kept in mind that we now know that genetic problems are not only inherited. Disturbances and/or distortions in gene structure are also induced or created by exposure to radiation. That radiation could be accidental exposure to radioactive material, it could be exposure to excessive diagnostic or therapeutic x-ray, or anything in between these two extreme examples. There is some suspicion that exposure to electromagnetic fields can cause abnormal changes in gene structure. There is pretty good evidence to support the idea that excessive doses of vitamin A or retinoic acid can disturb genetic control of the formation of the fetal head and central nervous system. This problem may show itself as cleft palate, facial deformities and the like.

On the other side of the coin, we have the factors that interfere with or distort the developmental process of the embryo and/or the fetus during the period of gestation in the uterus. These problems are not related to disturbance in gene structure, but rather they present obstacles to the proper development of the embryo and/or fetus during that very delicate period when the cells of the developing body are very busy either dividing, specializing, migrating and/or whatever else they may be doing.

Viruses and Congenital Malformations

As examples of this kind of extrinsic interference, let's consider that the mother is infected by a virus that causes her to contract a case of German measles, or as it is known in medical circles, rubella. This virus is very much able to cross the placenta. Next, it becomes a matter of which parts of the child are developing when the infection occurs, as to which sort of congenital malformations may be present at birth. When the rubella virus invades the developing embryo or fetus, it is quite capable of distorting or stopping the development of specific tissues and/or organs.

For example, should the infection occur during the sixth week of gestation, the child will very likely be born with cataracts, because the lens of the eyes are in a critical phase of development at that time. If the virus invades during the ninth week of gestation, the most likely problem will be deafness. Heart defects are a common congenital malformation if the rubella virus invades anytime between the fifth and the tenth week of gestation, because the intricacies of the structures of the valves and the chambers of the heart are being laid down during those weeks. Central nervous system problems are common complications of rubella infection anytime between the fourth and the tenth weeks of gestation, and dental deformities are common concomitants of infection between the sixth and the ninth weeks of intrauterine development.

Other viruses also have favorite malformations that they can cause because it seems that, in addition to gestational age of infection, certain viruses have a liking or propensity to attack specific kinds of tissues. For example, the cytomegalovirus likes to attack the brain and the eyes, as well as the liver and spleen in more severe cases. Therefore, in cytomegalovirus infections, especially during the first trimester of a pregnancy, we see microcephaly, cerebral calcifications, blindness, chorioretinitis, and problems with the spleen and liver. The bile in the blood may go high enough (kernicterus) to cause death of the fetus or newborn.

The virus of herpes simplex also likes to invade the brain, the eyes, the liver and the spleen. Therefore, it too often produces microcephaly, microphthalmos, retinal problems and mental retardation. More severe cases also involve liver and spleen, but are not usually as deadly as these due to the cytomegalovirus.

These are but a few examples of what viruses can do to the developing fetus. The most irreversible damages to the brain are done by virus infection during the embryonic period of development, which is the first eight to ten weeks of gestation.

Topic 46

Other Factors That Cause Congenital Malformations

Other factors that can and do cause congenital malformations are: maternal exposure to radiation during the pregnancy; maternal exposure to drugs or chemicals; maternal anemia; respiratory diseases that reduce oxygen supply to the developing child; maternal nutritional deficiencies; maternal hormonal problems; and the fetus which is locked or compressed into an abnormal position in the uterus over an extended period of time. Bones do not grow well against resistance. For example, it is thought that club foot may be a bone malformation caused by a malposition of the lower extremity in the uterus that prevents normal development of the foot.

Drugs That Can Cause Congenital Malformations

Drugs that can cause congenital malformations include thalidomide, which achieved great notoriety a few decades ago. Thalidomide was reputed to be safe for pregnant women as a mild sedative. We were wrong. It caused marked deformity of the extremities in many of the children whose mothers used it during gestation. Thalidomide is probably the drug that, through its notoriety, caused the United States government to become much more strict about the use of a wide variety of drugs by pregnant women. The big "clamp down" occurred subsequent to the "Thalidomide Baby" scandal. At present, pregnant women are generally advised to avoid almost all medications, rather than take a chance of inducing a birth defect by the use of some drug that may have unpredictable side effects upon the fetus.

Many antidepressant medications have also been incriminated as causes of limb deformities. The appetite depressants are also considered unsafe. The old standby medications for malaria, quinine and the sulfa drugs, are now considered potentially dangerous for the fetus. They may produce liver problems which can raise blood bile levels high enough to cause brain damage. The antibiotic streptomycin has been implicated as a cause of deafness in the newborn when used by the mother during gestation. We could go on and on about medications and the risk they may impose upon the developing embryo and fetus when used by the pregnant mother.

More recent studies are linking alcohol and tobacco usage during pregnancy to low-birth-weight babies. Low birth weight reduces the chances of postpartum survival and increases the risk of multiple malformations ranging from brain problems to facial disfigurements. Until all the facts are known, I'm sure it is best to err on the side of safety. Once a malformed child is born, it is too late to wish that you had done things differently. Most often the malformed child will have to live with the results of the drug exposure throughout its lifetime. Obviously, there is a great potential for serious defects to the unborn child if the mother should use illegal drugs during the pregnancy.

Clearly, the use and abuse of cocaine and other street drugs is high. The impact that this drug problem will present to the future of our society is not yet fully appreciated, but it is of great concern.

Many people do not consider hormones as drugs. However, the track record for the use of hormone supplements during pregnancy is alarming. Witness the high incidence of cancer, mostly of the genital organs, in the children of women who, as late as the 1960s, were given a female hormone to avert possible miscarriage. That hormone was diethylstilbestrol. First, it was only the female children that seemed to be affected. Now some suspicion is arising that perhaps male genital organ cancer may result from this hormone. Progesterone hormones were also used during pregnancy at times to help continue a pregnancy that was perhaps in a precarious situation. These progestins, as the family of hormones is called, we now know often caused the masculinization of a female child's genitalia. The clitoris may become enlarged to the extent that, at birth, it more resembles a penis than a clitoris. What effect this may have on sexual identity later on is not as yet fully understood. It also appears that the use of cortisone and many of its related hormone compounds are statistically related to the presence of cleft palate at birth.

In maternal metabolic problems, the physician and the pregnant mother may often find themselves in a difficult dilemma. Let's say that the mother develops a severe case of overactive thyroid gland function, of which the most severe cases are known as thyrotoxicosis. Allowed to continue, this thyrotoxic condition can result in fetal death. On the other hand, the medications that will hopefully control the thyroid gland may cause birth defects. There is a chance that the fetus may live through the thyrotoxicosis. There is also a chance that the medication may not cause a birth defect. There is no perfect answer here. Either way there is risk.

Also, it is not a rare circumstance that the pregnant mother has a problem during pregnancy that interferes with her respiratory system. The fetus requires an excellent supply of oxygen in the uterus in order to develop a normally functioning brain. The medication to solve the mother's problem may induce a birth defect in the child. Once again, no matter which way the doctor and mother decide to go, the results could be disastrous. There is no foolproof answer to this kind of problem. Whatever path is followed, there is a risk. I raise these examples not to scare you, but to perhaps help you understand with more compassion some of the problems that confront the healthcare professionals. Modern medicine is good but it does not have all the answers. A bad outcome does not necessarily mean that a mistake has been made.

Neural Tube Development and Malformations

Now let's look at the development of the neural tube. Normally, the neural tube is closed by about the 28th day of gestation. As you may recall, the neural tube is formed in the embryonic plate. It is the forbearer of the development of the brain and spinal cord. If something happens during the time that the neural tube is closing (during the fourth week of gestation) that event may interfere with the closure process. The results of lack of closure can be either devastating or relatively minor, depending upon the location of the closure defect and when it happened.

Spina bifida is one of the problems that can result from neural tube closure defect. This condition occurs in the United States about once in every 1,000 live births. That amounts to about one-tenth of one percent of the time. There are several classifications of spina bifida, depending on the structures/tissues involved in the defect.

Spina bifida occulta simply means that the vertebra did not close at the posterior midline. That is, the spinous process of the involved vertebra is not sealed into one piece in the back. This bony defect can often be felt with the palpating finger. This is not a truly serious problem because neither the meningeal membrane nor the nerve tissue of the spinal cord are protruding out of the spinal canal into the opening provided by the non-fusion of the vertebra. Spina bifida occulta may cause back pain and possible increased vulnerability of the spine, but it won't cause functional problems of the central nervous system. The vertebra are normally closed or fused into one piece at the posterior midline by the end of the 12th week of gestation. Often the spina bifida occulta is noticeable because the bony defect leaves a dimple in the overlying skin. There may also be a skin discoloration and sometimes a tuft of hair over the involved vertebra.

A much more serious problem occurs when there are external protrusions of the meningeal membranes into a cyst-like structure which lies under the skin at the level of the vertebral fusion defect (**Fig. 6-11**). It gets even more serious if nerve tissue of the spinal cord also protrudes into the cyst formation. The name applied to this more complicated and serious defect is spina bifida cystica. When only the meningeal membranes protrude from the spinal canal into the cyst, the diagnostic label is spina bifida cystica with meningocele. If there is also nervous tissue from the spinal cord and/or spinal cord nerve roots protruding into the cyst, the condition is labeled spina bifida cystica with meningomyelocele.

The spina bifida cystica with meningomyelocele is often complicated further by a condition whereby the herniation of the spinal cord tissues into the cyst formation causes an abnormal pull or traction, which is projected up the spinal cord to the place where it joins the medulla oblongata.

This pulling from below causes the medulla oblongata to be pressed against the foramen magnum, which is the large opening in the base of the skull through which the spinal cord passes to get into the spinal canal. If the abnormal pull is strong enough, it can cause the medulla oblongata to herniate into the foramen magnum. If the abnormal pull is still stronger, it can cause the medulla oblongata and the other brain stem tissues which attach to it from above to herniate downward through the foramen magnum. This foramen magnum opening is not large enough to comfortably allow passage of the medulla oblongata and the other brain stem structures through it. This situation then begins to strangulate the brain stem. The infant's life is now in jeopardy unless corrective measures are taken in a timely manner.

Sometimes the herniation of the brain stem is not so severe that life is threatened, but a blood accumulation (hematoma) may occur which obstructs the passageway of the foramen magnum. This, in turn, interferes with the passage of cerebrospinal fluid into the spinal canal from inside of the skull. This obstruction of cerebrospinal fluid circulation can induce a hydrocephalus, which is a part of the Arnold-Chiari syndrome.

When surgical correction for spina bifida cystica is undertaken, there are some very significant risks and/or complications. For example, when a large meningeal cystic sac is removed, you have also removed a reservoir for cerebrospinal fluid. Unless precautions are taken, this can induce a hydrocephalus. If the cystic sac contains nervous tissue from the spinal cord and/or any of its nerve roots, the result may be significant neurological damage.

Spina bifida of any type is a result of neural tube closure defect in that part of the neural tube that will give rise to the spinal column and the spinal cord. When the failure to fuse is at the head of the neural tube, the result may be a condition which is called a cranium bifidum. This is a situation wherein a skull bone fails to close on the midline. Most commonly this occurs in the occipital bone. Usually in cranium bifidum a meningeal sac protrudes through the failed closure in the skull bone. The sac or cyst occupies space under the scalp and will usually contain a significant amount of cerebrospinal fluid. This problem is often accompanied by hydrocephalus. When brain substance also protrudes into the sac, the problem is called a cranium bifidum cystica with meningoencephalocele. Surgery is the only answer and the risk is high.

Another failure of the neural tube is when nothing happens at the head end of the tube. This is rare. There is no skull (cranial vault) and there is no brain. This is not compatible with life.

At the other end of the spectrum we have the failure of the neural tube to close at the tail end. This usually results in a pilonidal cyst, which in terms of severity pales by comparison to those conditions we have just described. Many people go through life with a pilonidal cyst and have no problem. Others may become infected and may need surgical drainage or excision. The pilonidal cyst will usually present with a tuft of hair as its landmark. The dermal sinus is the name applied to a sinus tract which communicates from the skin into the spinal canal. This also is a failure of neural tube closure, usually near the tail end of the tube.

Topic 49

The Causes of Neural Tube Closure Defects

Because neural tube closure defects can be so devastating, a great deal of investigative effort has gone into understanding the causes and prevention. At the present time the opinions are still varied. Some observations and theories are indicated below. You are going to have to draw your own conclusions:

1. There is a well-established, higher incidence of neural tube defects in lower socioeconomic populations.
2. In one study, folic acid vitamin supplements of 180 micrograms per day in 4,783 pregnant women reduced the incidence of neural tube defects to one. The expected rate of occurrence in a study this size would have been four or five.
3. Amniotic fluid levels of vitamin B12 were down in seven cases of neural tube defects which occurred in a population of 221 women.
4. Several studies have suggested that zinc deficiency may correlate to neural tube closure defect incidence. The problem here is what parts of the body we should use to measure the zinc. Blood levels don't agree with finger and toe-nail levels, or with muscle-tissue content, etc., etc., etc.
5. Maternal alcoholism increases incidence of neural tube closure defects. This could mean that alcohol is the cause, or it could mean that the alcoholic mothers tested didn't get enough nutrients in their diets.
6. Certainly there could be a chromosomal or genetic defect that causes neural tube defects.

At this point it looks like zinc, calcium and folic acid must be adequate in order to reduce the risk of spina bifida. The protein linkages that close the neural tube in the embryo are bridged by calcium, thereby indicating its importance.

In light of these observations, it is safe to say that an expectant mother may want to take extra zinc, calcium and folic acid, even though we don't have conclusive proof as yet.

Congenital Malformations of the Skull and Vertebral Column

For purposes and ease of classification, the skull is divided into two parts: the neurocranium and the viscerocranium. The neurocranium houses the brain and its related nerves, blood vessels, connective tissues and so on. The viscerocranium refers to the bony structures of the face.

The neurocranium is further divided into two subclassifications according to the type of tissue from which the skull bone originated. The floor of the skull vault upon which the brain rests is called the chondrocranium because these bony parts originally derived from cartilage. The sides, the front, the back and the top of the skull are referred to as the flat bones of the skull. These bones were formed from membrane which ossifies as the skull develops in utero. The fontanelles or soft spots in the newborn baby's head are examples of regions wherein the membrane has not yet ossified (calcified). Also, the areas where the edges of the membranous bones approximate or come close to each other do not ossify by the time of birth. This allows the bone edges to override each other so that the larger head can pass through the smaller birth canal during the delivery. Premature ossifications of these skull bone junctures can make the vaginal delivery much more difficult, if not impossible.

Let's look at some of the problems that can occur and present themselves as congenital malformations of the skull. Cranial synostosis is an abnormally early union of the bones of the skull, which may or may not be present at birth. When present, it prevents normal growth of the skull during the first year of life. Of course, if the skull can't grow fast enough, the brain doesn't have the room to grow either. The brain weight at birth is about 335 grams under normal circumstances. And at the end of the first year of life, that brain weight has usually nearly tripled to about 925 grams. By the end of the second year of life, the infant brain is approaching the adult size. It is the skull expansibility provided by the cranial sutures (joints) that allows the skull vault to enlarge so readily and accommodate this rapid brain growth. When the cranial sutures are fused at birth, the brain tries to grow but the skull won't expand. The result will most likely be brain dysfunction and/or damage. It is imperative that these prematurely closed sutures be opened as soon as possible so that the brain of the infant will not be irreversibly damaged.

Cranial synostosis often causes blindness because the increased internal pressure in the eye as the brain tries to expand may impair the development of the optic nerves. Cranial synostosis can also be the causative agent in epileptic or seizure disorders. It will also cause remarkable head pain and, of course, the newborn or infant has a difficult time telling you about the pain. Clearly, cranial synostosis can be the culprit in a multitude of brain and central nervous system problems.

Surgical correction is probably the best answer.

As I mentioned previously during the discussion on spina bifida, there can be congenital defects in the formation of skull bones. This defective bone formation is referred to as a cranioschisis if it is large. This problem is often accompanied by a smaller than normal brain, or by no brain at all. Clearly this problem can be genetic, or it can be secondary to something that occurred during the development and closure of the neural tube. This usually places the external cause within the first month of the pregnancy.

Congenital malformations of the vertebral column include the spina bifida problems which were previously discussed, as well as conditions where there are too many or too few vertebrae. Usually, this situation where the number of vertebrae is incorrect goes unnoticed until later in life when chronic back pain may emerge and x-rays are taken. Sometimes, due to unknown causes, two successive vertebrae may be fused together at birth. Once again, this condition often goes unnoticed until back problems develop later in life. Less often a newborn presents with either the right or the left side of a vertebrae completely missing. This may be discovered more easily during the newborn evaluation because there will be a noticeable soft area where a bone is supposed to be. This condition makes the spinal column more vulnerable to dysfunction than do the other situations wherein there is an incorrect number of spinal vertebrae, or when two vertebrae are abnormally fused together.

Topic 51

Scoliosis

At this time I should like to present a personal opinion on the subject of scoliosis, and how I believe that the scoliotic process may be started during the obstetrical delivery. Scoliosis is simply a spinal curvature which goes sideways. It can be a "C" curve or an "S" curve, and it can be markedly rotated or less obviously so, although some rotation to accommodate for the sideways bending is required. Thus, we have the name "rotoscoliosis" by which this condition is also known (**Fig. 7-1**).

I have mentioned this condition and our ideas about cause previously. But rather than have you interrupt your reading in order to turn back and find this discussion, I will briefly reiterate the concept here. Scoliosis can be caused by a number of factors. Most of them are things that happen later in life, incidents that cause pelvic imbalances and the like. However, we suggest that, when there is interference with the normal passage through the birth canal, an imbalance in the craniosacral system may be established, which sets the scene for scoliosis or spinal curvature as the child grows up.

The interference to which I refer may be a forceps-assisted delivery, a prolonged labor or a very quick delivery, a breech delivery, and whatever else may significantly modify the nature-intended journey through the birth canal. The reason that these interferences with the natural delivery become potential contributing factors for scoliosis is as follows. When the child is delivered normally, head-first looking down, at a moderate rate of speed through the birth canal, this journey represents its first spinal manipulation and its first craniosacral treatment. The birth canal is so designed that a passage through it may well be intended to mobilize each joint in the pelvis, each joint between two vertebrae, each joint between a rib and a vertebra, and all of the joints or sutures of the skull. The mobilization of each of these joints requires time. If the journey is too fast, some of the joints may not have time to mobilize. If the journey is too slow, the forces may be placed upon joints for an inordinate amount of time and induce a strain on those joints. This, in turn, may create fibrotic changes that immobilize the joint and contribute to an abnormal spinal configuration.

A similar situation may occur when a suction cup or forceps are used to exert abnormal traction upon the newborn's head against a resistance to the passage through the birth canal. Strain, fibrosis and loss of joint mobility may result. The same is true of strains of the newborn's body that are induced by abnormal position, such as breech or face upwards, as the child passes through a birth canal that was designed for a different mode of delivery.

Craniosacral system problems may arise from an abnormal locking of the newborn head in the mother's pelvis, from the aggressive use of forceps and suction devices, from breech deliveries and so on. When the bones of the cranial vault are dysfunctional and unbalanced, the dura mater membrane system that travels down the spinal canal may reflect that imbalance. This dural tube (dura mater membrane system) imbalance may then place excess tension on spinal cord nerve roots which, in turn, may cause an imbalance in tonus of the muscles that influence the positions of the vertebrae and the ribs. This imbalance in muscle tone is often the cause of scoliosis as the newborn begins to develop an erect posture.

All of this could be avoided by good and prudent mobilization of the newborn spine and ribs, as well as mobilization and balancing of the craniosacral system. This work could be done during the first few days after delivery without significant risk to the infant.

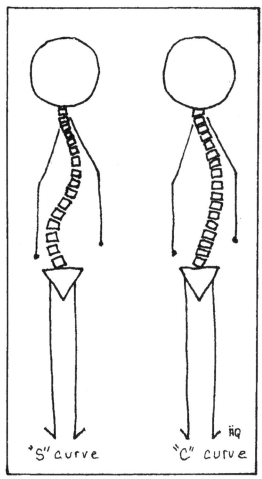

Fig. 7-1
Spinal Curvatures:
As shown in the illustration, spinal curvatures
can take either an "S" or a "C" shape.
There is always some degree of compensatory
rotation. There is also a wedge-shaped
deformity of one or more vertebral body shapes,
which is common as the problem progresses.
See text for details.

Congenital Hydrocephalus

Hydrocephalus may be congenital or acquired. The term hydrocephalus refers to a condition which is marked by a significant dilation (enlargement) of the ventricles of the brain. This ventricular dilation is most often due to an obstruction of cerebrospinal fluid flow in one or more of its exit pathways, which causes accumulation of that fluid within the brain.

In the craniosacral system model, it is put forth that hydrocephalus may also be caused by a dysfunction of the control system that governs the rate and quantity of cerebrospinal fluid which is manufactured within the ventricular system of the brain. Or, there may be a dysfunction of the cerebrospinal fluid reabsorption system, which is comprised of the arachnoid villi within the venous sinuses of the skull.

A functional classification has been made which divides congenital hydrocephalus into communicating and non-communicating. In communicating hydrocephalus, a dye that is injected into one of the lateral ventricles of the brain is seen to travel into the subarachnoid space from the ventricular system of the brain and show up down low in the lumbar region of the spinal canal inside the subarachnoid space. In non-communicating hydrocephalus, the dye injected into one of the lateral ventricles of the brain does not get into the subarachnoid space. This means that the cerebrospinal fluid cannot escape from the ventricular system.

Another method of classification involves use of the term obstructive hydrocephalus, which refers to any obstruction to cerebrospinal fluid flow either within or outside of the brain's ventricular system. The obstruction prevents communication between the ventricular system of the brain and the subarachnoid space that surrounds the brain and the spinal cord.

Obstructive hydrocephalus is the most common form. When the obstruction is within the brain, the ventricles on the fluid-production side (proximal side) of the obstruction will dilate. On the other side of the obstruction, the ventricle size is normal. This situation makes for ease of diagnosis. Obstructions may occur at the foramen of Monro, which connects the lateral ventricles on each side to the third ventricle. In this case, one of the lateral ventricles will be dilated and the rest of the system may appear normal. When the obstruction is in the third ventricle itself, both of the lateral ventricles will be dilated because they both drain into this third ventricle.

The cerebral aqueduct of Sylvius connects the third ventricle with the fourth ventricle. Cerebrospinal fluid flows from the third ventricle, via the cerebral aqueduct, into the fourth ventricle. When the cerebral aqueduct is not functioning properly, both lateral and the third ventricles will be dilated.

The outflow from the fourth ventricle into the subarachnoid space is through the foramina of

Luschka and Magendie. When these foramina are incompetent, the fluid cannot get out into the subarachnoid space. All four ventricles of the brain will be dilated. Many malformations of the ventricular system of the brain which result in obstructive hydrocephalus are due to infections, such as intrauterine meningitis. These infections involve the fetus. They may not be discernable in the mother.

Congenital hydrocephalus occurs in about one to three newborns per 2,000 deliveries, depending on whose data you accept. The causes of congenital hydrocephalus, in addition to the aforementioned intrauterine infections, may also include intracranial hemorrhage due to birth trauma/injury, premature delivery and genetic causes. Probably, incompetency of the cerebral aqueduct of Sylvius is most often the cause of congenital hydrocephalus. Improper formation of the arachnoid villi, which impairs cerebrospinal fluid reabsorption, is among the least common causes. If the hydrocephalus is severe enough to warrant concern about brain development against the excessive fluid volume, surgery is definitely indicated. A shunt should be installed.

Topic 53

Congenital Malformations of the Eye and the Ear

The critical period of development for the eye and ear is the third through the sixth week of gestation. The lens of the eye is in its developmental stages during the fourth, fifth and sixth weeks. Therefore, congenital cataracts are usually due to problems during this period of the pregnancy. The most common cause of cataracts is still thought to be maternal infection with rubella (German measles). However, cataracts may also be caused by other infections, toxic problems, or by genetic defects.

Congenital deafness is also most often linked to maternal infection with rubella, although it too may be secondary to other infections, toxic problems or genetic defects. The most common cause of congenital deafness is a problem with the function of the tiny bones (ossicles called the hammer, anvil and stapes) that conduct sound from the ear drum through the middle ear chamber into the inner ear, where sound wave is converted into nerve impulse.

Topic 54

Brain Function and Dysfunction

We've talked a good bit about structural malformations of the central nervous system and its related tissues. Now let's look at brain function and what sort of things can happen. Most congenital malformations of the structure of the brain originate during the third, fourth and/or fifth week of gestation. This is when the nuclei of most of the fundamental brain structures present themselves. After these basic brain-part origins have been laid down, they spend the rest of their time developing so that they can efficiently function when they are called upon.

As we have said before, there are many things that can happen during the pregnancy, during the delivery, or very shortly after delivery that cause problems. Brain-function problems are most often secondary to other problems that occur during these times. Certainly, we have to look seriously at the effects of infection and drugs during these brain development times. Also, we have to consider lack of oxygen to the brain that can be related to an umbilical cord wrapped tightly around the child's neck, and other causes of fetal distress in the uterus. Most of these causes relate to maternal health problems and/or problems that relate to failing placental attachment to the uterine wall, or failure of the placenta to deliver adequate blood supply to the fetus.

Other problems that result in brain dysfunction include delivery trauma, which may result in intracranial bleeding or hemorrhaging in the newborn. The "bleed" can be beneath the dura mater membrane (subdural), between the arachnoid membrane and the pia mater (subarachnoid), within the brain tissue itself, and/or within the ventricular system of the brain. The seriousness of the bleed depends upon where it occurs, and the quantity of the blood which has leaked out of the blood vessels.

Brains are sometimes contused or bruised. These bruises involve smaller leakages (extravasations) of blood than do the frank bleeds or hemorrhages. However, any blood cells that escape from the blood vessels and make their way into brain tissue present potential brain-function problems. This is because, as the blood cells break down or deteriorate, the byproducts are very irritating molecules. These molecules are the result of catabolism. (Catabolism is the breaking down of more complex substances into less complex substances or molecules.)

During the catabolism of red blood cells, some of the byproducts are actually bile salts. If you have ever tasted bile, you know how irritating it can be to your tongue. Imagine how irritating it can be to brain cells. The response of the brain tissue to these irritating foreign molecules is to fibrose. That is, some of the (glial) cells of the brain, not the neurons, multiply, stiffen and contract, forming a fiber network that interferes with normal neuronal conduction of electrical impulses. So essentially, this part of the brain may become unable to function normally. If it happens to be a speech area, the development of speech will be subnormal. If it is a motor area to the right hand that has been involved in the degradation of red blood cells and fibrosed, the motor control of the right hand will be impaired, and so on.

It also strikes me that energy is always produced as a product of catabolism. I have not seen it written anywhere, but it seems reasonable that this abnormal source of energy in brain tissue could produce seizures. In any case, bleeds, brain bruises and contusions should always be taken seriously. My experience has strongly suggested to me that properly and judiciously applied CranioSacral Therapy can help the irritating molecules to be more quickly carried away from the site of a bleed, bruise or contusion, thus minimizing the degree of fibrosis that occurs. Also, it seems that the effect of an established fibrosis can be reduced by CranioSacral Therapy, thus enhancing the function of the involved area of the brain. I believe that these beneficial effects are obtained because CranioSacral Therapy enhances the flow of all bodily fluids within the skull. In so doing, it helps to shorten the time of brain tissue exposure to irritants. Also, it increases fresh blood flow, thus reducing the stifling effect of fibrosis upon the circulation of fresh blood to a specific area of brain tissue.

In addition to those problems we have just considered that impair the development of proper brain function in the newborn, we also have a list of metabolic problems that can and often do compromise the functional activity of the brain. Among these problems are an elevation of blood bile in the fetus and/or newborn. This is called kernicterus. This situation occurs when there is an Rh problem between mother and fetus, or when there is any kind of serious liver or gall bladder problem in the fetus and/or newborn. Other blood-destructive problems can also cause kernicterus. Remember, the degradation or catabolism of red blood cells produces bile salts. If the newborn infant's blood contains elevated levels of bile salts for a long enough time, the brain will become irritated. It will fibrose in response to the irritation, and we may now have a total brain that has difficulty with capillary blood circulation and the conduction of electrical impulses.

Another metabolic problem that can result in the dysfunction of a normally structured brain is low blood sugar. If the mother has low blood sugar (hypoglycemia), the fetus will have low blood sugar. If the fetus has this problem for more than a few minutes, the neurons of the fetal brain begin to die of starvation. The degree of brain dysfunction that we see in the child relates to how many neurons in the brain have starved to death. The same situation holds true for oxygen deprivation for more than a few minutes.

There is also a long list of genetically inherited biochemical problems that impair the function of a normally structured and developed brain. Some of these problems are correctable and, if discovered and treated in time, will not cause permanent brain dysfunction. Among these genetically related biochemical problems are such conditions as phenylketonuria, maple syrup urine disease, tyrosinosis, hyperprolinemia, hydroxyprolinemia, histidinuria, citrullinuria, homocystinuria and many, many more. These are all biochemically very complicated problems which we will not delve into beyond simply naming some of them in order to give you a feel for the possibilities for error in metabolism.

Topic 55

Cerebral Palsy

Cerebral palsy may be defined as a persisting qualitative motor dysfunction that appears before the age of three years. It is due to a non-progressive damage to the brain, which can be due to any one of a number of causes. When the palsy is manifest as a stiffness and spasticity of muscle, it may be known as Little's disease. Spasticity suggests that the pyramidal tracts are involved in the damage. However, my own experience suggests that spastic cerebral palsy may also occur secondary to problems with the motor cortex. Some of these problems may be correctable, or at least show improvement with the use of CranioSacral Therapy. It would appear that some of these spastic palsies are due to abnormal tensions of the dura mater membrane and/or jamming of some of the sutures of the skull vault.

The problems that are causally related to cerebral palsy may be incurred in the uterus, during the delivery or in the early post-delivery period. Cerebral palsy may be caused by developmental defects of the central nervous system. It can also be caused by intrauterine infections such as meningitis or encephalitis. Cerebral palsy can also be caused by kernicterus, oxygen deprivation, strokes, or accidents and trauma that injure brain tissue.

By this overview of some of the potential causes of cerebral palsy, it becomes clear that the diagnosis indicates that something is wrong that is causing a motor dysfunction, but it says almost nothing about the cause. Many parents who bring in their cerebral palsied children for treatment have the mistaken idea that cerebral palsy is a specific disease. It is not. Cerebral palsy is a name that describes a set of symptoms. The cause for each case of cerebral palsy must be determined. It is through this determination of cause that something may be found as good treatment. Most people think that cerebral palsy is for life. I have had a few patients who have broken this rule and recovered.

It should also be emphasized that the cerebral palsied child may have a normally functioning intellect. Mental retardation is not usually a part of cerebral palsy although, because speech is frequently impaired to some degree, it may appear that the cerebral palsy patient has an intellectual defect as well.

Section VIII

The Triune Brain: A Model
by Paul D. MacLean

Our brains serve us as detectors and perceivers; as amplifiers and dampeners; and as analyzers, decision makers and commanders. Our brains tell us what is going on around us and in us. They dictate what we feel, how we like or dislike those feelings, and they tell us what we will do about all of these feelings. Then, as if that weren't enough, they tell us how to do it and, based on remembered past experience, they almost always provide a probability prediction about the success or failure of our choices, therein often letting us know why we choose to take a certain action.

Without the services rendered to us by our brains, we would not be able to adapt to and survive in the changing worlds, both around us and inside of us.

Paul D. MacLean, M.D., is a perpetual student, an expert, an experienced observer, an objective scientist and a philosopher of rare ability. Dr. MacLean has spent much of his life in the in-depth study of the interrelationships between the anatomical structures and the physiological functions of brains, and of the behaviors of the owners of these brains. He has studied and observed the brains and behaviors of the animal kingdom, from lizards to humans. He has done these studies with a high degree of objectivity. However, his objectivity did not cause him to sacrifice his ability to interpret on a subjective level. He has done his work in great depth.

I find MacLean's model of the triune brain an extremely fascinating and useful one. It is fascinating in its display of the ingenious ways in which he has integrated the several academic disciplines in which he has expertise. It is useful in that it helps us to understand why people and animals do what they do. It also helps us to predict what they will do in a variety of circumstances.

For all the accolades I could heap upon MacLean and his Triune Brain Model, remember that a model is still a model. In science, models are not laws, nor are they inflexible. A model is put forth as a temporary explanation that can be used to explain why things are as they are. It attempts to tell us what responses we might expect when we put in certain stimuli, and where things might be going from there. Clearly, the model is a way of freeing ourselves from dogma. A model is either changed or discarded when it does not satisfactorily explain things as they happen within the system to which that model has been applied. MacLean's model is not perfect. It is a model that provides a framework or matrix upon which we can base further thought and investigation about brains, behaviors, and evolutionary relationships between all creatures that possess central nervous systems. MacLean's model answers some questions. It raises more questions that take the place of those it answers.

Topic 56

The Foundation of the Triune Brain Model

In order to more easily comprehend MacLean's triune brain model, I should like to briefly review the in utero development of the human brain.

As you may recall from our previous discussions, at the gestational age of four weeks, when the fetus is about four millimeters long, there is a neural tube that has developed. This neural tube will become the brain and spinal cord of the child. At the head end of this neural tube three vesicles have developed. These vesicles are arranged longitudinally along the neural tube. They are not side to side. A vesicle can be defined in this situation as a small bladder-like cavity that is most often, and is for our purposes, filled with fluid. These three vesicles are destined to develop into the forebrain, the midbrain and the hindbrain. The neural tube will, within another two weeks, at six weeks gestational age, attain an embryonic length of about six millimeters, and the forebrain will further subdivide into two vesicles. These vesicles will develop into the telencephalon, which is close to the extreme head end of the embryo, and the diencephalon, which is right behind the telencephalon.

The midbrain is directly behind the diencephalon, and the hindbrain is right behind the midbrain as we look from the head end towards the tail end of the neural tube. The vesicle that will be the midbrain does not further subdivide into more vesicles. The hindbrain, at about the same time that the forebrain is subdividing, also subdivides into two vesicles. These two vesicles will become the metencephalon, which is right behind the midbrain, and the myelencephalon, which is next in line looking from head to tail. The neural tube, as it extends tailward from the myelencephalon, will become the spinal cord.

MacLean's triune brain model deals only with the forebrain. Everything behind the diencephalon (the tailward subdivision of the forebrain vesicle) is considered as a "neural chassis" by MacLean. This neural chassis takes care of vital life functions, reflexive physiological activities like breathing, digestion, heart beating and so on. MacLean's model does not consider that the neural chassis has much to do with behavior which is beyond the vegetative state.

In his model, MacLean conceives of three separate but functionally and structurally integrated brains that cap the neural chassis. These three brains, in the order of the phylogenetic as well as intrauterine appearance or development are: (1) the reptilian brain, which he equates closely with the R-Complex, (2) the mammalian brain, which is pretty much what we know as the limbic system and (3) the neocortex. I shall try to explain how MacLean uses these three brains to explain both brain development and behavioral interrelationships between all vertebrates. Just in case there is any doubt, a vertebrate is any animal that has a spinal column/vertebral column. The vertebrate is a member of the subdivision vertebrata, of the phylum Chordata. Vertebrates include all mammals, birds, reptiles, amphibians and fishes. Chordata is the phylum that includes all animals that have had a notochord at any stage of their embryological development.

All vertebrates have a neural chassis. In the uterus, including the human embryo, the neural chassis develops first. Then, if the embryo is destined to develop at least to the level of reptile, the reptilian brain of MacLean develops functionally as a cap which would be placed upon the head of the neural chassis. Remember that the neural chassis ends at the top of the midbrain. Essentially then, the neural chassis is almost the same as the brain stem, although some authorities do not include all or part of the midbrain in the brain stem.

MacLean stresses the idea that the neural chassis remains intact. It is capped by, and not replaced by, the reptilian brain, but is significantly under the influence of the reptilian brain. If the embryo is destined to be a reptile, this is as far as the brain development goes. When the embryo of the reptile is born, it has a neural chassis and a reptilian brain cap. If the embryo was to be a fish, it would have been born with just the neural chassis and no reptilian brain cap. If, on the other hand, the embryo was destined to be a lower order of mammal, subsequent to the development of the reptilian brain cap, another cap would develop on top of the reptilian brain. This second cap in MacLean's model would be the mammalian brain cap. This mammalian brain cap then exerts influence and some control over both the reptilian brain cap and the neural chassis. Now let's consider that the embryo is destined to become a human or another higher mammal, such as a dolphin or a whale. Should this be the case, a third cap would develop after the completion of the development of the mammalian brain cap. This third cap is the neocortex. The neocortex has further refined abilities and functions. It exerts some modicum of control and influence over the mammalian brain cap as well as the reptilian brain cap and the neural chassis.

At this point you may say, "So what's the big deal?" The "big deal" is this: All of the instincts, reflexes, perceptions, responses, etc., that reside in the neural chassis, the reptilian brain cap and the mammalian brain cap, are present deep inside of the brain of the most refined and intelligent human being. To be sure, these lower animal instincts may be very well controlled or suppressed, but they are there and they require energy to be controlled. Based on this concept, a lot of the "neurotic" behaviors, such as compulsions, obsessions, phobias, rituals and the like, can be explained. These behaviors may be located in one of our deeper brain caps or in our neural chassis.

We will consider each of these MacLean "brains" in greater detail in a moment, but for the sake of clarity let's look at a few simple examples. The neural chassis is concerned with vital life functions, like breathing, heart pumping and so on. Consider that you cannot hold your breath until you suffocate yourself to death. Your neocortex may say yes, you want to do this, but you will pass out first and recommence breathing again unless there is some pathological condition that kills you as you are holding your breath. Further, as you run low on oxygen you get this powerful reflexive urge to breathe. Your diaphragm starts pumping away and it is all you can do to keep yourself from breathing. This strong urge to breathe that you may or may not be able to overcome is the little debate going on inside between your neocortex that wants you to hold your breath and your neural chassis that wants you to breathe. Ultimately, the neural chassis will win. You may have to lose consciousness, but you will breathe. The neural chassis is more primitive and powerful in the area of vital life forces.

The reptilian brain is ritualistic, deceptive, territorial and survivalistic. The mammalian brain is the seat of altruism, sense of family, motherhood and apple pie, emotion, play and the like. The neocortex is, of course, the intellect. The person who has too many martinis or too much ethanol (alcohol) in any kind of fancy or palatable presentation, demonstrates perfectly how the uppermost cap controls and influences the brain caps beneath it. Alcohol anesthetizes the brain from the higher centers downward to the neural chassis. So, let's look at our drinker. First, the neocortex is rendered dysfunctional. The good decisions disappear. As the mammalian brain cap becomes the highest functionally operating cap, the drinker becomes emotional, loyal, backslapping, gregarious, overly expansive, etc. He buys a drink for the house. His wife is the best little woman in the world, and so on. As he continues drinking more alcohol, perhaps because his neocortical judgment is numbed, this gregarious, friendly, loving person may well change. His mammalian brain cap is getting numbed. Now the reptilian brain cap takes charge. Territoriality becomes apparent. "Hey, get off of my bar stool or I'll knock you flat," and so on. He displays rituals, and if you get in the way he may try to attack you. He won't usually bother you if you are not in his proclaimed territory. If he continues to imbibe he will anesthetize his reptilian brain cap. Now he'll just pass out and his neural chassis will keep him alive until the alcohol is metabolized from his brain. He may not know what he did, because the neocortex is a significant factor in conscious memory. The other two caps have some memory function, but each has a little different quality as the memory relates to consciousness.

I recall floating in an isolation tank and becoming aware that my body was moving like a fish. My neural chassis remembered how fish swim, but I certainly did not remember on a conscious level.

In addition to alcohol causing the various MacLean brains to become dysfunctional, I believe it is fairly obvious that stress, fear, anger, lust for power and so on can have similar effects. When nations go through the times of colonizing other lands, or when they fight over international boundaries, this may be a manifestation to some degree of failed neocortical influence over the reptilian brain. When you get angry and it won't go away and you start grinding your teeth in your sleep, this may be a manifestation of loss of neocortical control over the mammalian brain cap. Lower mammals fight, hunt and survive in their world largely by their jaws and by their teeth. Reptiles are deceptive. That is part of how they survive. When a human is particularly deceptive and untrustworthy, we sometimes call that human a "snake." This could be a more appropriate name calling than we realize. Consider that the poorly controlled reptilian brain may well manifest itself with deceptive behavior.

We could go on and on, but I'm sure that you get the idea.

The Reptilian Brain

In MacLean's model the reptilian brain, which is the most primitive of his three brains, caps the neural chassis. It makes up about 75 percent of the gray matter of the center of the brain. This means it has a preponderance of neuron cell bodies and other nonmyelinated structures.

Contained within MacLean's reptilian brain are the basal ganglia. These basal ganglia are large masses of gray matter located deep in the basal regions of the cerebral hemispheres. They contribute part of the walls of the lateral ventricles. Functionally, the basal ganglia represent the cerebral limb of the extrapyramidal motor system. This motor system is largely responsible for the more automatic and largely non-conscious aspects of posture and locomotion.

The substantia nigra is sometimes the name used to mean the basal ganglia, even though the substantia nigra is only one of the components.   The name substantia nigra means "black substance." This name has been applied because of the dark color of this area of brain tissue. The dark color is due to a higher concentration of melanin pigment in these tissues.

Classical anatomists, as is common, have some disagreement about which brain structures shall be included as basal ganglia components. However, they are in agreement that the following structures are within the general category:

1. Corpus Striatum
    a. Globus Pallidus
    b. Caudate Nucleus
    c. Putamen
2. Subthalamic Nucleus
3. Red Nucleus
4. Substantia Nigra
5. All of the above structures have interconnections with the reticular formation, the cerebellum and the cerebrum. Some authorities include these interconnections as parts of the basal ganglia and some don't. It's your choice.

Also, we find that authorities disagree upon whether or not the amygdaloid bodies are part of the basal ganglia. MacLean places these amygdaloid bodies in the mammalian brain. Therefore, he does not consider them as part of the basal ganglia. There is also disagreement about the classification of the vestibular nuclei and even the cerebellum. A few authorities would place these structures within the basal ganglia.

MacLean uses the terms reptilian brain, striatal complex and R-Complex almost interchangeably. He divides his reptilian brain into four main categories according to their output of nerve impulses:

1. Olfactostriatum, which offers most of its output to the hypothalamus and the midbrain.
2. Corpus Striatum, which offers most of its output to the globus pallidus and the substantia nigra.
3. Globus pallidus, which offers most of its output to the subthalamic nucleus, the thalamus, and to the tegmentum of both the subthalamus and the midbrain.
4. Substantia innominata, which offers most of its output to the hypothalamus.

In MacLean's model, most of the nerve impulses that go into the basal ganglia come from the reticular system, the limbic system (especially the amygdala and the cingulate cortex), and from widespread areas of the neocortex.

Reptilian Brain Function

The functions of the reptilian brain according to MacLean are not only motor, as many authorities assert. The reptilian brain does indeed seem to be involved in higher motor reflexes, and in the motor activities related to speech. Most authorities are in agreement up to this point. But beyond these motor functions, the argument begins.

MacLean has studied the behavior patterns of a wide variety of reptiles. These reptiles do not possess the next brain cap. There is no mammalian brain. The highest order of brain tissue that they possess is the reptilian brain cap, which is also known as the R-Complex, and includes little more than the basal ganglia. Yet MacLean, in his studies, has observed reptiles to exhibit grooming behavior. They rub themselves against the ground in order to remove objects which may be attached to their skin. They breed by copulation, preceded by some ritualistic behavior, but actually very little compared to the mating dances of the mammals. They are very territorial. That is, they mark off an area that is theirs, and they will attack and fight to keep it. They do very little migration in groups or flocks. Reptiles are much more alone than are mammals, but in severe cold weather they do group together. A dominant reptile will often harass a submissive reptile to the death. Reptiles will either avoid or attack unfamiliar creatures or objects. Whether the reptile in question chooses to avoid or attack is extremely unpredictable.

Reptiles follow routines on a day-to-day basis. For example, a typical day in the life of a reptile such as a lizard might look like this: The reptile emerges from its shelter and basks in the sun for a while. Then the reptile defecates and begins feeding within its own territory. This morning feeding process goes on for as much as four hours. Next comes an afternoon siesta. The siesta is followed by an afternoon feeding. During this second feeding of the day, the reptile may become adventurous and search for food outside of its own territory. After filling the stomach, the reptile basks in the sun again within its own territory. It then returns to its shelter for the night. This is not unlike humans, when performance pressure is relaxed or removed entirely.

Woven within the matrix of the aforementioned master routine for the day are several behavioral characteristics. Some of these characteristics will seem familiar to you if you observe your own behaviors, and those of your friends and neighbors. There are powerful suggestions in human activities that we all still possess active reptilian brain caps. You will probably see examples of isopraxic behavior, which simply means that there is a lot of imitation going on. Humans, like reptiles, respond in positive or negative ways to most stimuli without first reasoning which way to respond. Both species manifest many reflex responses. Madison Avenue takes advantage of this behavior pattern when it markets various products. We all do lots of repetitious behaviors. You can "people watch" in a mall or "lizard watch" in your local lizard hangout to see this.

Reptiles do a lot of deceptive behaviors. Deception is a way of life which is necessary for the reptile's survival. Deceptive practices are rooted in the reptilian brain cap, and if you people watch, you need not look far to see that this reptilian brain cap activity is still there in many, many people. In fact, one might consider that the best tennis stars, the best basketball players, and the best quarterbacks and receivers and runners in football are the best at deception or "faking."

Reptiles also have signature behaviors. In our backyard there is a rather large colony of small lizards. These lizards are continually doing "push-ups" and puffing out the large red throat areas. MacLean interprets these signature behaviors as warnings to other lizards not to be aggressive. These behaviors are also used to attract females. (It is only the males that do the "push-ups" and the red-throat displays.) When one male lizard is intimidated by another male lizard, he turns around and gets as small and tight to the ground as he can.

Lots of people do similar things. Macho men flex their muscles and build their bodies. We see displays of muscle power on television in Mr. Universe contests. We see women on display in beauty pageants. Some of what you see is almost certainly a manifestation of the reptilian brain cap. It is signature behavior; it says, "Look at who I am."

Yes, we all have reptilian brain caps, which are suppressed in their activities to some extent by the mammalian brain cap and the neocortex. But the suppression is not complete, and the reptilian brain shows through to variable extents at different times and in different persons.

Some of the diseases of humans that affect MacLean's reptilian brain cap are such things as Parkinson's disease, Huntington's disease, Sydenham's chorea and so on. These are all diseases that affect motor control and result in repetitive, purposeless motion. MacLean also suggests the possibility that autism and schizophrenia, because of the repetitive movements, may be problems related to the human reptilian brain cap.

The Mammalian Brain

MacLean's mammalian brain cap is formed as a cap which covers or overlies the reptilian brain cap. In utero, the mammalian brain cap develops after the reptilian brain cap has formed over the neural chassis. If the embryo is destined to become a mammal, it remains in the uterus beyond the time when the reptile would have been born, in order to further develop the mammalian brain cap and thus, supposedly, have more intelligence than the reptile.

MacLean's mammalian brain is pretty much synonymous with the limbic system as it is classically described. Anatomically, the limbic system sort of wraps around the brain stem. It forms a sort of boundary around the brain stem. According to MacLean, the limbic system or mammalian brain cap has no overlap or representation in the reptilian brain. However, a few authorities would place the amygdaloid bodies, which are part of MacLean's limbic system, within the basal ganglia. If this confuses you, don't worry. You are not alone.

The mammalian brain cap provides mammals with three main distinctions that are not found in reptiles. First, mammals nurse their offspring and provide maternal care. Reptiles let the newborn fend for themselves. Second, mammals have audiovocal communication between mother and offspring. This may take the form of almost any sound you can imagine, but it works. Reptiles have no audiovocal communication. Third, mammals play with each other. Parents play with offspring in various ways, and they teach as they play. Siblings play with each other and they develop many skills needed for survival in this way. Reptiles do not play. They seem to rely upon inborn survival instincts. The mammalian brain cap is the place where the concept of family and altruism is housed. It is the home of maternal and paternal instinct, and of sibling love. The neocortex may say that a particular parent has been hateful to a child. But it is a major chore for the neocortex to suppress the instinctive mammalian brain love of the child for the abusive parent. It is difficult to overcome the love instinct, even though it makes good neocortical sense not to love. It can be done, but it takes a good bit of energy to turn against a parent or a sibling or your own child.

The limbic system, or mammalian brain cap, is divided into three main subdivisions. These are: (1) the amygdalar, (2) the septal and (3) the thalamocingulate subdivisions. The hippocampus is included in the amygdalar subdivision according to some authorities, and others put the hippocampus within the septal subdivision. For our purposes it matters little which authorities you favor, because we will look at the limbic system as the mammalian brain cap, and will be most interested in its function.

The mammalian brain is both interoceptive and exteroceptive. Interoceptive refers to the fact that it receives information from various sources within the body. Exteroceptive refers to the fact that it also receives information from the environment outside of the body.

On the interoceptive side, the mammalian brain cap receives nerve impulse input from the senses of taste and smell. It receives sensations from the mouth, the throat (esophagus), the stomach, the duodenum (beginning of the small bowel at the end of the stomach), the colon, and from all of the organs located in the pelvis. It receives many of the sensual sensations from the pelvis which relate to sexual activity.

The mammalian brain cap also receives a lot of input from the hypothalamus, which has a lot to do with emotional feelings. It also receives interoceptive input from the midbrain. The midbrain relays and forwards information to the mammalian brain cap that is related to the conditions inside the body, such as the tension in muscles, the condition of internal organs and the like.

The exteroceptive input to the mammalian brain cap is largely from olfactory, visual and auditory stimuli. Clearly, the mammalian brain cap of MacLean is a place that receives a lot of input related to survival.

Topic 60

What the Mammalian Brain Does For You

In general, the mammalian brain cap is the place where all the activities related to food take place. This includes hunting, killing prey, searching out vegetable foods, protecting food once obtained and so on. It also is the seat of sexual and procreative activities, as well as maternal care for offspring such as nursing, protection and so on. It is the seat of play between parents and offspring, and between siblings. The mammalian brain cap is the place that makes us aware of danger, gives us fear, gives us the anger and/or courage to attack.

The mammalian brain cap is also the seat of emotion. It remembers and re-presents various emotional responses, especially to smells. It is the source of our romantic and/or sexual responses to these various smells. Without the mammalian brain cap, there would probably not be a perfume industry, nor would we use deodorants.

The mammalian brain cap has the ability to turn the volume of emotional response either up or down. When you control your emotions, your neocortex is probably requesting your mammalian brain cap to reduce the intensity to a lower level, or perhaps even to keep the emotional response at a non-conscious level.

The mammalian brain cap is also where we have our sense of self. Without this mammalian brain cap, we would look in a mirror and not know ourselves. It is largely in the hippocampus where sense of self resides.

The mammalian brain gives us ongoing memory for recent events. When this mammalian brain cap is damaged, the individual may not be able to remember any present events, but they may easily recall childhood, etc. It would be the extreme of absent-mindedness.

Seizures

Psychomotor epilepsy, temporal lobe seizures and limbic seizures are all names for the same condition. MacLean might call them mammalian brain cap seizures. These are seizures that involve emotion with physiological concomitants. That is, during the mammalian brain cap seizure the patient might experience the extreme of a wide range of emotions. He/she might experience uncontrollable rage or terror or ecstasy, or even sexual orgasm. Or he/she might experience anything in between these extremes, or a combination of emotions, depending upon which regions of the mammalian brain cap are affected. Concurrently, almost any internal organ response might occur. The heart could race to the point where you feel like it will explode and stop. Or you could become extremely short of breath, or your bowel could cramp and so on. The possibilities are almost endless.

MacLean presents a theory of one way that mammalian brain seizures could be caused. He feels that, since the mammalian brain cap is largely within the temporal lobes of the brain, the damage could easily be caused during the birthing process.

MacLean paints the following scenario as a possible causal event. The temporal lobes of the brain rest upon a relatively horizontal meningeal membrane of dura mater called the tentorium cerebelli. This horizontal membrane has an opening in its center which allows the passage of the brain stem to go down towards its spinal cord connection. MacLean theorizes that, when the top of the infant's head is compressed by its passage through the birth canal, it might cause a partial and temporary herniation of the brain hemispheres through this opening in the tentorium cerebelli. This situation, or even a prolonged excessive pressure of the undersurface of the cerebral hemispheres of the brain upon the tentorium cerebelli, could cause a bruising of the underside of the temporal lobes. This is because the lobes would be the parts of the cerebral hemispheres that contact the free border of the opening of the tentorium cerebelli. Also, it seems quite possible that the blood supply to the temporal lobes of the brain could be damaged by this pressure or herniation. In either case, bruising of the brain tissue or compromise of blood supply, or a combination of the two, might result in irritation of brain tissue due to very tiny areas of blood cells escaping from capillaries into brain tissue. This extravasated blood (escaped from the blood vessels) sets up an irritation in the brain tissue which worsens as the extravasated blood cells deteriorate. The irritation causes some brain cells to turn into fibrous tissue (similar to scar tissue) which, in turn, hardens to sclerotic tissue. This tissue both irritates the normal brain tissue and interferes with the delivery of fresh arterial blood to the nearby brain tissues. The result of either or both of these situations might well be a seizure disorder.

As a practitioner of CranioSacral Therapy, I find this theory to be quite feasible. I also know that the problem could most likely be corrected by a good CranioSacral Therapist during the first few days after delivery.

The Neocortex

It appears to me that the major focus of MacLean's detailed personal study has been more upon the reptilian and mammalian brain caps. For his concepts of the neocortex, he relies more upon the work of others, especially upon the observations and reports of neurosurgeons.

MacLean puts forth the concept that, not only does the neocortex influence the reptilian and the mammalian brain caps, but these two "brains" also influence the neocortex. He also seems convinced that the two-way influencing involves mostly the frontal areas of the neocortex. He speaks very little about interrelationships between the parietal, temporal and/or occipital cortical regions and the reptilian and mammalian brain caps. I would not rule out the possibilities of more widespread interrelationships with the whole neocortex. It seems only that the investigatory work had not been done at the time that MacLean published his triune brain concept/model in 1990.

In his writing, MacLean uses the terms protomentation and emotionalmentation. Protomentation refers to the intercommunications and influences upon each other by the neocortex and the reptilian brain cap. This protomentation refers to what we do when we start thinking about our routines and begin evaluating and perhaps changing them. In reverse, it refers to our awareness of how much we are captives of our own routines and rituals.

Emotionalmentation refers to the interrelationships and influences between the neocortex and the mammalian brain cap. This process of emotionalmentation lets us know how strong an emotional response might be, and how difficult it may be to control or dampen that emotional response. In reverse, we may be thinking of a certain thing which stimulates the communication between the neocortex and the mammalian brain cap. This, too, is emotionalmentation. Clearly, the mammalian brain is the structure that gives us humans our feelings of empathy and altruism.

MacLean sights many cases that support his model of interrelationships between the three brains. When the neocortex is not present in a human due to surgical removal, tumor, accident, etc., it is often observed that the person will lie, cheat, deceive, etc. These behaviors are not premeditated according to MacLean, but rather are manifestations of the reptilian brain in the act of providing survival behaviors without moderation or influence of the neocortex. If the person is very ingratiating and yet very deceptive (and you have probably met some of these people), MacLean feels that the ingratiating manner is also part of the reptilian brain survival-skills activity. The deceptive actions are moment-to-moment survival activities. They are not premeditated.

Also, it has been observed quite often that a lack of the frontal neocortex correlates to a lack of anxiety. MacLean considers anxiety to be that unpleasant and uneasy feeling that sometimes accompanies the anticipation of coming or future events. The same person, however, can and does experience immediate fear when tangible danger is present.

Without our neocortex, we simply would not envision a future. We would live day to day without long-range goals or objectives. The mammalian brain cap likes to play, and without the neocortex to influence it, we would seek more immediate pleasure and fun. Also, without the neocortex to moderate mammalian brain cap activity, we would laugh and cry a lot more. And we might do it at times that neocortically endowed persons would surely consider most inappropriate.

The neocortex is also very necessary for problem solving, mathematics and the like. I'm sure that by now you get the idea. I have presented this synopsis of MacLean's triune brain model because I believe it does indeed shed light upon behaviors and behavior disorders that may relate to various brain structure abnormalities, and to the ways in which our behaviors may appear inconsistent when we are placed in certain stressful situations. It isn't a perfect model, but I have found it to be quite helpful.

Section IX

The Whole Is Greater Than the Sum of Its Parts

The Whole

By the whole, I mean our consciousness, our behaviors and our responses. When I say consciousness, I mean all levels of consciousness. There are several levels of consciousness of which we are aware, and there are many, many levels of consciousness of which we are unaware. At the present time, we are just beginning to scratch the surface of a true understanding of consciousness at any of its levels. There have been many theories of consciousness which have turned out to be invalid. The problem is so difficult to research, partially because we have to use our own consciousness to research consciousness. Our own consciousness is largely dependent upon our perceptions of our internal and external influences and environments. Since there probably are not two people who perceive exactly the same, it becomes very difficult, if not impossible, to be objective about consciousness in general, as well as its components.

How do you make the jump from increased electrical impulses and increased neurotransmitter (biochemical) activity within a neurocircuit in the brain to the perceived image of a beautiful glowing sunset that elicits feelings of peace, tranquillity and joy? After all, what happened in the brain is increased electrical and chemical activity in specific areas, and yet, we perceive a warm glow of peace and love going through our whole body as we look at this beautiful sunset. How does this happen? It doesn't happen without a brain. At least, we don't think it does. But how do we know that the brainless animal does not feel a rush of warmth and peace and love in the presence of the same sunset? (Decerebration is a much-used experimental method.) On the other hand, if you are a night creature you might perceive the same sunset as a signal to get up and get going, a signal to find food, to hunt down a prey, to find a mate and so on. We have lots of raccoons in our neighborhood. They sleep all day, they frolic at night. They are very, very smart, if I can gauge their intelligence by their ability to outwit me when I wanted them out of the attic of our house. For several weeks, every morning at about four a.m. they would return to our dormers and run and jump. They were like an alarm clock. I put about 100 mothballs in the overhead of our house because I reasoned that the unpleasant smell would discourage the raccoons from continued occupancy above our ceilings. Not so. They threw the mothballs out and continued occupancy. Finally, I realized that the family — mother and three little ones — left every evening at sundown and returned at about four a.m. So, I put heavy-duty screening across the entryway after I saw them leave. They came back and I was up to greet them. Mother raccoon tried to get through the screening, and she was very good at finding the weak spots. I became concerned so I went out and spoke with her. I told her she had to find another home. She listened. After about ten minutes of conversing, she chattered at her little ones and they left. They never returned. What sort of consciousness do raccoons have? What feeling do they get when they see a sunset?

Some more puzzlements about consciousness arise from experience with hypnosis. What is the consciousness of hypnosis? I have done this and still wonder how it works. I have induced a patient into a deep hypnotic trance. Then I have burned the back of the right hand with a lighted cigarette. I told the patient that I was burning the back of the left hand. The patient felt the burn on the back of the left hand and a blister was raised on the back of the left hand. This patient's consciousness became convinced by my words that the burn was on the opposite hand from the contact with the lighted cigarette. And the body responded physiologically with blister formation to the mistaken conscious perception. Can we reliably study consciousness with consciousness?

How many times have you suddenly, hours later, realized that you did something of which you were unaware at the time? Just recently I was leaving a hotel after giving some lectures. I flew home. When I awakened the next morning, I could clearly see my vitamin chest left on the counter top in the hotel bathroom. I had not unpacked, and when I looked in my suitcase there was no vitamin chest. I called the hotel and they had my vitamin chest in the housekeeping department's lost and found. I saw the vitamin chest clearly, just as I had left it the day before. Yet at the time I left the hotel room, I thought that I had packed it. What part of my consciousness recorded my error and told me about it later? How do electrochemical phenomena get transposed into awareness, not at the time but hours later? I have this type of experience at least once a month. If you think about it, you probably have had similar experiences.

How many times do you go to bed with a question on your mind and wake up with the answer? I have come to rely upon this phenomenon. In writing this very chapter, I have puzzled over how to approach this question of consciousness for several days. Then one night as I was about to go to sleep, I said to myself that it was time to get to it. I awakened at six a.m. with the title for the section and a general outline of the approach to the problem. It is this outline and approach that you are now reading. How do brain cells intercommunicate during sleep, send out electrical impulses, act out biochemical reactions, and have me awaken with a new concept that was created by my brain while I was in another state of consciousness which we call sleep? Yes, we can describe some of the electrical and the biochemical phenomena that accompany an insight or the beginning of a new creative concept, but how do we get from the observed electrochemical activities to an image which is unfamiliar to us? An image which has been newly created by a bunch of electrical and biochemical actions and reactions.

Another one that I find puzzling is the person who has had one too many alcohol-containing libations. They black out. They get from the bar and wake up in bed in the morning with a horrible headache and no recollection of how they got home. A good friend of mine who does not often overindulge in spirits fermenti had this experience just recently. What happened in terms of consciousness and brain function?

For decades the majority of neuroscientists and medical practitioners have accepted the dogma that sets forth the proposition that the "intelligence" of the animal or human is positively correlated with the size of the brain. Some carried this idea a step further and stated that the level of "intelligence" is positively correlated with the thickness of the cerebral cortex. With modern technology comes evidence that these dogmatic ideas are obsolete and incorrect. Recently, studies have been done on above-average and academically inclined individuals. These studies show that even microcephalics are quite capable of being honor students. In fact, a significant percentage of the honors mathematics majors at a California University who were studied turned out to be microcephalic. One particular patient studied by a neurosurgeon in England had an IQ score of over 120 and was an accomplished mathematician. Tests showed that the brain tissue outside of the ventricular system (this includes the cerebral cortex and some subcortical tissue) was generally less than 1 millimeter in thickness. A millimeter is a bit less than 1/16 of an inch. There goes the theory that brain size and cortical thickness determines the level of intelligence. It will probably take several years before the dogma is overthrown, but in the meantime there is plenty of room for hope with microcephalics and hydrocephalics with enlarged ventricles.

So what are awarenesses, instincts, intuitive thoughts, precognitions, synchronous thoughts and images, perceptions, memories, feelings, generalizations, problem-solving skills, insights, strokes of genius, creative abilities, innate talents, and so on and on and on. To be very honest, we don't know. We can talk about some of the physical phenomena that accompany some of these conscious or unconscious phenomena. But we cannot as yet, and may never be able to, explain how some tiny nerve impulses at a given place in the brain can make you feel so good, or make you feel so bad, or make you see a picture of a tree, or make an equation pop into your head that solves a problem, or make you see where you lost your car keys. The mystery remains. The whole is definitely much greater than the sum of its parts.

The Parts

The parts of the nervous system in its entirety have been under study for several decades. Recent discoveries have shown how various parts are structured and how they function. But the jump from how the parts work so that they present us with the ideas, perceptions and feelings that we experience, is a great jump indeed. Nonetheless, we will take a brief look at several of the parts that comprise the nervous system, especially the brain and the spinal cord.

I am sure that, by the time we finish our brief look at these components, you will appreciate that the intelligence that designed the nervous system must possess true genius. Included in the designer's areas of expertise and genius would be architectural design, electrical engineering, biochemistry, pharmacology, physics, biology, psychology, computer design, technology and programming, theory of chaos, embryology, statistics and so on. It is a humbling experience to realize that one of us might spend a lifetime of study in order to gain just a fraction of the wisdom in a single one of these areas that the designer of the human brain employed to build such a beautifully functional and mysterious organ.

Topic 65

Neurons, Synapses and Glial Cells

The cells in the nervous system are neurons and glial cells. The neurons are the cells that, until recently, have received most of the attention of the researchers. This is because the neurons were considered to be the most important. After all, it is the neuron that conducts the electrical impulses to the central nervous system from the sensory receptors. It is the neurons that decide what, if anything, to do about the information that is coming into the spinal cord and the brain. Once the neurons have decided upon which actions to take, they then conduct the electrical impulses to the effector organs.

When one neuron has to communicate with another neuron, it does so across a synapse. A synapse is the junction between two neurons. It is hard to believe, but a single neuron may have as many as 10,000 synaptic connections with other neurons. That is, a single neuron in the brain may functionally communicate with 10,000 other neurons. This makes the potential choices for messages going in different directions through the brain at any given instant a number that is beyond my own comprehension. That number is in the billions. Is it any wonder that once in a while we have to take a moment or two to "think about it?"

The neuron is composed of a cell body, an axon, and one or more dendrites. The axon and the dendrites are microscopic projections of cytoplasm from the cell body. The dendrites receive impulses or messages from other neurons and take them into the cell body of the receiving neuron. The axon is usually singular, and is most often longer than a dendrite. There is usually only one axon, and one cell body, for each neuron (**Fig. 9-1**). The number of dendrites per cell body is variable, but there are usually more than one, and there may be hundreds.

The axon is the sending organ of the neuron. The electrical impulse, which is the neuronal message, goes away from the cell body via the axon. The axon transmits the message either to another neuron or to an end organ, such as a gland or a muscle. The transmission of the electrical impulse along the axon is dependent primarily upon the movement of electrically charged particles called ions. The ions move in a controlled fashion through the membrane that encloses the axon. The principal ions that are important in the transmission of electrical impulses from one end of the neuron to the other are sodium, potassium, calcium, chloride and, to a more limited extent, magnesium.

The neuron cell body does many things. It includes the nucleus which has the DNA, or genetic material, that tells the neuron in general what it can and can't do. The neuronal cell body also has mitochondria, which make protein molecules. Each of these molecules has very specific functions. These protein molecules are often sent down the axon to a destination in order to help

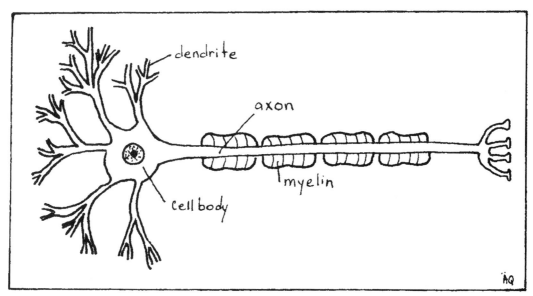

Fig. 9-1
A Typical Neuron:
Dendrites receive nerve impulses from other neurons. These impulses are conducted into the cell body and out the axon to their destinations, which could be to other neurons or end organs, such as muscle fibers, glands, etc.

keep the effector organ vital, or to assist in the function of the synapse. The cell body may have several other inclusions in it, but the ones that have received the most attention from researchers thus far are the nucleus and the mitochondria. The matrix of the cell body is cytoplasm, which is more or less the viscous fluid that fills the membrane and, along with the cytoskeleton of the cell body, gives the body its shape. As I previously mentioned, the axon extends either to another neuron or to an effector or end organ. The junction at the end of the axon is always the synapse.

Usually, the synaptic communication is biochemical. There is a space between the axon and the next neuron or the effector organ in the biochemical synapse. Another less common type of synapse is the gap junction synapse. In the gap junction synapse, there is no biochemical substance (neurotransmitter) required for the electrical impulse to go on to the next neuron. These gap junction synapses have a much smaller space between the delivering axon and the receiving neuron or dendrite. The electrical impulse is conducted directly from the axon to the next dendrite across protein bridge molecules or connectors.

In the gap junction synapse, the electrical current can flow in only one direction. In the regular biochemical or neurotransmitter synapses, the electrical impulse sometimes moves in a retrograde direction. The two neurons involved in a gap junction synapse must be of similar size for the electrical impulse to cross the cleft between them.

Regular synapses are synapses that convert the electrical impulse to biochemical activity in order to cross the cleft between the delivering axon and the next neuron or end organ, and they are much more numerous. The cleft space across this synapse is about 10 times wider than the gap junction synapse. The biochemicals that enable the message to cross the regular synapses are known as neurotransmitters.

Before we talk about neurotransmitters, let's look at the types of regular synapses. There are essentially three types (**Fig. 9-2**). The regular synaptic types are named appropriately according to their components. The most common type of the regular synapse is called the axodendritic synapse. This synaptic type is formed when the impulse delivering axon participates with an impulse receiving dendrite to form the synapse.

The second type is called the axosomatic synapse. As you might guess, this type of synapse is formed by an impulse-delivering axon and an impulse-receiving cell body. The axon via the synapse sends its impulse directly into the cell body. It does not fool around with the dendrite.

The third type of synapse is the axoaxonic synapse. In this case, the impulse-delivery axon delivers its impulse via the synapse to another axon which is presynaptic. That is, the impulse-receiving axon is headed for another synapse and receives this impulse before it gets to its own intended synapse. The effect of this axoaxonic synapse on the impulse-receiving axon is usually one of inhibition. That is, it reduces the delivery potential of the post-axoaxonic synapse axon to deliver its own message impulse to its intended destination synapse. This does not mean that the axon in question can't deliver. It simply means that it requires a stronger or longer stimulus to make it deliver. Another name for the axoaxonic synapse is the presynaptic synapse.

The glial cells have been the most neglected cells of the nervous system. There are about twice as many glial cells as there are neurons. Many of the functions of the glial cells are still in question and under investigation. All of the cells in the nervous system that are not neurons are called glial cells, except for the cells that are related to blood vessels.

Some of the known functions of the glial cells are as follows.

1. They provide mechanical support for neurons.
2. They produce myelin sheathing. In the central nervous system, it is the oligodendroglial cells (a subdivision of glial cells) that produces the myelin. In the peripheral nervous system, it is the Schwann cells (another subdivision of glial cells) that are responsible for myelination.
3. They function in the rapid uptake and inactivation of neurotransmitter substance that has been discharged into the synaptic cleft.
4. They form the scar tissue after brain and/or spinal cord injury.
5. They remove waste products and tissue debris after neuronal or other cell death.
6. They provide the filter system between blood and neurons.
7. They help control the concentration of the electrically charged ions in the fluid outside of the cells in which the neurons are bathed. Therefore, they help provide the correct levels of sodium, potassium, calcium, chloride and magnesium that are required for the neurons to do their work of electrical impulse conduction.

In addition to these known functions, there is some evidence to support the idea that glial cells help to guide the migrating neurons to the right places as the embryonic nervous system is developing.

The glial cells are divided into large cells (macroglia) and small cells (microglia). The system further divides and subdivides until it gets quite confusing. The classification of glial cells is constantly changing as new discoveries are being made. This further adds to the confusion. So we won't go into all the details and names. Suffice it that you know that astrocytes are the largest glial cells. These are the cells that make up the astrocytoma tumors, which are the most common of the brain tumors. The oligodendroglia that do the myelination in the brain are in the microglia glial cell family.

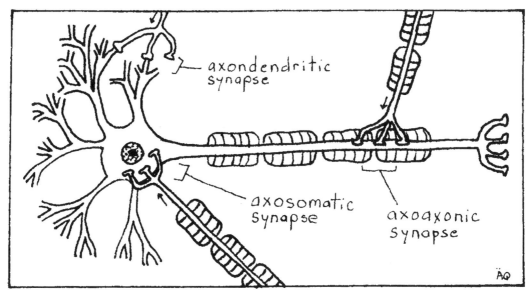

Fig. 9-2
Types of Synapses:
The axodendritic synapse is most common. The impulse comes into the dendrite from the axon
of another neuron. The other two types are the axosomatic and the axoaxonic, wherein axon
impulses go into the nerve cell body and the axon, respectively, from the axon of another neuron.
Axoaxonic synapses usually function in an inhibitory manner by reducing the impulse conduction
of the axon to which they connect.

The most recent research results are suggesting that glial cells may assist neurons more directly in electrical communication. Glutamine, one of the neurotransmitters, is manufactured inside of glial cells. The glutamine is then somehow transmitted into the neurons by the glial cells. Who knows where the study of glial cells will take us? A hundred years ago they were considered second-class citizens in the nervous system. It was thought that all they did was fill space and offer support to neurons.

The Neurotransmitters

The regular synapse is structured so that there are tiny vesicles or bubbles in the terminal end of the axon, very near the synapse. These vesicles are full of neurotransmitter chemicals. There is only one type of neurotransmitter in each vesicle, and usually there is only one type of neurotransmitter at a given synapse, even though there are many vesicles full of neurotransmitter in a given axon ending.

The neurotransmitter in the vesicle is a liquid that has specific chemical properties that can activate receptor sites on the other side of the synaptic cleft. All the neurotransmitter has to do is get to the other side of the synaptic cleft. When the electrical impulse comes down the axon as it nears the synapse, the vesicles, full of neurotransmitter solution, move to the synaptic surface of the impulse-delivering axon. The vesicles rupture and the molecules of neurotransmitter are discharged into the synaptic cleft. The synaptic cleft is the name given to the space between the surface of the impulse-delivering axon and the receiving structure, whatever it may be, on the other side of the synapse. When the neurotransmitter is discharged into the synaptic cleft, its molecules cross the cleft space and activate the receptors on the other side. The receiving neuron or end organ immediately converts this chemical energy into electrical energy, which the neuron then turns into an impulse of electricity. This impulse, in turn, travels out its axon to the next synapse. If the receptor is in a muscle, the neurotransmitter-delivered chemical energy is converted to electrical energy once again and causes the muscle to contract. So, you can see that neurotransmitters are chemical-energy carriers that serve to carry electrical messages from the sender to the receiver across a space between the two. The space is called the synaptic cleft and the whole unit is called the synapse.

To date, there are many neurotransmitters, and there are more being discovered almost monthly. The first two neurotransmitters to be discovered were acetylcholine and norepinephrine. Up until the 1950s, life with neurotransmitters was simple. Acetylcholine was considered to be the neurotransmitter that served muscle at its junction with the motor nerves. It was also the dominant neurotransmitter used by the parasympathetic division of the autonomic nervous system. This is the division that runs the restorative activities of the body by aiding digestion, kidney function, bladder and bowel evacuation, slowing heart rate, aiding liver and gall bladder function and the like.

Norepinephrine was the neurotransmitter that enabled us to run, to fight, to perform super-human acts that might save our lives or the lives of others in time of crisis. It stimulated the adrenal glands to do their thing, increased heart action, increased blood flow to muscles, opened your bronchi so you could get more oxygen, and shut down such things as digestive processes and so on. Life was so simple then. Today, there are over 32 newly discovered possible neurotransmitters. The functions of acetylcholine and norepinephrine are not nearly so straightforward as they were.

The next two neurotransmitters to be discovered after acetylcholine and norepinephrine were dopamine and serotonin. The confusion they caused mounted in the 1950s. Dopamine, as you probably know, is deficient in Parkinson's disease. This deficiency causes the shaking and lack of smooth unintentional movement that is so obvious in Parkinson's patients. Serotonin somehow may be related to mental problems. We know that it is related to mood problems of depression and psychosis. You get agitated when serotonin levels are high, and conversely you can get the blues when they are low.

Now we have many more neurotransmitters in the protein and amino acid category. There are still questions, but we do know some facts: (1) glutamate and aspartate excite the nervous system. (2) GABA and glycine inhibit the nervous system. (3) nicotine antagonizes acetylcholine. Therefore, it reduces brain and muscle action somewhat. Since the early ideas about acetylcholine, we have found that it is extremely important in brain function. It makes you think and remember. Hence, the tranquilizing effect of a "smoke," especially if you are hooked on nicotine. The endorphins are a natural opiate. You can get addicted to your own endorphins. This may be why you can go too far with an exaggerated exercise program and actually feel good while you physically hurt your body by giving it too much work to do.

Myelin

Myelin is a substance produced by the glial cells. It is produced by the oligodendroglia in the central nervous system, and by the Schwann cells in the peripheral nervous system. Myelin insulates the nerve axons and enables them to conduct electrical impulses more rapidly, and without short circuiting. If myelin breaks down or is destroyed, the impulses can leak out of the axon and the muscle does not get the intended message. The problem is very similar to a bare wire in your home or your car. Things just stop working right.

Sometimes children just don't make myelin. Then they have problems. Sometimes diseases like multiple sclerosis come along, which destroy myelin sheathing. These are usually autoimmune diseases which, for one reason or another, cause our own cells to digest our myelin. This leaves defects in the insulation and allows the nerve fibers to "short-circuit" or to "leak" their electrical impulses into the surrounding fluids and tissues. Incidentally, myelin is about 40 percent cholesterol. So cholesterol does do some good for us.

Topic 68

Closing Thought

This coverage of the finished product is far from inclusive of all we know or don't know about brains and how they work. But it should give you a background and a feel for things, so that you have a better chance of keeping abreast of some of the advances in neuroscience, and how they can affect you and your loved ones, and/or your patients and clients.

Section X

Treatment of the Brain and Spinal Cord

Thus far in my career, I have had five books published and have contributed a couple of chapters in books that have been compendiums by multiple authors. If my memory serves me correctly in areas of patient integration, I have never written about any technique in which I was not personally experienced. I believe I should continue this approach, for it has served me well. Therefore, I shall in this book write only about treatment techniques for the brain and spinal cord with which I have had personal experience.

The treatment approach with which I have had the most experience by far is CranioSacral Therapy. I have often coupled CranioSacral Therapy with SomatoEmotional Release^sm, with Therapeutic Imagery and Dialogue, with Acupuncture, with a variety of bone and joint manipulation techniques, with a variety of connective tissue release techniques, with hypnosis and with some pharmaceutical agents. I am committed to an eclectic approach and, in all honesty, do not have a personal investment in any one of these approaches. It is true that I use CranioSacral Therapy and SomatoEmotional Release^sm with Therapeutic Imagery and Dialogue the most. The reason for this predominance of usage is that, in my hands, this combination of techniques has given me the best results. In fact, I wrote my first textbook on CranioSacral Therapy for the purposes of recording my research and clinical experiences on paper. I did this in order to discharge my responsibilities to the healthcare professions and to the patient populations. My purpose was to make available to all those who desired it everything that I knew about the craniosacral system, its evaluation, its effect on patient health and its treatment. My plan after the book was published was to move on into other fields of research. If you look at my history, it becomes clear at a glance that the last part of my life plan was thwarted. I kept returning to CranioSacral Therapy because I found it to be the approach that gave me the best results with patients. And very shortly, CranioSacral Therapy led me into SomatoEmotional Release^sm. In a short time, it became clear that CranioSacral Therapy and SomatoEmotional Release^sm would be inextricably intertwined and complementary to each other. Then came the discovery that patients experienced spontaneous mental images during the treatment sessions which combined CranioSacral Therapy and SomatoEmotional Release^sm. It seemed obvious to me that these images might well be attempts by the levels of consciousness of which we are unaware to communicate with the conscious awareness. I began to call these levels of consciousness of which we are unaware the "nonconscious," so as not to confuse my concept with the "subconscious" of Sigmund Freud and others. I reasoned that, somehow, the nonconscious was trying to communicate with the patient's conscious awareness by the use of images and symbols. It also seemed reasonable that these attempts at communication by the nonconscious were stimulated, provoked or facilitated by the hands-on work that we were doing with CranioSacral Therapy and SomatoEmotional Release^{sm}. If an image or symbol came forward, it seemed important that we "milk" every bit of meaning possible from it. What better way to do this than to start a conversation with it. This was the beginning of Therapeutic Imagery and Dialogue. Soon, the three methodologies of CranioSacral Therapy, SomatoEmotional Release^{sm} and Therapeutic Imagery and Dialogue were all blended together, and could never again in good conscience be separated. I found myself totally involved in this rather complex and yet straightforward approach to patient healing. It soon became patient self-healing, and the therapist became the facilitator to the self-healing process.

I had done a lot of acupuncture work and a wide variety of bone, joint and connective tissue work for several years before the craniosacral system presented itself to me. So it was quite natural to incorporate these techniques with the aforementioned CranioSacral Therapy, SomatoEmotional Release^{sm} and Therapeutic Imagery and Dialogue trilogy. The same is true of my previous work with hypnosis and so this technique, although seldom indicated, was incorporated where it seemed appropriate.

Since I practiced general osteopathic medicine and some surgery for over 11 years before entering the Michigan State University faculty as a clinician-researcher, it was also quite natural that some of the methods that I had used in this previous practice, like medication and surgical procedures, would also be incorporated. In actual fact, about the only medications I use anymore are those that will correct edematous swelling of the meningeal membranes, some pain medication, and an occasional sedative or muscle relaxant. And the number of times I actually use pharmaceutical agents as part of patient care is very small. CranioSacral Therapy and the rest of it have shown me how to assist the patient's self-corrective mechanisms which are inherent in their bodies. This approach works so well that I probably give a prescription for medication or an injection to less than five percent of the patients that I work with. I have almost completely forsaken any type of surgical procedure.

After all this chatter, I think I owe you a reasonable but brief description of CranioSacral Therapy, SomatoEmotional Release^{sm} and Therapeutic Imagery and Dialogue.

CranioSacral Therapy

CranioSacral Therapy is a system of evaluation and treatment that deals with the rather recently recognized craniosacral system. This system is a semi-closed hydraulic system. This means that it has a fluid inside of a watertight container. The fluid within the container has a controlled inflow and a controlled outflow of fluid. In this case, the fluid in the system is the cerebrospinal fluid. The watertight container is formed by the tough and watertight dura mater. The dura mater is the outermost membrane layer of the three-layered meningeal membranes that enclose the brain, the spinal cord, some major closely related nerve trunks, and the related blood vascular system.

It is of significance that the dura mater (watertight container for our semi-closed hydraulic system) is tightly attached to the internal surfaces of the bones that form the skull/cranial vault. It is also noteworthy that the dura mater enjoys relative freedom to glide up and down within the spinal canal. Its only normal restrictive attachments within the spinal canal are in the front part of the canal in the upper neck to the posterior bodies of the second and third cervical vertebrae, and in the low back at the second sacral segment. This latter segment is lower than the end of the lumbar spine by about two inches, depending on the size of the patient.

These bony attachments of the dura mater allow us to use the bones of the skull, the upper cervical vertebrae, and the sacrum at the lower end of the spine as handles which enable us to manipulate the dura mater, and thus to affect change in the function of the craniosacral system.

The cerebrospinal fluid inflow is furnished by the choroid plexuses, which are located within the walls of the ventricular system of the brain. The outflow of cerebrospinal fluid from our semi-closed hydraulic system is via the arachnoid villi and the arachnoid granulation bodies. These are found largely in the venous drainage sinuses within the confines of the dura mater membrane, but separated from the venous blood circulation.

Actually, the choroid plexuses extract the cerebrospinal fluid from the blood. They then deposit this fluid in our craniosacral system which, as you recall, is the semi-closed hydraulic system. The arachnoid villi and granulation bodies return the cerebrospinal fluid to the blood system. In order to accomplish these tasks, both the choroid plexuses and the arachnoid villi and granulation bodies must have one side exposed to the blood system and the other side exposed to the inside of the craniosacral system, which contains the cerebrospinal fluid.

What seems to be the case is that the cerebrospinal fluid input into the craniosacral system is not constant, but pulsatile. In the usual and normal individual, the inflow goes on for about three seconds, then it stops for about three seconds and repeats. The total cycle then is three seconds of inflow of cerebrospinal fluid, plus three seconds of rest, which makes a total of six seconds for a complete cycle of activity by the choroid plexuses. Thus, on the average there are about 10 cycles of fluid input per minute. (One cycle per six-second period = 10 cycles per 60 seconds.)

On the outflow side, it would seem that the return of cerebrospinal fluid into the venous blood system by the arachnoid villi and granulation bodies is constant. Therefore, in order for the craniosacral system to maintain a constant range of fluid volume, the rate of return of cerebrospinal fluid into the blood system must be about half the rate of the inflow during its three seconds of activity in each cycle of the craniosacral system.

The control of rate of inflow into the craniosacral system seems to be accomplished by nerve reflex circuits that read the amount of stretch alternating with the amount of compression within the sagittal suture of the skull between the two parietal bones. As the stretch reaches the threshold level, the nerves telegraph the choroid plexuses to stop the inflow of cerebrospinal fluid into the craniosacral system. Since the outflow of fluid is constant, the volume of fluid diminishes while the inflow is interrupted. As the volume diminishes, the sagittal suture begins to compress. When the compression level reaches its threshold, the nerves signal the choroid plexuses to resume the inflow of fluid into our craniosacral system. The cycle repeats rhythmically.

The outflow of cerebrospinal fluid back into the blood system is modulated by nerves which read the tension within specific areas of the dura mater which forms our watertight container for the craniosacral system. Outflow is constant, but is regulated up or down rather gradually as the tensions in the dura mater indicate it should be done.

CranioSacral Therapy makes use of the hands of the therapist, which have been sensitively trained to locate abnormal restrictions or abnormal tension patterns in the dura mater membrane as the pulsatile activity of the craniosacral system is evaluated. When restrictions and/or abnormal tension patterns are found, the therapist has to design a method whereby the pulsatile activity of the system can be used to self-correct the problem. This is also done exclusively by the use of very light pressures and touches by the therapist's hands.

The same type of evaluative process is used to locate the origin of the skull bone and sutural restrictions, and/or abnormal membrane tension patterns. More often than not, the origin may be found outside of the craniosacral system in the less severe cases. In the case of head or spinal trauma, the origin of the problem may be within the craniosacral system. In either case, the origin or primary cause must be found and corrected.

SomatoEmotional Release^{sm}

More often than not, the problems within the craniosacral system are related to trauma which occurred either within that system originally, or trauma which is being reflected into the craniosacral system from outside of its boundaries. In either case, the trauma frequently has an emotional component. The trauma could be only emotional or only physical. However, most often it is a combination of both. Release of the trauma and correction of its effects upon the craniosacral system usually results in a release of suppressed emotion which relates to the trauma in question. This release, in turn, may lead to the release of a chain of traumatic experiences, all of which will have both emotional and physical components. There is usually a common thread that runs through all of these related trauma. This thread of commonality guides the facilitative treatment process on into the next problem just as the last problem is being resolved. It is as though the patient's body has an inner wisdom/intelligence that leads the process on until the patient has reached his/her saturation point for a given treatment session. Most of this release is accomplished by hands-on body-positioning work by the therapist.

Topic 71

Therapeutic Imagery and Dialogue

When we incorporate the recognition of the mental images that form, and then talk with these images, we multiply the power of the facilitative treatment and self-healing process by at least a factor of two. The incorporation of image recruitment and talking with the image may be, at first, awkward for both patient and therapist. But once it is begun, it almost always flows smoothly. This is not psychotherapy or psychiatry. The therapist simply supports and mildly encourages the patient's nonconscious to come forward and let the patient know what goes on beneath the surface. The therapist is encouraging the patient to embark upon a process of self-realization and integration.

I have truly seen what seem to be miracles happen with the reasonably effective use of this treatment trilogy. The main issue for the therapist is to avoid leading, guiding, judging and directing. The therapist is along for the ride. The therapist makes it happen, but he/she does not know what will happen. I often use the analogy that the therapist and the patient are driving a car. The therapist has his/her foot on the gas pedal, while the patient steers.

In Closing

I have explained in brief form how I work with patients. I have trained several teachers and we, as an Institute, continue to train more and more therapists in the techniques I have just described. At present (1995), we number about 20,000 in the United States, Canada, Europe, Japan, Australia and New Zealand. I am happy that CranioSacral Therapy would not turn me loose. I have seen it help a wide variety of problems related to dysfunction of the brain, the spinal cord, the peripheral nervous system, the musculoskeletal system, the myofacial system, the endocrine system and the immune system. I have seen it help chronic pain, chronic fatigue, weakness, paralysis and severe Post Traumatic Stress Disorder of many types, from child abuse to Vietnam War veterans with terrors and night sweats. The real beauty is that the treatment trilogy to which I abide is virtually risk-free.

Thanks for listening.

John E. Upledger, D.O., O.M.M.

References

Abeles, M. 1991. *Corticonics - Neural Circuits of the Cerebral Cortex.* Cambridge University Press.

Ackerman, Diane. 1990. *A Natural History of the Senses.* Random House.

Aidley, David J. 1989. *The Physiology of Excitable Cells.* Cambridge University Press.

Allen, Delmas J.; Budd, G. C.; Pansky, B. 1988. *Review of Neuroscience.* Macmillan Publishing Co.

Anderson, James E. 1978. *Grants Atlas of Anatomy.* Williams & Wilkins, Co.

Barondes, Samuel H. 1993. *Molecules and Mental Illness.* Scientific American Library.

Barr, Murray L. 1979. *The Human Nervous System: An Anatomic Viewpoint.* Harper & Row, Publishers, Inc.

Becker, Robert O.; Selden, Gary. 1985. *The Body Electric.* William Morrow and Co.

Bloom, Floyd E.; Lazerson, Arlyne. 1988. *Brain, Mind and Behavior.* WH Freeman and Co.

Bolles, Edmund Blair. 1991. *A Second Way of Knowing.* Prentice-Hall Press.

Boyd, J.D.; Hamilton, W.J.; Mossman, H.W. 1959. *Human Embryology, Prenatal Development of Form and Function.* W. Heffer and Sons, Ltd.

Bradford, H.F. 1986. *Chemical Neurobiology.* W.H. Freeman and Company.

Breig, Alf. 1978. *Adverse Mechanical Tension in the Central Nervous System.* John Wiley and Son.

Brown, M.C.; Hopkins, W.G., Keynes, R.J. 1991. *Essentials of Neural Development.* Cambridge University Press.

Chusid, J.G. 1982. *Correlative Neuroanatomy and Functional Neurology.* Lange Medical Publications.

Clemente, Carmine D. 1985. *Gray's Anatomy, 30th American Edition.* Lea and Febiger.

Collins, R. Douglas. 1982. *Illustrated Manual of Neurologic Diagnosis.* J.B. Lippencott.

Dawkins, Richard. 1989. *The Selfish Gene.* Oxford University Press.

DeArmond, Stephen J; Fusco, Madeline M.; Dewey, Maynard M. 1989. *Structure of the Human Brain - A Photographic Atlas.* Oxford University Press.

Diamond, Marian C.; Elson, Lawrence M;Schiebel, Arnold B. 1985. *The Human Brain Coloring Book.* Barnes & Noble Books, Division of Harper and Row.

Dowling, John E. 1988. *The Retina.* Harvard University Press.

Edelman, Gerald M. 1987. *Neural Darwinism.* Basic Books.

Edelman, Gerald M. 1988. *Topobiology.* Basic Books.

Edelman, Gerald M. 1989. *The Remembered Present.* Basic Books.

Edelman, Gerald M. 1992. *Bright Air, Brilliant Fire.* Basic Books.

Edited by: Abbott, N.J. 1991. *Glial-Neuronal Interaction.* New York Academy of Science, Volume 633.

Edited by: Bjornsson, Johannes; Carp, Richard I.; Love, Arthur; Wisniewski, Henryk M. 1994. *Slow Infections of the Central Nervous System.* New York Academy of Science, Volume 724.

Edited by: Cseit, Helen F. 1986. *The Neuronal Microenvironment.* New York Academy of Sciences.

Edited by: Das, Dipak K. 1994. Cellular, *Biochemical and Molecular Aspects of Reperfusion Injury.* New York Academy of Science, Volume 723.

Edited by: Duncan, I.D.; Skoff, R.P.;; Colman, D. 1990. *Myelination and Dysmyelination.* New York Academy of Sciences, Volume 605.

Edited by: Ganong, W.F.; Dallman, M.F.; Roberts, J.L. 1987. *The Hypothalamic-Pituitary-Adrenal Axis Revisited.* New York Academy of Science, Volume 510.

Edited by: Hall, Zach W. 1992. *An Introduction to Molecular Neurobiology.* Sinauer and Associates.

Edited by: Khachaturian, Zaven S.; Cotman, Carl W.; Pettegrew, Jay W. 1989. *Calcium, Membranes, Aging and Alzheimer's Disease.* New York Academy of Science, Volume 568.

Edited by: Kummerow, Fred A.; Benga, Gheorghe; Holmes, Ross P. 1983. *Biomembranes and Cell Function.* New York Academy of Science, Volume 414.

Edited by: Margulis, Lynn; Fester, René. 1991. *Symbiosis as a Source of Evolutionary Innovation.* Massachusetts Institute of Technology.

Edited by: Rowland, Lewis P. 1984. *Merritt's Textbook of Neurology.* Lea and Febiger.

Edited by: Salama, Andre. 1984. *Presynaptic Modulation of Post Synaptic Receptors in Mental Diseases.* New York Academy of Sciences, Volume 430.

Edited by: Shepard, Gordon M. 1990. *The Synaptic Organization of the Brain.* Oxford University Press.

Edited by: Warwick, R.; Williams, P.L. *Gray's Anatomy, 35th British Edition.* 1973. W. B. Saunders Co.

Edited by: Wolpaw, Jonathon; Schmidt, John T.; Vaughan, Theresa M. 1991. *Activity Drives CNS Changes in Learning and Development.* New York Academy of Sciences, Volume 627.

Elson, Lawrence M.; Kapit, Wynn. 1977. *The Anatomy Coloring Book.* Canfield Press/Barnes & Noble, Department of Harper & Row Publishing, Inc.

Finger, Stanley. 1994. *Origins of Neuroscience.* Oxford University Press.

Flanagan, Owen. 1992. *Consciousness Reconsidered.* Bradford Book - MIT Press.

Fox, Sidney. 1988. *The Emergence of Life.* Basic Books.

Goodsell, David S. 1993. *The Machinery of Life.* Springer-Verlag.

Gould, Carol G.; Gould, James L. 1994. *The Animal Mind.* Scientific American Library.

Green, Elmer and Alyce. 1977. *Beyond Biofeedback.* Delacort Press.

Haines, Duane E. 1991. *Neuroanatomy - An Atlas of Structures, Sections and Systems.* Urban and Schwarzenberg.

Heimer, Lennart. 1983. *The Human Brain and Spinal Cord.* Springer-Verlag.

Hellige, Joseph B. 1993. *Hemispheric Asymmetry.* President and Fellows of Harvard College.

Hille, Bertil. 1992. *Ionic Channels of Excitable Membranes.* Sinauer Associates.

Hobson, J. Allan. 1989. *Sleep.* Scientific American Library.

Hofer, Myron A. 1981. *The Roots of Human Behavior.* W.H. Freeman and Co.

Hooper, Judith; Teresi, Dick. 1986. *The 3-Pound Universe.* Dell Publishing.

Hubel, David H. 1988. *Eye Brain and Vision.* Scientific American Library.

Jones, H. Royden. 1985. *Diseases of the Peripheral Motor Sensory Unit.* Ciba Geigy, Volume 37, Number 2.

Kandel, Eric R.; Schwartz, James H.; Jessell, Thomas M. 1991. *Principles of Neuroscience.* Appleton and Lange.

Keim, Hugo A.; Hensinger, Robert N. 1989. *Spinal Deformities.* Ciba Geigy, Volume 41, Number 4.

Konner, Melvin. 1982. *The Tangled Wing.* Holt-Rinehart-Winston.

Konner, Melvin. 1990. *Why the Reckless Survive.* Viking.

Kosslyn, Stephen M.; Koenig, Olivier. 1992. *Wet Mind.* The Free Press - MacMillan.

Langman, J. 1975. Medical Embryology: *Human Development - Normal and Abnormal.* The Williams and Wilkins Co.

Levitan, Irwin B.; Kaczmarek, Leonard. 1991. *The Neuron-Cell and Molecular Biology.* Oxford University Press.

Lewin, Roger. 1993. *Origin of Modern Humans.* Scientific American Library.

Lewontin, Richard. 1982. *Human Diversity.* Scientific American Library.

Luciano, Dorothy S.; Sherman, James H.; Vander, Arthur J.1975. *Human Physiology: The Mechanisms of Body Function.* McGraw-Hill Book Co.

MacLean, Paul D. 1990. *The Triune Brain in Evolution.* Plenum Press.

Mandel, Peter. 1986. *Energy Emission Analysis.* Synthesis Publishing Co., Siegmar Gerken.

Moore, Keith L. 1988. *The Developing Human: Clinically Oriented Embryology.* W.B. Sanders Co., Harcourt Brace Jovanovich, Inc.

Moore, Keith. 1974. *Before We Are Born: Basic Embryology and Birth Defects.* W. B. Saunders Co.

Netter, Frank H. 1958. *The Ciba Collection of Medical Illustrations, Volume I: Nervous System.* Ciba.

Netter, Frank H. 1983. *The Ciba Collection - The Nervous System, Volume I.* Ciba Pharmaceutical Co.

Nicholls, John H.; Martin, A. Robert; Wallace, Bruce G. 1992. *From Neuron to Brain.* Sinauer Associates, Inc.

Nilsson, Lennart. 1985. *The Body Victorious.* Delacort Press.

O'Doherty, Neil. 1979. *Atlas of the Newborn.* J.B. Lippincott Co.

Oldfield, Harry; Coghill, Roger. 1988. *The Dark Side of the Brain.* Element Books.

Ornstein, Robert; Thompson, Richard F. 1984. *The Amazing Brain.* Houghton Mifflin Co.

Partridge, Lloyd D.; Partridge, L. Donald. 1993. *The Nervous System.* Bradford Books - MIT Press.

Patten, Leslie; Patten, Terry. 1988. *Biocircuits.* H.J. Kramer, Inc.

Peters, Alan; Palay, Sanford L.; Webster, Henry. 1991. *The Five Structures of the Nervous System.* Oxford University Press.

Posner, Michael I.; Raichle, Marcus E. 1994. *Images of Mind.* Oxford University Press.

Prochiantz, Alain. 1948. *How the Brain Evolved.* McGraw-Hill.

Purvis, Dale. 1988. *Body and Brain.* Harvard University Press.

Restak, Richard. 1984. *The Brain.* Bantam.

Restak, Richard. 1988. *The Mind.* Bantam Books.

Rock, Irvin. 1984. *Perception.* Scientific American Library.

Rohen, J.W.; Yokochi, Chihiro. 1983. *Color Atlas of Anatomy: A Photographic Study of the Human Body.* Igaku-Shoid, Ltd.

Roper, Stephen D.; Atema, Jelle. 1987. *Olfaction and Taste IX.* New York Academy of Science, Volume 510.

Rosenfield, Israel. 1988. *The Invention of Memory.* Basic Books.

Upledger, John E. 1987. *CranioSacral Therapy II, Beyond the Dura.* Eastland Press.

Upledger, John E. 1990. *SomatoEmotional Release^{sm} and Beyond.* UI Publishing.

Upledger, John E. 1991. *Your Inner Physician and You.* UI Enterprises / North Atlantic Books.

Upledger, John E.; Vredevoogd, Jon D. 1983. *CranioSacral Therapy.* Eastland Press.

Ward, Milton. 1977. *The Brilliant Function of Pain.* Optimus Books.

Wild, Gaynor C.; Benzel, Edward C. 1994. *Essentials of Neurochemistry.* Jones and Burtlett Publishers.

Wills, Christopher. 1989. *The Wisdom of the Genes.* Basic Books.

Wills, Christopher. 1993. *The Runaway Brain.* Basic Books.

Winfree, Arthur T. 1987. *The Timing of Biological Clocks.* Scientific American Library.

Wolf, John K. 1981. *Segmental Neurology.* University Park Press - Baltimore.

Wolpert, Lewis. 1991. *The Triumph of the Embryo.* Oxford University Press.

Zeki, Semir. 1993. *A Vision of the Brain.* Blackwell Scientific Publications.

Glossary

Abducent Cranial Nerve (VI) - Controls the lateral rectus muscles that prevent cross-eyedness.

Accessory Cranial Nerve (XI) - Gives motor supply to the sternocleidomastoideus and trapezius muscles of the neck.

Acetylcholine - An acetic compound of choline, which is a neurotransmitter at cholinergic synapses in the central, sympathetic and parasympathetic nervous systems, and at the myoneural junctions.

Achromatic Spindle Fibers - Precursors of the microtubules that will form during the second stage of cell division (metaphase). The microtubules guide the chromatids to the correct positions for mitotic cell division.

Acoustic Cranial Nerve (VIII) - Also known as the vestibulocochlear nerve or the auditory nerve, it controls the senses of equilibrium, balance and hearing.

Acrosome - Located on the sperm head, the acrosome is a cup-like membrane that covers the front part of the head of the sperm. This membrane cap contains enzymes that help dissolve the protective membrane of the ovum/egg for sperm entry and fertilization.

ACTH (Adrenocorticotropic Hormone) - A hormone secreted by the anterior pituitary gland that stimulates release of the glucocorticoid, cortisol and corticosteroid hormones from the adrenal cortex.

Active Conduction - Refers to the mechanism whereby certain substances or molecules are temporarily combined with other substances that actively conduct them through cell membranes.

Allantois Membrane - One of the membrane layers that surround the embryo, it is where the blood vessels that connect mother to embryo are developed. It arises from the yolk sac on about the 15th day of gestation.

Amnion - The innermost membrane enveloping the embryo within the uterus. It is filled with amniotic fluid.

Amniotic Fluid - A liquid within the amnion that surrounds the fetus and protects it from injury. It contains fetal urine, and it fills the fetal lungs and gastrointestinal tract.

Amygdala - Walnut-sized masses of gray nerve cells located on each side of the brain. They are involved in aggressive behavior, fear reactions and conditioned fear responses. They are also, in part, responsible for self-preservation activities, and they are critical sites for learning, especially when related to environment adaptation.

Anabolism - That aspect of metabolism that is the building up or synthesizing stage of activity. It is the opposite of catabolism, which is the degrading, tearing down or using up stage of metabolism.

Anaphase - Occurs when the two groups of daughter chromosomes (chromatids) separate and move along the spindle fibers to one centriole pole or the other. The anaphase takes approximately three minutes.

Anterior Commissure - The neuronal fibers that interconnect structures which are located in opposite hemispheres of the forwardmost regions of the brain. They are located in the subcortical white matter. Also known as the rostral commissure.

Anus - The opening of the rectum on the body surface; the distal orifice of the alimentary canal.

Aorta - The great artery arising from the left ventricle, being the main trunk from which the systemic arterial system proceeds.

Aortic Valve - The valve that prevents the retrograde flow of blood from the aorta into the left ventricle while that ventricle is at rest and is being refilled with blood from the left atrium. This rest period is called diastole.

Apgar Rating - Evaluation of a newborn infant's physical status by assigning numerical values (0 to 2) to each of five criteria: heart rate, respiratory effort, muscle tone, skin color and response to stimulation.

Apoptosis - A type of neuronal cell death that occurs during the development of neural circuitry. It is a natural phenomenon not related to a pathological process within the involved cell.

Aqueduct of Sylvius - The connecting passageway between the third and fourth ventricles of the brain through which cerebrospinal fluid passes. Also known as the cerebral aqueduct.

Arachnoid Granulation Bodies - They function as a part of the reabsorption mechanism of the cerebrospinal fluid as it is constantly being taken back into the blood vascular system. They connect on one side with the subarachnoid space and on the other side with the venous system.

Arachnoid Membrane - The middle layer of the three membranes in the meningeal membrane system. The three layers, from central to peripheral, are the pia mater, the arachnoid membrane and the dura mater.

Arachnoid Villi - Once it has bathed the brain tissue, cerebrospinal fluid is reabsorbed back into the blood stream by structures called arachnoid villi. They are located throughout the entire venous sinus system, with special concentrations in the sagittal and straight sinuses.

Arnold-Chiari Syndrome - Herniation and molding of brain stem and cerebellar tissues into a deformed and narrowed foramen magnum. It is the result of a congenital deformity of the occiput and upper cervical spine.

Aspartate - An amino-acid neurotransmitter. It contains four carbon atoms and acts in an excitatory way similar to glutamate, but is less powerful.

Aster - The centriole with its attached spindle fibers on which groups of daughter chromosomes (chromatids) move to one centriole pole or the other.

Astrocytes - A type of glial cell located in the central nervous system that provides architectural support for the neurons. Astrocytes send out projections from the central nervous system tissues into the pia mater membrane. These projections serve to attach the pia mater closely to the brain, spinal cord and enveloped nerve roots.

Atlanto-Occipital Membrane - A fibrous membrane that connects the atlas (first cervical vertebra) with the occiput.

Atlas - The first cervical vertebra.

Atrophy - A wasting away; a diminishing in the size of a cell, tissue, organ or part.

Auditory Cranial Nerve (VIII) - Also known as the acoustic cranial nerve or the vestibulocochlear nerve, it controls the senses of equilibrium, balance and hearing.

Auricle of the Heart - The ear-shaped appendage of either atrium of the heart. Formerly, this word was used to designate the whole atrium. This usage is now obsolete.

Autoimmune Disease - Any of a group of disorders in which tissue injury is associated with humoral or cell-mediated responses to the body's own constituents; they may be systemic or organ-specific. The body's immune system does not recognize some part or system of the body as part of itself, and attacks it.

Autonomic Ganglia - Aggregations of nerve cell bodies related to the autonomic nervous system and located outside of the central nervous system. These ganglia direct nerve impulses in proper directions after information comes in from the sensory end organs. They appear to make some decisions without relying on higher centers of the central nervous system. These ganglia relate mostly to the internal organs and glandular structures.

Autonomic Nervous System - The normally involuntary or "unconscious" division of the peripheral nervous system. The autonomic nervous system is believed to be exclusively motor in its function. That is, it sends out impulses to various organs, glands and systems so that the body can function automatically without conscious control. Biofeedback is used to bring autonomic function under conscious control.

Axis - A line through a body about which a structure revolves; a line around which body parts are arranged. Also, the second cervical vertebra.

Basal Ganglia - Functionally, the basal ganglia represent the cerebral limb of the extrapyramidal motor system. This motor system is largely responsible for the more automatic and largely non-conscious aspects of posture and locomotion.

Basal Plate - Forms the floor or base of the skull.

Basilar Artery - Located at the midline of the body within the skull, where the right and left vertebral arteries join. It drains into the circle of Willis.

Blast - An immature stage in cellular development before the appearance of the definitive characteristics of the cell.

Blastocyst - The mammalian embryo following the early division of the zygote. It resembles a ball with a central cavity, within which there is a cluster of cells called the embryoblast. The outer surface cells are called the trophoblast. The blastocyst occurs at about the fourth day of gestation.

Blood-Brain Barrier - A network provided by glial cells that develops shortly after birth. It integrates with the capillary system and serves to selectively pass or reject various substances from blood to brain.

Brachial Arches - Brachial arches are present by the third gestational week of embryonic life. In fish, the brachial arches would become gills. In the human embryo, they will form many of the head and neck structures.

Brain Stem - The stem-like portion of the brain connecting the cerebral hemispheres with the spinal cord, and comprising the pons, medulla oblongata and midbrain; considered by some to include the diencephalon.

Brieg, Alf - A Swedish neurosurgeon and author of the book entitled "Adverse Mechanical Tension in the Central Nervous System." He offers a unique hypothesis that explains spinal cord injury in terms of hydraulic forces.

Broca's Area - Named after French surgeon Paul Pierre Broca, who discovered that these specific areas of the brain's cortex were essential for speech.

Bruit - A sound or murmur heard in the body, especially when the sound is abnormal.

Capillary - One of the minute vessels connecting the arterioles and venules, the walls of which act as a semipermeable membrane for interchange of various substances between the blood and tissue fluid.

Carotid Body - These two small tissue masses are types of chemical analysis stations. There is one located adjacent to the bifurcation of the carotid artery into its internal and external branches on each side of the neck. They send information about oxygen concentration and blood pH to the brain on a moment-to-moment basis.

Carotid Canal - A hole in the petrous part of the skull's temporal bone through which the internal carotid artery passes. Inside the skull, this internal carotid artery runs for a short distance between two layers of dura mater membrane.

Cartilage - A specialized, fibrous connective tissue which forms the temporary skeleton in the embryo. It provides the model upon which the bones develop, and constitutes a part of the organism's growth mechanism. It is also present in adults, especially as a connector substance between bones.

Catabolism - The degrading aspect of metabolism during which larger molecules in living organisms are broken down into smaller molecules.

Cauda Equina - The collection of spinal roots descending from the lower spinal cord and occupying the vertebral canal below the cord's end.

Caudate Nucleus - One of the structures included in the basal ganglia, which are interconnected gray masses located deep in the cerebral hemispheres. Basal ganglia are involved with the cerebellum in the modulation, control and coordination of all body movements.

Cavernous Sinus - The areas located between the two layers of dura mater membrane on each side of the body of the sphenoid bone within the skull. They communicate with each other across the midline of the skull in front of and behind the stalk of the hypophysis (pituitary gland).

Centrioles - The two cylindrical organelles located in the centrosome and containing nine triplets of microtubules arrayed around their edges; centrioles migrate to opposite poles of the cell during cell division and serve to organize spindles. They are capable of independent replication and of migrating to form basal bodies.

Centrosome - A specialized area of condensed cytoplasm containing the centrioles and playing an important part in mitosis.

Centrum Semiovale - The white matter that's visible when you remove the top of the brain at the level of the corpus callosum.

Cephalhematoma - Also known as cephalohematoma, it is a subperiosteal hemorrhage which is limited to one cranial vault bone. It is usually benign and is a result of birth trauma.

Cephalic Flexure - The flexure that allows the forebrain (forward part of the brain) to bend forward over the front end of the notochord.

Cerebellum - The large posterior brain mass lying above the pons and medulla and beneath the posterior portion of the cerebrum; consists of two lateral hemispheres united by a narrow middle portion, the vermis. Its major function is in motor coordination and the memory of movement patterns.

Cerebral Aqueduct - A narrow channel in the midbrain connecting the third and fourth ventricles. Also known as the aqueduct of Sylvius.

Cerebral Hemispheres - The two major divisions of the brain, left and right, which are separated by the longitudinal cerebral fissure. The falx cerebri maintains the hemispheric separation. The hemispheres are functionally cross-connected by the commissures.

Cerebral Palsy - A persisting qualitative motor dysfunction that appears before the age of three years. It is due to non-progressive damage to the brain, which in turn could be due to any one of a number of causes.

Cerebral Peduncles - The two cerebral peduncles are located on each side of the ventral surface (underside) of the midbrain. They primarily contain connecting fibers that descend from the cerebral cortex down to the midbrain and the spinal cord.

Cerebral Steal - The appropriation of energy from the rest of the brain by one brain system or component for its own use. This occurs because there is a limited supply of energy available for total brain function. Thus, it is budgeted out to various systems and components based on demand, need and priority.

Cerebroside - A general designation for sphingolipids in which sphingosine is combined with galactose or glucose; found chiefly in nervous tissue.

Cerebrospinal Fluid - The plasmalike fluid that is extracted from blood by the choroid plexus within the brain's ventricular system. It is contained within the compartment formed by the dura mater. The functions of cerebrospinal fluid still offer several mysteries to modern science. We know that it offers a hydraulic cushion for the brain to soften the blows of the delicate brain and spinal cord against their bony containers during accidents and so on. Also, the cerebrospinal fluid supplies some nutrition, removes some waste, and perhaps provides some acid-alkaline balance stability for the brain and spinal cord. There is also some conjecture that it contains an inherent energy.

Cerebrum - The main portion of the brain, occupying the upper part of the cranial cavity; its two hemispheres, united by the corpus callosum and other less prominent commissures, form the largest part of the central nervous system in mankind. The term is sometimes applied to the postembryonic forebrain and midbrain together, or to the entire brain.

Cholesterol - A steroid alcohol molecule which is often combined with fatty acids. It is found in animal fats, bile, blood, brain tissue, milk, egg yolk, myelin sheaths of nerve fibers, liver, kidneys and adrenal glands. It constitutes a large part of most gallstones and occurs in the atheromata of the arteries, in various cysts, and in carcinomatous tissue. It is a precursor of bile acids and is important in the synthesis of steroid hormones.

Chondroblast - An immature cartilage-producing cell.

Chondrocranium - The cartilaginous cranial structure of the embryo. This cartilage serves as precursor to the bones of the cranial base.

Choroid Plexus - A system that extracts cerebrospinal fluid from blood, it relies largely upon the principles of osmotic pressure and selective conduction mechanisms. It is formed by glial cells and capillaries.

Chromatid - Initially, there are two parallel spiral filaments joined at the centromere that make up a chromosome. During embryonic development, the chromosome divides to produce two chromatids, one of which will form the new chromosome in each of the two daughter cells of the dividing cell.

Chromatin - The substance of chromosomes. It is made up largely of DNA with some RNA. When the cell chromosomes become active, a larger amount of RNA is present. RNA molecules serve as messengers that distribute the instructions of the DNA to the organelles of the cell within which the DNA resides.

Chromosome - In animal cells, a structure in the nucleus containing a linear thread of DNA that transmits genetic information and is associated with RNA and histones; during cell division, the material composing the chromosome is compactly coiled, making it visible with appropriate staining. The coiling permits movement in the cell with minimal entanglement.

Cingulate Cortex - Gray matter that constitutes a cortex or cortical layer covering the central lobes, which are buried deep in the lateral cerebral fissures.

Cingulate Gyrus - Much like a girdle, it encircles the v-shaped limbic system seated on top of the brain stem beneath the diencephalon.

Circadian Rhythm - Lightness and darkness seem to influence the pineal gland's level of activity, which in turn influences our levels of hormones and neurotransmitters, and how these levels fluctuate during certain times of the day or night. Circadian rhythm is the term applied to these light-and-dark-influenced rhythmical physiological fluctuations, and to many other cyclic patterns which are emerging as research continues.

Cisterna - Considered to be reservoirs for cerebrospinal fluid. In some cases they are located between the lower structures of the brain and the base of the skull.

Cloaca - A common passage for fecal, urinary and reproductive discharge in most lower vertebrates. Also, the terminal end of the hindgut before division into rectum, bladder and genital primordia in mammal embryos.

Clonic Seizures - A type of grand mal seizure in which the muscles alternately contract and relax.

Coccyx - Triangular bone formed by fusion of the last four (sometimes three or five) vertebrae at the extreme lower end of the spinal column during fetal development.

Colliculi - Located in the midbrain, they are relay stations for our senses of sound and sight.

Commissure - A bundle of nerve fibers passing from one side to the other in the brain or spinal cord. Commissures form functional connections between the two sides of the brain and spinal cord.

Common Carotid Artery - All of the freshly oxygenated and nutrient-rich blood that gets to the brain is pumped from the left ventricle of the heart into the aorta. The aorta gives off its major branches to the brain early on. These branches are called the common carotid arteries. On the right side a large artery called the innominate is interposed between the aorta and the common carotid artery for a short distance.

Congenital - Present at and existing from the time of birth.

Coronal - The transverse suture of the skull which separates the posterior aspect of the frontal bone from the anterior aspects of the two parietal bones.

Corpora Quadrigemina - Four aggregations of nerve cell bodies with synapses located in the tectum. The corpora quadrigemina are then subdivided into the two superior colliculi and two inferior colliculi.

Corpus Callosum - The major crossover connection between the right and left cerebral hemispheres. It contains about 200 million crossover fibers, and is located deep in the brain at the bottom of the sagittal fissure. It is this fissure that divides the brain into its two separate hemispheres. The sagittal fissure is also known as the longitudinal cerebral fissure.

Cortex - Outer layer of an organ as distinguished from its inner substance. The cerebral cortex is the outermost layer of the brain. Its surface area is expanded by an intricate pattern of sulci and gyri. It is made up of neuronal cell bodies which are not myelinated. It is therefore gray in color.

Cortisol - An adrenal cortex hormone that stimulates uterine contractions and the onset of labor when it enters the maternal blood stream of sheep and probably humans. Among its many functions is stress, anti-inflammatory action, etc.

Cranial Nerves - The 12 pairs of nerves that either exit or enter the brain rather than the spinal cord.

Cranial Synostosis - The abnormal union of two skull bones by ossification of the suture between them.

Craniopharyngioma - A tumor composed of epithelial-lined cysts derived from the infundibulum of the hypophysis or Rathke's pouch. When the craniopharyngeal canal persists (is not reabsorbed) after the hypophysis has passed from the oral cavity through this canal to the underside of the brain during embryonic development, the craniopharyngioma is formed.

Cranioschisis - A congenital fissure of the skull.

Craniotabes - The reduction in mineralization of the skull with abnormal softness of the bone, usually affecting the occipital and parietal bones along the lambdoid sutures.

Cretinism - Arrested physical and mental development with dystrophy of bones and soft tissues, due to congenital lack of thyroid secretion.

Cri Du Chat - A hereditary congenital syndrome characterized by hypertelorism, microcephaly, severe mental deficiency, and a plaintive cat-like cry. It is due to the deletion of the short arm of chromosome 5.

Crista Galli - A thick, triangular process projecting upward from the cribriform plate of the ethmoid bone.

Crus Cerebri - A structure made up of fiber tracts descending from the cerebral cortex to the various nuclei of the brain stem, especially to the pons and the spinal cord. The crus cerebri are located in the ventral part of the brain, and they run longitudinally for the most part.

Cyanosis - A bluish discoloration of skin and mucous membranes due to excessive concentration of reduced hemoglobin in the blood. Reduced hemoglobin is secondary to a deficiency of available oxygen for any reason. In this definition, "reduced" means the opposite of oxygenated. There may also be a reduced or insufficient quantity of hemoglobin which causes cyanosis. Insufficient quantities of hemoglobin are most often due to nutritional deficiencies.

Cytokinesis - The division of the cytoplasm during the division of eukaryotic cells.

Cytoplasm - The protoplasm of a cell exclusive of that which is within the nucleus (nucleoplasm).

Daughter Cells - Cells arising from cell division by the parent cell during mitosis.

Decerebrate Posture - A rigid posture which displays an exaggerated tonus or rigidity of the extensor muscles. It results from the loss of modulatory influence by the motor cortex upon the stretch reflexes of the extensors which are mediated largely in the spinal cord.

Decussation - The situation wherein nerves from the right side of the brain cross over to control the left side of the body and vice versa. The major decussation in the adult human is called the pyramidal tract, located largely in the medulla oblongata.

Dens - A tooth or tooth-like structure.

Dermatome - One of three divisions produced by each somite, in addition to the sclerotome and myotome. The dermatome is the part of the somite that produces skin.

Diaphragma Sellae - The opening in the dura mater membrane which allows passage of the stalk of the pituitary gland. It is located in the space which is four posted by the clinoid processes of the sphenoid bone.

Diaster - Also known as amphiaster, it is the figure formed by the achromatin fibers during the nuclear division stage of mitosis. The figure resembles two stars, which are the poles, joined by a spindle of the fibers.

Diencephalon - The posterior of the two brain vesicles formed by specialization during embryonic development of the prosencephalon. It consists of 5 divisions: (1) epithalamus, (2) metathalamus, (3) subthalamus, (4) hypothalamus and (5) thalamus.

Diffusion - The process of becoming diffused, or widely spread. It occurs when different concentrations of substances in liquids mix together and reach an equilibrium.

Diploid - Having two sets of chromosomes, as normally found in the somatic cells.

DNA (Deoxyribonucleic Acid) - A nucleic acid that on hydrolysis yields adenine, guanine, cytosine, thymine, deoxyribose and phosphoric acid; it is the carrier of genetic information for all organisms except RNA viruses.

Dopamine - A neurotransmitter in the central nervous system, it is classified as a catecholamine and it is a precursor in the synthesis of norepinephrine and epinephrine. It is deficient in Parkinson's disease. The major areas of concentration are in the basal ganglia, specifically in the substantia nigra.

Duct of Müller - Also known as paramesonephric ducts, they are present in embryonic development. In the male they atrophy. In the female they contribute to the formation of the uterus and the vagina.

Ductus Arteriosus - A short tube which connects the pulmonary artery with the aorta. In the fetus it provides a channel for blood leaving the right ventricle of the heart to go directly to the aorta and to short circuit the lungs. This is because the lungs do not function as such until after delivery. The ductus arteriosus closes shortly after delivery. If it does not close appropriately, surgery may be indicated.

Dura Mater - Also known as the dural membrane, it is the outermost, toughest of the three meninges (membranes) which form the sac or envelope which contains the brain and spinal cord.

Dural Tube - The dura mater layer of the meninges within the spinal canal which extends from the foramen magnum to the sacral hiatus.

Ectoderm - The outer layer of cells in the embryo after the establishment of the primary germ layers. From it are derived the epidermis (skin) and epidermic tissues, such as the nails, hair and glands of the skin; the nervous system; the external sense organs and mucous membranes of the mouth and anus.

Embryo - In animals, those derivatives of the fertilized ovum that eventually become the offspring, during their period of most rapid growth, i.e., after the long axis appears and until all major structures are represented. In humans, it is the developing organism from fertilization to the end of the eighth week. After the eighth week the embryo becomes known as the fetus.

Embryonic Disc - Once blastocyst implantation has occurred and the rudimentary placenta is established, some of the cells within the blastocyst flatten out to form the embryonic disc. This three-layered disc extends out from the wall of the blastocyst into its cavity. The part of the disc that remains attached to the wall of the blastocyst will become the tail end of the embryo. The part that protrudes out into the cavity will become the head end of the embryo.

Embryonic Period - The developing organism from conception until approximately the end of the eighth week.

Endocrine System - System of glands and other structures that elaborate internal secretions (hormones), which are released directly into the circulatory system, influencing metabolism and other body processes.

Endoderm - Sometimes called entoderm, it is the innermost of the three primary germ layers of the embryo. From it are derived the cellular linings of the pharynx, respiratory tract (except the nose), digestive tract, bladder and urethra.

Endoplasmic Reticulum - A network of tubules and Nissl bodies located in the cytoplasm (perikaryon) of the neuron, involved in the movement, and perhaps the synthesis of proteins which are constantly being transported through the cytoplasm to and from the nucleus, and into and out of the perikaryon from the outside of the cell.

Endorphin - Any of a group of endogenous polypeptide brain substances that bind to opiate receptors in various areas of the brain and thereby raise the pain threshold.

Enkephalins - Along with endorphins, enkephalins are included in a class of molecules called peptides, which exert great influence upon the function of the internal organs and organ systems. Most known peptides function as neurotransmitters.

Entoderm - Sometimes called endoderm, it is the innermost of the three primitive germ layers of the embryo; from it are derived the epithelium of the pharynx, respiratory tract (except the nose), digestive tract, bladder and urethra.

Ependymal Cells - The choroid plexus is a system that extracts cerebrospinal fluid from blood. The specialized cells from which the choroid plexus is formed are called the ependymal cells. These ependymal cells are a specialized subdivision of the epithelial cells.

Epithalamus - The part of the diencephalon just superior and posterior to the thalamus, comprising the pineal body and adjacent structures.

Erythroblastosis Fetalis - Hemolytic anemia of the fetus or newborn due to transplacental transmission of maternally formed antibody against the fetus' erythrocytes, usually secondary to an incompatibility between the mother's Rh blood group and that of her offspring.

Estrogen - Hormone of the body largely responsible for the development of female secondary sex characteristics. During the menstrual cycle it acts on the female genitalia to produce an environment suitable for the successful passage of sperm through the vagina and cervix so that fertilization can take place.

Eustachian Tube - The tube that runs from your middle ear cavity into the pharyngeal cavity. It is the tube that sometimes requires time to equalize pressures when you get off of an airplane and you can't hear very well.

External Carotid Artery - At the level of, or just below the level of your Adam's Apple, the common carotid arteries on both sides of your throat/neck divide into the internal and external carotid arteries. The external carotid arteries deliver blood to the exterior part of the head, face and the greater part of the neck.

Extrapyramidal System - A system of nerve fiber tracts that pass through the medulla oblongata without decussating and work in coordination with other neural structures to exert great influence and control over posture, movement and coordination.

Facial Cranial Nerve (VII) - It passes out of the skull through the stylomastoid foramen, a little canal that is located below and behind the ear on each side of the head. As an infant ages, this nerve is protected by the mastoid process of the temporal bone of the skull. It provides motor innervation to most of the facial muscles.

Facilitated Segment - The spinal cord has vertical or longitudinal connections running from head to tail and vice versa. These connections pass through a series of horizontal or transverse segments. Impulses going up and down the spinal cord might be thought of as elevators going up and down within a tall building. If a passenger gets off of the elevator on a given floor, that passenger can then go to any subdivision of that floor (just as a nerve impulse can go to a selected muscle or other end organ). If a lot of passengers go to the same floor, the crowd may overload and affect everything on that floor. The same sort of overload of nerve impulses occurs within a given spinal cord segment. When this kind of spinal segment impulse overload occurs, we call this segment "facilitated." A facilitated spinal cord segment loses some of its innervational specificity and control. It becomes overly responsive, hypersensitive to smaller stimuli and very irritable. It then causes all of its effector tissues to be overactive, i.e., muscle spasms, hypertonus, etc.

Fallopian Tube - There are two of them, one extending from each side of the uterus. They collect the eggs released by the ovaries during ovulation and deliver them to the uterus. One egg per month is the general rule, usually from alternating ovaries. Thus, each fallopian tube is called upon to deliver one egg every other month.

Falx Cerebelli - A fold of dura mater separating the two cerebellar hemispheres; it extends vertically down from the tentorium cerebelli which separates the cerebellum below from the cerebrum above.

Falx Cerebri - The fold of dura mater in the longitudinal fissure separating the cerebral hemispheres; it extends vertically up and forward from the tentorium cerebelli.

Fetal Period - The product of conception from the end of the eighth week until the moment of birth.

Fibroblast - An immature fiber-producing cell of connective tissue capable of differentiating into chondroblast, collagenoblast or osteoblast, the cells of which produce cartilage, collagen and bone, respectively.

Fibrosis - The formation of fibrous (containing fibers) tissue as a reparative or reactive tissue process.

Fimbria - Fringe borders or edges such as those seen at the distal ends of the fallopian tubes where the released ova are collected.

Flexion Posture - A normal newborn posture in which the upper arms and thighs are abducted (away from the central line of the body) at the shoulders and hips. The elbows, wrists, knees and ankles are all flexed. While the fingers are also flexed, the thumbs are positioned in the palms of the hands. This flexion posture occurs when the newborn is placed upon his/her back in the supine position.

Follicle - A sac or a pouch-like depression or cavity.

Fontanel (Fontanelle) - A soft spot; one of the membrane-covered spaces remaining at the junction of the sutures in the incompletely ossified skull of the fetus or infant.

Foramen of Luschka - Along with the foramen of Magendie, it is one of the apertures of the fourth ventricle of the brain. The foramen of Luschka is partially responsible for the delivery of cerebrospinal fluid to the subarachnoid spaces.

Foramen of Magendie - Along with the foramen of Luschka, it is one of the apertures of the fourth ventricle of the brain. The foramen of Magendie is partially responsible for delivering cerebrospinal fluid to the subarachnoid spaces and penetrating canals to interact with the brain, spinal cord and nerve roots.

Foramen Magnum - A large opening in the anterior inferior part of the occipital bone between the cranial cavity and vertebral canal.

Foramen of Monro - In the forward part of the brain, the foramina of Monro connect the lateral ventricles to the third ventricle. There are two of these foramina, one on each side of the third ventricle.

Forebrain - The part of the brain developed from the anterior of the three primary brain vesicles, comprising the diencephalon and telencephalon.

Fornix - An arch-like structure or the vault-like space created by such a structure.

Fornix Commissure - Commissures are nerve-fiber tracts that cross over from one side of the brain to the other and function to integrate right and left-sided brain activities. One group of crossover nerve fibers are called the fornix commissure. This commissure connects the right and left sides of the hippocampus in the diencephalon area of the brain.

Fourth Ventricle of the Brain - The lowermost ventricle of the brain. It receives cerebrospinal fluid from the third ventricle and distributes this fluid via the foramina of Magendie and Luschka to the subarachnoid spaces and into the spinal canal located within the spinal cord.

Frontal Cortices - The cerebral cortices of the frontal lobes of the brain are involved in many functions: movement control of the body, including gross and fine motor control of muscles and muscle coordination; involuntary control of postural stance; eye movement and focusing; thought processes, such as insight, memory and decision-making; our responses to emotional messages; attentiveness; the ability to categorize and organize information; and the ability to generalize learned responses from one situation to another. There is also an area of the frontal cortex that relates to our ability to discriminate between various sound pitches.

FSH - Follicle-stimulating hormone released by the pituitary gland and which causes the ovum-containing follicle to be formed in the ovary in preparation for ovulation.

Ganglia - Plural of ganglion.

Ganglion - A knot, or knot-like mass; in neuroanatomy, a group of nerve cell bodies located outside the central nervous system; occasionally applied to certain nuclear groups within the brain or spinal cord.

Genetic Hypertelorism - A type of facial malformation wherein the paired structures are abnormally distant from each other.

Geniculate Bodies (Medial and Lateral) - The medial geniculate bodies are small, paired and oval-shaped. They serve as relay stations for input coming in via our auditory sensory system. The lateral geniculate bodies are small, paired, oval-shaped projections on the rear ends of the metathalami on both sides. They contain nerve cell aggregations that relay visual stimuli to the occipital cortex for organization and interpretation into the visual images we perceive.

Gestation - The period of development from the time of fertilization until the reference time under consideration, for example, four weeks gestation. Sometimes gestation is used to indicate the time for implantation rather than for fertilization.

Globus Pallidus - The pale interior spherical mass of the lenticular nucleus.

Glossopharyngeal Cranial Nerve (IX) - The paired cranial nerves that pass through the jugular foramina along with the vagus and the accessory cranial nerves. They send branches to the tongue, the ears, the salivary glands and the stylopharyngeus muscles. They participate in taste sensation, sensation from the ears, salivation and muscle contraction.

Glycine - A two-carbon amino acid that is involved in the nervous system as an inhibitory neurotransmitter.

Golgi Complexes - Assemblies of vesicles and folded membranes within the cytoplasm of cells. They store and transport biochemical products such as enzymes and hormones. The Golgi complexes and their related materials often contribute to the formation of cell walls. In the case of the ovum, they seem to be involved in cell division.

Gonads -A usually paired organ in animals that produces reproductive cells such as sperm in the male human and ova in the female. The gonads also produce sex hormones.

Graafian Follicles - Vesicular ovarian follicles. They contain the ova that are to be released during the ovulation times of the menstrual cycles.

Grand Mal Seizures - Grand mal seizures, when they occur, are of two types: tonic and clonic. The tonic seizure means that muscles contract and continuously maintain their contraction. The clonic seizure is one in which the muscles alternately contract and relax. The grand mal seizure involves all of or the greater portion of the total body.

GRH - Gonadotropic-releasing hormone is released by the hypothalamus into the specialized portal blood system between it and the anterior pituitary gland where GRH then stimulates that gland to secrete gonadotropic hormone.

Gyri - The folds or convolutions formed by the grooves in the brain.

Habenular Trigone - A small, depressed triangular area related to the sense of smell. It overlays the habenular nuclei. The habenular structures connect the sense of smell with the limbic system, which results in memories and emotions being stirred by certain odors.

Haploid - Having half the number of chromosomes characteristically found in the somatic (diploid) cells of an organism; typical of the gametes of a species whose union restores the diploid number.

Hensen's Node - In notochord formation, a primitive node of cells occurs in the ectoderm layer near the cranial or head end of the primitive streak. This node is called Hensen's node as well as the primitive node. Cells grow forward from this node to extend the developing central nervous system towards the head end.

Hindbrain - The part of the brain developed from the posterior of the three primary brain vesicles, comprising the metencephalon and myelencephalon.

Hippocampus - A curved elevation in the floor of the inferior horn of the lateral ventricle. It is a functional component of the limbic system. It serves a triage function in the memory system.

Horse's Tail - The roots that extend from the end of the spinal cord to the exits from the vertebral canal down at the lower lumbar and sacral end of the spinal column are called the cauda equina. This is Latin for horse's tail.

Hydrocephalus - A congenital or acquired condition marked by dilation of the cerebral ventricles, usually occurring secondarily to obstruction of the cerebrospinal fluid pathways, and accompanied by an accumulation of cerebrospinal fluid within the skull. Typically, there is enlargement of the head, prominence of the forehead, brain atrophy, mental deterioration and convulsions. Hydrocephalus may also occur when there is a positive imbalance between cerebrospinal fluid production and its reabsorption.

Hypoglossal Canal - A canal through the bone of the occiput deep (internal) to the occipital condyle on each side through which the hypoglossal nerve passes.

Hypoglossal Cranial Nerve (XII) - The nerve that controls the muscles of the tongue.

Hypoglycemia - Deficiency of glucose (sugar) in the blood, which may lead to nervousness, hypothermia, headaches, confusion, unconsciousness and, when prolonged and severe, may lead to convulsions, coma and even death.

Hypothalamus - Prominently involved in the functions of the autonomic nervous system and the nervous mechanisms underlying moods and motivational states. This is one of the smallest brain structures, and yet it has almost the widest variety of controls and functions.

Hypotonia - Diminished tone of muscles. It commonly refers to skeletal muscle but may also refer to the smooth muscles of the gastrointestinal tract, and other internal organs and sphincters.

Hypoxia - Reduction of oxygen supply to a tissue below normal levels for any reason. Often refers to oxygen deficit to brain tissue.

Icterus - A yellow color of skin and sclera due to excess bile pigment in the blood stream for any reason.

Implantation - Also called nidation, it occurs as the blastocyst enters the uterine cavity, makes contact and integrates into the wall of the uterus.

Incus - Middle ossicle of the three-bone chain in the middle ear, so named because of its resemblance to an anvil. Incus is Latin for anvil.

Infundibulum - A funnel-shaped passage; the word is used in many situations, such as in relation to the hypothalamus, the uterus, the nasal passages, etc.

Insula - A triangular area of the cerebral cortex forming the floor of the lateral cerebral fossa on each side of the brain.

Internal Acoustic Meatus - The opening in the inner skull (temporal bone) through which the facial and vestibulocochlear nerves pass towards the periphery.

Internal Capsule - A fan-like mass of white (myelinated) fibers. It connects the cerebral cortex to many subcortical (lower) brain centers. The internal capsule is the most frequent location of adult stroke because its blood supply is extremely vulnerable. It is considered a component of the basal ganglia system. When damaged, it causes problems with motor coordination, if not full paralysis. It's also related to sight and hearing, and may be involved in problems of the newborn related to these senses.

Internal Carotid Artery - Begins at the bifurcation of the common carotid artery in the neck at the level of the upper border of the thyroid cartilage. It travels almost completely vertically from its origin to the base of the skull. It enters the skull through the carotid canal, which is a hole in the petrous part of the temporal bone. The artery then runs for a short distance between two layers of dura mater membrane. This particular area between the two layers of membrane is called the cavernous sinus. After passing through the cavernous sinus, the internal carotid artery enters the cavity within the skull that is enclosed by the two layers of the dura mater. Thus, the artery is now fully within the craniosacral system. The internal carotid arteries then contribute to an ingenious design that nature has placed within the skull in order to insure adequate survival blood supplies to the brain in case one of the carotid arteries becomes obstructed. This system is called the circle of Willis.

Internuncial Neurons - The many nerve cells that connect the left and right sides at every segmental level of the spinal cord, and which make short intersegmental connections ipsilaterally. The term is less often used to designate the short neurons that function as interconnectors in the brain.

Interstitial Fluid - The fluid that is outside of the cells and not within the vascular or lymphatic systems. It bathes the cells, and delivers substances into and receives them from within the cells, respectively.

Interventricular Foramina - Each hemisphere of developed brain has a "lateral" cavity or chamber within it. These two lateral ventricles connect by way of openings on their medial sides to a third ventricle located at the midline of the midbrain. These connecting openings are named the interventricular foramina. These foramina allow cerebrospinal fluid to drain from the lateral ventricles into the third ventricle.

Interventricular System - The name for the design of the system of brain ventricles and their interconnections.

Intervertebral Disc - Lies between each two vertebral bodies. It is a fluid-filled sac that acts as a cushion or shock absorber, and allows motion between the vertebrae. The fluid within the sac is quite viscous.

Ischium - The most posterior of the three bones that make up the pelvic girdle. The other two bones are the ilium and the pubes.

Jaundice - Yellowness of the skin, sclera, mucous membranes and excretions due to hyperbilirubinemia and deposition of bile pigments.

Jugular Foramen - The opening on each side of the base of the skull through which the jugular veins and the glossopharyngeal, the vagus and the accessory cranial nerves pass.

Kernicterus - A condition with severe neural symptoms associated with high levels of bilirubin in the blood. It has the potential for causing serious brain damage.

Krebs Cycle - A high energy-producing metabolic cycle of biochemical reactions that is fundamental to all aerobic animals. It is also known as the citric acid cycle and the tricarboxylic acid cycle.

Lacrimal Glands - The tear glands.

Lacunar Bone Deformity - A condition in which the cells that produce bone (osteoblasts) convert to or become outnumbered by cells that absorb bone (osteoclasts), and the bone begins to reabsorb. The result is a defect in the bone.

Lamina Terminalis - A thin plate that originates during embryonic development from the telencephalon. It is the forwardmost part of the neural tube. Ultimately, it forms the forwardmost (anterior) wall of the third ventricle. At birth it connects the two hemispheres of the brain and runs vertically between the roof plate of the diencephalon and the optic chiasm. It separates the telencephalon from the diencephalon.

Lanugo - The fine hair on the body of the fetus.

Lateral Ventricles - The forebrain divides into two hemispheres, so the ventricular derivatives of the neural tube within the forebrain duplicate and each of these hemispheres gets one ventricle. These two paired ventricles are called the lateral ventricles. They connect through openings on their medial sides to a third ventricle which is located at the midline of the midbrain.

Limbic System - A group of brain structures which are associated with olfaction (smell), memory, autonomic functions (involuntary), and certain aspects of emotion and behavior. It includes the amygdala, the hippocampus, the fornix, and some authorities include the hypothalamus. It is found in all mammals.

Little's Disease - Cerebral palsy may be defined as a persisting qualitative motor dysfunction that appears before the age of three years. It is due to a non-progressive damage to the brain, which in turn can be due to any number of causes. When the palsy is manifest as a stiffness and spasticity of muscle, it may be known as Little's Disease.

Locus Ceruleus - A very small pigmented structure in the pons where it forms a part of the floor of the fourth ventricle. The locus ceruleus manufactures the great majority of the norepinephrine that is made in the brain tissue. It has powerful influence in the process of emotional arousal, and appears to be a key factor in the sense of pleasure, anger and aggression. In addition, it's essential in learning, memory and sleep.

Lumen - The cavity or channel within a tube or tubular organ.

Luteinizing Hormone - In the female, the anterior pituitary gland's response to the gonadotropic releasing hormone from the hypothalamus is the production and release of two hormones into the blood stream: follicle stimulating hormone and luteinizing hormone. Luteinizing hormone in males stimulates the production of androgens by the testes. In females it stimulates ovulation, corpus luteum formation and the production of progesterone.

Lymph - A fluid extract of blood that carries varying numbers of white blood cells and a few red blood cells. It is active in immune responses and fluid movement throughout the body. It collects micro-organisms and debris, and deposits them in the lymph glands that act as filters. Lymph is ultimately returned to the venous blood system.

Lysosomes - Membrane sacs found in the cytoplasm of animal cells. They contain digestive enzymes that react with food in preparation for metabolism. These enzymes also digest debris from bacteria, viruses and dead cells.

Malleus - The most lateral ossicle of the chain in middle ear, so named because of its resemblance to a hammer. Malleus is Latin for hammer.

Mantle Layer - There are three layers of cells or tissue that develop around the spinal canal. The layer of cells right next to the spinal canal becomes the neuroepithelial layer. Moving outward through the neuroepithelial layer we encounter the mantle layer and then the marginal layer.

Marginal Layer - The third layer of cells or tissue that develops around the spinal canal.

Medulla - The innermost part or central tissue of various organs such as the kidneys, the adrenal glands, the spinal cord, etc.

Medulla Oblongata - Located in the myelencephalon division of the hindbrain, it connects the spinal cord below with the pons above. The decussation of nerve fibers, wherein the nerves from the right side of the brain cross over to control the left side of the body and vice versa, occurs in the medulla oblongata. The medulla oblongata also contains several nuclei that are primarily related to basic physiological functions such as swallowing, breathing, blood pressure control, heart rate and the even occurrence of heart rhythm. It contains much of the sensory neuronal network that functions in the receipt of sensory input from the head and neck, as well as the sensory input from the special senses of hearing, seeing and proprioception. The medulla oblongata acts as a relay station for nerve messages between the cerebral cortex motor control areas and the cerebellum.

Meningeal - Relating to the meninges.

Meninges - The three membranes covering the brain and spinal cord: dura mater, arachnoid membrane and pia mater.

Menses or Menstruation - The cyclic, physiologic discharge through the vagina of blood and mucosal tissues from the non-pregnant uterus; it is under hormonal control and normally recurs at approximately four-week intervals throughout the reproductive period (puberty through menopause), except during pregnancy and lactation.

Mesencephalon - The midbrain.

Mesoderm - The middle of the three primary germ layers of the embryo. From it are derived the connective tissues, bone, cartilage, muscle, blood, blood vessels, lymphatics, lymphoid organs, notochord, pleura, pericardium, peritoneum, kidneys and gonads.

Mesonephros - The excretory organ of the embryo, arising caudad to the pronephric rudiments or the pronephros and using its ducts.

Metabolism - The sum of all the physical and chemical processes by which living organized substance is produced and maintained (anabolism), and also the transformation by which energy is made available for the uses of the organism (catabolism).

Metaphase - The second stage of cell division (mitosis or meiosis), in which the chromosomes, each consisting of two chromatids, are arranged in the equatorial plane of the spindle prior to separation.

Metathalamus - The part of the diencephalon composed of the medial and lateral geniculate bodies; often considered to be part of the thalamus.

Metencephalon - The division of the brain that includes the pons, cerebellum, aqueduct of Sylvius, and the hindmost or posterior part of the third ventricle.

Metopic Suture - In the newborn, it divides the frontal skull bone into right and left halves. The metopic suture is one of the few sutures of the skull that almost totally disappears as we begin to grow up.

Microcephaly - An abnormal smallness of the head, often related to mental retardation and a variety of neurological deficits.

Midbrain - The part of the brain developed from the middle of the three primary brain vesicles, comprising the tectum and the cerebral peduncles, and traversed by the aqueduct of Sylvius.

Mitochondria - Small, spherical to rod-shaped cytoplasmic organelles enclosed by two membranes separated by an intramembranous space; the inner membrane is folded in, forming a series of projections. Mitochondria are the principal sites of the ATP synthesis. They contain enzymes of the citric acid cycle, and for fatty oxidation, oxidative phosphorylation, and many other biochemical pathways. They contain their own RNA and ribosomes, replicate independently, and synthesize some of their own proteins.

Mitosis - A method of indirect cell division in which two daughter nuclei normally receive exactly the same chromosomes and DNA content as that of the original cell.

Mitral Valve - The valve through which oxygenated blood passes from the upper chamber (atrium) on the left side of the heart to the lower chamber (ventricle) on the left side.

Molding - The adjusting of the shape and size of the fetal head to the birth canal during labor.

Monaster - The single star-shaped figure at the end of prophase in mitosis.

Moro (Startle) Reflex - Flexion of an infant's thighs and knees, fanning and clenching of fingers, with arms first thrown outward and then brought together as though embracing something; produced by a sudden stimulus and seen normally in the newborn.

Motor Cortex - The area of the brain that generates commands to be transmitted to the various muscles and other effector organs of the body.

Myelencephalon - The posterior of the two vesicles comprising the hindbrain in embryonic development of the hindbrain. It ultimately forms the medulla oblongata and the lower part of the fourth ventricle.

Myelin - The sheath surrounding the axon of myelinated nerve fibers. It is primarily composed of lipid material and serves as an insulator which prevents neuronal (axonal) "cross-talk" or short circuits.

Myelin-Producing Cells - The Schwann cells in the peripheral nervous system and oligodendroglial cells in the central nervous system. Both types fall under the general heading as glial cells.

Myotome - The muscle plate or portion of a somite from which voluntary muscles develop.

Nervous System - The organ system which, along with the endocrine system, correlates the majority adjustments and reactions of the organism to its internal and external environment. It includes the brain, the spinal cord, the nerve roots and all of the peripheral ganglia, nerves and receptors.

Neural Arch - Also called arcus vertebrae and neural arch of the vertebra. It is the arch created by the laminae and the pedicles of a vertebra through which the spinal cord passes.

Neural Chassis - Everything behind the diencephalon (the tailward subdivision of the forebrain vesicle) is considered a neural chassis by Paul D. MacLean, M.D., who has spent much of his life studying the interrelationships between the brain's anatomical structures and physiological functions and behaviors. The neural chassis takes care of reflexive vital life functions, such as breathing, digestion and heart beating. MacLean's model does not consider that the neural chassis has much to do with behavior beyond the vegetative state.

Neural Crest - Located between the ectodermal surface and the neural tube, and formed as the cells within the neural folds specialize. These neural crest cells form all of the nerve cell ganglia located along the spinal cord and in the head. Neural crest cells will also migrate all over the body to form other nerve cells and ganglia located near the various internal organs, glands and blood vessels.

Neural Tube - The tube within the embryo from which the nervous system develops.

Neuroblast - An embryonic cell from which nervous tissue is formed.

Neuroenteric Canal - Connects the embryonic neural tube and the archenteron, which is the primitive digestive cavity.

Neuroepithelial Layer - The layer of cells right next to the spinal canal. It is one of three layers of cells or tissue that develop around the spinal canal. Moving outward through the neuroepithelial layer we next encounter the mantle layer and then the marginal layer.

Neuromere - Any of a series of transitory segmental elevations in the wall of the neural tube in the developing embryo; also, such elevations in the wall of the mature rhombencephalon.

Neurons - Nerve cells which conduct electrical impulses, not to be confused with glial cells which do not conduct electrical impulses but provide other necessary functions in the nervous system.

Neuropores - The openings at both ends of the embryonic neural tube. Failure of closure during in utero development may result in a variety of congenital abnormalities, such as pilonidal cyst, meningocele, etc.

Neurotransmitter - A biochemical substance released from the axon terminal of a presynaptic neuron upon excitation, which diffuses across the synaptic cleft to either excite or inhibit the target cell.

Neurulation - In the early embryo, this is the process of the formation of the neural plate, which then becomes the neural groove and ultimately develops into the neural tube. This neural tube is the precursor to the fetal brain and spinal cord.

Neutrino - A particle in the nucleus of an atom that has no mass or electrical charge that we know of as yet.

Nidation - Also called implantation, it occurs as the blastocyst enters the uterine cavity, makes contact with the wall of the uterus, makes a cavity within that wall and functionally integrates with it.

Norepinephrine - A biochemical produced as a hormone by the adrenal medulla (inner part of the adrenal gland) and as a neurotransmitter by neurons within the central nervous system. It is one of the catecholamines and is deeply involved in the "fight or flight" response to emergency situations.

Notochord - The rod-shaped cord of cells below the primitive groove of the embryo, defining the initial axis of the body. It acts as a stimulus to the development of the spinal cord and the vertebral column. Once the development of these structures has been established, the notochord disappears.

Notochordal Canal - The canal through which food from an embryo's yolk sac is distributed to the rapidly multiplying cells geographically related to it.

Notochordal Process - In an embryo, the extension cells from the primitive node to the prechordal plate are called the notochordal process. It delineates the axis of the embryo.

Nuclear Membrane - The membrane that forms the sac within which the cell nucleus is located.

Nucleolus - A rounded refractile body within the nucleus of most cells, which is the site of synthesis of ribosomal RNA.

Nucleoplasm - The protoplasm of the nucleus of a cell.

Nucleus - The most prominent structure or organelle within the neuron or other type of cell. It usually is spheroid in shape, enclosed within a membrane sac, and it rotates slowly within the cell. It contains the cell's DNA within its chromosomes, a generous quantity of RNA, and an inclusion body called a nucleolus.

Nucleus Pulposus - A semifluid mass contained within a membrane of fine white and elastic fibers. It is the center of an intervertebral disk.

Occipital Condyles - The two rounded projections from the inferior side of the occiput that are that bone's contributions to the atlanto-occipital joints. The hypoglossal cranial nerves XII pass through foramina beneath these condyles. Jamming of these joints can interfere with hypoglossal nerve function, which presents itself as lack of control of muscles of the tongue.

Occiput - The back part of the head. Also used to denote the occipital bone, which forms the posterior part of the skull vault and part of the floor of the skull cavity.

Oculomotor Cranial Nerve (III) - Supplies several muscles of the eyeballs: the superior rectus muscles, inferior rectus muscles, medial rectus muscles and inferior oblique muscles. It also controls the levator palpebrae muscles. In addition, the oculomotor nerves control constriction of the eye pupils through the circular muscles in the irises, and accommodation of the lenses, which relates to thickening and thinning of the lenses in order to focus on objects at variable distances.

Olfactory Bulbs - The rhinencephalon includes the smell receptors in the nose. The fibers of these receptors pass up through tiny holes in the ethmoid bone to the olfactory bulbs which lie above this bone. From there the stimuli created by the smells are conducted along the underside of the brain through the olfactory tracts to several connections in the brain which coordinate smells with memories, emotions, whetting or diminishing of the appetite, etc.

Olfactory Lobes - The forwardmost part of the brain, the telencephalon, produces the olfactory lobes that will ultimately produce the limbic lobes, also called the rhinencephalon. This brain area, in conjunction with the sensory-receptor system, gives us our sense of smell.

Oligodendroglia - Neuroglia cells differentiate into astrocytes and oligodendroglia gliocytes. Oligodendroglia cells myelinate the brain nerve cells, and they provide structural support to the neurons.

Oligodendroglia Gliocytes - Neuroglia cells differentiate into astrocytes and oligodendroglia gliocytes. These cells serve to support the nerve cells, and they produce myelin.

Optic Chiasm - The optic chiasm is a crossover structure that sends some of the visual messages from the right eye to the left side of the brain and vice-versa. This system helps integrate the total picture that we see with both eyes. It provides our stereoscopic visual perception.

Organelle - A generalized word used to describe such things as mitochondria, Golgi complexes, lysosomes, endoplasmic reticulum, ribosomes, centrioles and other microscopically visible structures within the cell and its nucleus.

Organs of the Corti - Located in the inner ears, these organs are involved in the sense of hearing, especially that of sound-pitch discrimination.

Osmosis - The passage of pure solvent from a solution of lesser to one of greater solute concentration, when the two solutions are separated by a membrane that selectively prevents the passage of solute molecules but is permeable to the solvent.

Ossification - The formation of bone or bony substance from cartilage, membrane or other precursor materials.

Ossification Points - The areas in a future bone where the cartilage or membrane begins to calcify and form bone. The bone formation then spreads out radially from the point of ossification.

Osteoblast - A cell arising from a fibroblast which, as it matures, becomes specialized in bone production.

Ovarian Follicle - The ovum and its encasing cells at any stage of its development. The stages of its development are spoken of as primordial and vesicular as it matures.

Ovary - The female gonad; either of the paired female sexual glands in which ova are formed.

Overriding - The overriding of skull edges, known as head-molding, allows the fetal head to collapse as it passes through the birth canal. The fetal head can then gain access to the outside world without too much damage to either mother or child.

Ovum - An egg; the female reproductive or germ cell which, after fertilization, is capable of developing into a new member of the same species.

Palate - Roof of the mouth; the partition separating the nasal and oral (mouth) cavities.

Paraphysis - Sometimes there is an abnormal formation in the roof of the diencephalon. It sags and causes an obstruction to cerebrospinal fluid flow from the lateral ventricles into the third ventricle of the brain. This is called a paraphysis. If this problem presents itself after birth, it can cause a form of hydrocephalus.

Parasympathetic Division of the Autonomic Nervous System - Provides motor innervation to certain visceral structures. It is a trophotropic system, i.e., it regulates those functions that are necessary for long-term survival. It is not involved in the stress or emergency responses governed by the sympathetic system.

Paraventricular Nuclei - As parts of the fetal hypothalamus, they receive signals from the fetal organ systems that they're ready to begin life independent from the maternal placental and intrauterine systems.

Parent Cells - Those cells which undergo mitosis or meiosis and give rise to "daughter" cells; cells which produce a progeny during developmental stages of the organism.

Pericardium - The membrane around the heart.

Perineurium - The sheath that surrounds each bundle of nerve fibers that form the peripheral nerves. Once each of these bundles passes through its individual intervertebral foramen, it is considered a part of the peripheral nervous system.

Periosteum - A specialized connective tissue covering all bones and having bone-forming potential.

Peristalsis - The worm-like movement by which the alimentary canal or other tubular organs propel their contents; consists of waves of contraction passing along the tube for variable distances.

Peritoneum - The lining of the abdominal cavity.

Pharynx - The throat; the musculomembranous cavity behind the nasal cavities, mouth and larynx. It communicates with them and with the esophagus.

Phylogeny - The complete developmental history of a race or group of organisms.

Pilonidal Cyst - When present, this cyst is located at the lower end of the spine. It may travel under the skin and open near the lower end of the tailbone (coccyx). It contains hair and is classified as a dermoid cyst.

Pineal Gland - A small cone-shaped gland attached by a stalk to the posterior wall of the third ventricle. It secretes melatonin, which is a hormone that influences sexual maturation, circadian rhythms, and is now thought to be anti-aging and anti-carcinogenic.

Pituitary Gland - Also called the hypophysis, it has anterior and posterior lobes. The anterior lobe is glandular and the posterior lobe is neurogenic. It is suspended by a stalk from the hypothalamus. The large anterior lobe releases into systemic circulation any one (or combination) of a variety of tropic hormones, each of which activates the corresponding endocrine gland and triggers the release of its hormone. The posterior lobe relates to fluid balance and the regulation of uterine contractions during labor.

Placenta - The organ of metabolic interchange between fetus and mother. There is no direct mixing of fetal and maternal blood under normal circumstances. However, the intervening placental membrane is sufficiently thin to permit the absorption of nutritional materials, oxygen, and some harmful substances like viruses into the fetal blood. The placenta also releases carbon dioxide and nitrogenous waste from the fetus.

Planum Temporale Cortex - The brain area that seems most involved in the selection of the words we use to verbally express an idea.

Plasticity of the Brain - The state in which a brain area may show the ability to take over some of the function of another area that has been damaged. Until recently, brain plasticity was considered impossible in humans.

Pleura - A double membrane which lines the thoracic cavity and covers the surfaces of the lungs. There is a small space between the two membrane layers which contains a serous lubricating fluid.

Pons - Any slip of tissue connecting two parts of an organ. Usually it refers to the pons varolii, which is a thick tract of nerve fibers that functionally connects the midbrain to the medulla oblongata in the brain.

Pontine Flexure - One of three flexures between the brain and spinal cord, the pontine flexure bends backward. It helps compensate for the two forward flexures that occur initially during embryonic development.

Positron Emission Tomography - Also known as a PET scan, this is a technique in which radioactive tracers are given to a subject under study, and the emission of positrons is recorded by instrumentation. A positron is a positively charged particle in the nucleus of an atom that has about the same mass as an electron. The electron is negatively charged. In the positron emission process, an atomic nucleus ejects both a positron and a neutrino at the same time. A neutrino is a particle that has no mass and no known electrical charge.

Prechordal Plate - As the primitive streak proliferates, a protective plate forms across the head end of the embryonic disc. This plate, called the prechordal plate, will prevent primitive streak mesodermal cells from passing into the head end of the embryonic disc. The plate will also become the source for many of the tissues of the mouth and throat.

Premotor Cortex - A portion of the cortex involved in motor control, it is located in the anterior wall of the central gyrus.

Prepuce - The foreskin; a cutaneous fold over the glans penis.

Primitive Body Segments - During the third week of gestation as the neural folds grow, a multitude of mesodermal cells present themselves along the sides of the notochord and the neural folds. This expanding mass of mesoderm organizes into paired blocks that lie on either side of the neural folds and the notochord just underneath the ectoderm. These paired blocks are initially called primitive body segments. Ultimately, these primitive body segments will give origin to somites.

Primitive Streak - It runs from the attachment of the embryonic disc at the inner wall of the blastocyst out to the edge that protrudes the furthest into the blastocyst cavity. The primitive streak is actually a line of rapidly proliferating cells at the bottom of a groove that has formed in the embryonic disc. The proliferation of the primitive streak cells contributes to the mesoderm layer that interposes between the ectoderm and the entoderm.

Progesterone - Hormone of the female body. Its function is to prepare the uterus for the reception and development of the fertilized egg.

Prophase - The first stage in cell reduplication in either meiosis or mitosis.

Proprioception System - That subdivision of the sensory nervous system which provides information about a body part's position in space and its positional relationship to other body parts. These positions are both static and dynamic.

Proprioceptor - Any of the sensory nerve endings that give information concerning movements and position of the body; they occur chiefly in muscles, tendons and the labyrinth.

Prosencephalon - The forebrain.

Protoplasm - A viscid, translucent colloid material which is an essential constituent of the living cell. It refers to both cytoplasm and nucleoplasm.

Pupillary Reflex - Reflexes that help us accommodate to light by changing the size of the opening of the pupil of the eyeball. The pupil constricts in response to brighter light and it dilates in response to darkening.

Putamen - One of the structures included in the basal ganglia.

Pyramidal Tracts - The motor nerve tracts that cross over in the medulla.

Raphe Nuclei - The neurons along the midline of the pons. Serotonin is one of the most important neurotransmitters in the entire central nervous system. Its highest concentration is located within the neurons that have their cell bodies within these raphe nuclei.

Serotonin distribution to the rest of the central nervous system is largely by way of the neuronal projections of the raphe nuclei.

Rathke's Pouch - A diverticulation in the primitive oral cavity that appears during the third week of embryonic life. By the end of the sixth week of gestation, Rathke's pouch will have become the anterior division of the pituitary gland.

Refractile - A condition in which the direction of light waves is diverted.

REM Sleep - The stage of sleep in which rapid eye movements take place.

Reticular Formation - A system of reticular or net-like substance which is found in the spinal cord and brain stem. It then passes through the midbrain in its tegmental region, and communicates particularly with the nuclei of the motor nerves to the eye and with the substantia nigra. The reticular formation helps the eyes to reflexively track and accommodate in "fight or flight" circumstances. It also plays a major role in emotional responses and in alertness. It is an alarm system which prepares us for action when the threat of any potentially dangerous circumstance presents itself.

Rhinencephalon - This brain area, in conjunction with the olfactory receptor system, gives us our sense of smell.

Rhombencephalic Flexure - It occurs at the juncture between the brain and the spinal cord. This bend extends about 90 degrees, allowing the brain to tilt forward on the spinal cord.

Rhombencephalon - The hindbrain.

Ribosome - Any of the intracellular ribonucleoprotein particles concerned with protein synthesis; they consist of reversibly dissociable units and are found either bound to cell membranes or free in the cytoplasm. They may occur singly or in clusters.

RNA (Ribonucleic Acid) - A complex organic chemical compound concerned with the manufacture of the protein molecules that are essential for life. It frequently acts as a messenger molecule between DNA and mitochondria and/or other organelles, especially those concerned with protein synthesis.

Sclerotome - The area of a bone innervated from a single spinal segment, or that mass of embryonic mesenchyme separated from the ventromedial somite which will eventually produce the vertebra and ribs of that segment.

Seizures - Tonic/Clonic (Grand Mal) - Grand mal seizures, when they occur, are of two types, tonic and clonic. The tonic seizure means that muscles contract and continuously maintain their contraction. The clonic seizure is one of which the muscles alternately contract and relax. Other types of seizures are petit mal (lapses in consciousness), Jacksonian (specific body parts/regions), and limbic or temporal lobe, which are emotional and/or autonomic.

Sella Turcica - The place where the pituitary gland drops into the skull floor. It is located in the body of the sphenoid bone and relates to the clinoid processes of that bone.

Semipermeable Membrane - A membrane that allows solvents to pass through freely, but is selective about which molecules or particles of solute are allowed passage.

Septum Pellucidum - A thin walled structure situated between the fornix and the corpus callosum, the septum pellucidum is a part of the limbic system that receives nerve impulses or messages from the hippocampus by way of the fornix. It then sends impulses to the hypothalamus. It appears that the septum is significant in mating activities, copulation and procreation.

Serotonin - One of the most important of the neurotransmitters in the entire central nervous system. Its highest concentration is located within the neurons that have their cell bodies within the raphe nuclei.

Skull Base - The floor of the skull, formed by a cartilaginous bone.

Skull Vault - The roof and walls of the skull, formed mostly from membranous bone.

Somesthesia (Somatesthesia) - Body consciousness, awareness or sensibility.

Somesthetic Cortex - One of the major areas of cerebral cortex, it is involved primarily in sensory perceptions.

Somite - One of the paired, block-like masses of mesoderm arranged segmentally alongside the neural tube of the embryo. They form the vertebral column and segmental musculature.

Sphenoid Bone - One of the major bones of the skull. It forms a cross structure in the floor of the cranial vault behind the frontal bone and forward of the temporal and occipital bones. Its lateral aspects form part of the side walls of the vault right behind the frontal bone. The sphenoid bone forms the sella turcica, which houses the pituitary gland.

Sphingomyelin - An important substance in myelin.

Spina Bifida - A developmental anomaly marked by defective closure of the vertebral bony encasement of the spinal cord through which the meninges and spinal cord may or may not protrude.

Spina Bifida Cystica - A serious case of spina bifida in which there are external protrusions of the meningeal membranes into a cyst-like structure that lies under the skin at the level of the vertebral fusion defect. In even more serious situations, nerve tissue of the spinal cord also protrudes into the cyst formation.

Spina Bifida Cystica Meningocele - A case of spina bifida cystica in which only the meningeal membranes protrude from the spinal canal into the cyst.

Spina Cystica Meningomyelocele - In spina bifida cystica, if there is also nervous tissue from the spinal cord and/or spinal cord nerve roots protruding into the cyst, the condition is labeled spina bifida cystica with meningomyelocele.

Spinal Canal - Also called the vertebral canal, it is the canal within the vertebral spine within which the spinal cord is formed, housed and protected as it passes from the foramen magnum to the sacral hiatus.

Spinal Cord Nerve Roots - The major nerve roots that exit from the spinal cord. In the lower spinal area these roots descend within the canal after the spinal cord has ended. These roots are called the cauda equina, which means horse's tail in Latin.

Spinal Manipulation - Refers to manual treatment of the spinal column in order to "correct" its mobility, supposed malalignments and/or functional problems. This work is done primarily by chiropractors and osteopaths. It is also known to have been used, especially in the far East, by many health practitioners for centuries.

Spinal Reflexes - They provide the means by which our bodies can react to something before our brains get the message. The impulses come in via the dorsal nerve roots and are transmitted to the ventral (motor) nerve roots (lower motor neurons) by internuncial neurons.

Spinothalamic Tracts - Several nerve tracts or bundles within the spinal cord and brain that connect the spinal nerve roots with the thalamus for triage and relay to higher brain centers.

Sternum - The elongated flat bone forming the anterior wall of the chest.

Strabismus - Squint; deviation of the eye that the patient cannot voluntarily overcome or control.

Striatum - A commonly used abbreviated name for corpus striatum, which is a subcortical mass located anterior to, and lateral to, the thalamus in both brain hemispheres.

Stylomastoid Foramen - A small canal located below and behind the ear. It passes the facial cranial nerve (VII) and the stylomastoid artery.

Substantia Nigra - It separates the crus cerebri from the tegmentum of the midbrain. The substantia nigra also connects several higher brain centers with the lower centers of the brain stem. It gets its name from its color, which is dark brown to black. It is a part of the basal ganglia. The substantia nigra secretes dopamine, which is a neurotransmitter related to depression and possibly schizophrenia when deficient in quantity.

Subthalamus - A transitional region of the diencephalon interposed between the (dorsal) thalamus, the hypothalamus, and the tegmentum of the mesencephalon (midbrain).

Sulcus Limitans - In an embryo's developing spinal cord, it is a limiting membrane that develops in a vertical, transverse direction in such a way that it cuts across the mid-section of the spinal cord. The sulcus limitans essentially divides the spinal cord into an anterior (front) longitudinal half and a posterior (back) longitudinal half. The front half will function as the motor or outflow part of the spinal cord. The back half will serve as the sensory or input part of the spinal cord

Suture - A stitch or series of stitches made to secure apposition of the edges of a surgical or traumatic wound. Also, the joint between two skull bones. Skull sutures are slightly moveable throughout life except under pathological conditions. Sutural mobility is one of the corner stones of CranioSacral Therapy.

Sympathetic Division of the Autonomic Nervous System - The part that takes care of emergency responses. It has little or no concern with the long-term effects of its demands. (It only wants to get you through the moment.)

Synapse - The junction between the processes of two neurons where neural impulses are transmitted by electrical or chemical means.

Synaptic Cleft - The space between the surface of an impulse-delivering axon and whatever the receiving structure may be on the receiving neuron or other effector cell.

Tectum - Usually the roof of the midbrain. It may also refer to the roof of almost any structure, especially in the brain.

Tegmentum - The roof of the pons.

Telencephalon - The forwardmost division of the brain.

Telophase - The last of the four stages of mitosis and the two divisions of meiosis, in which the chromosomes arrive at the poles of the cell and the cytoplasm divides.

Tentorium Cerebelli - A fold of dura mater supporting the occipital lobes and covering the cerebellum. Often referred to as the "tent," it is more horizontal than vertical.

Terminal Lamina - See lamina terminalis.

Tetany - A syndrome manifested by sharp flexion of the wrist and ankle joints, muscle twitching, cramps and convulsions, sometimes with attacks of stridor; due to hyperexcitability of nerves and muscles often caused by a decrease in the concentration by extracellular ionized calcium; occurring in parathyroid hypofunction, vitamin D deficiency, alkalosis, and as a result of excessive ingestion of alkaline salts.

Thalamus - Either of two large ovoid masses consisting chiefly of gray substance, situated one on either side of and forming part of the lateral wall of the third ventricle. It is divided into dorsal and ventral parts. The term thalamus without a modifier usually refers to the dorsal thalamus, which functions as a relay center for sensory impulses to the cerebral cortex.

Third Ventricle of the Brain - A ventricle located at the midline of the midbrain that connects to the lateral ventricles from which it receives cerebrospinal fluid. It drains this fluid into the fourth ventricle of the brain through the aqueduct of Sylvius, which connects these (the third and the fourth) two ventricles.

Thoracolumbar Division - This usually refers to the sympathetic division of the autonomic nervous system.

Thyroid Cartilage - The shield-shaped cartilage of the anterior throat, which protects and is a part of the larynx (voice box). It is popularly known as the Adam's apple.

Thyrotoxicosis - A morbid condition due to overactivity of the thyroid gland.

Tonic Seizures - A type of grand mal seizure in which the muscles contract and continuously maintain their contraction.

Tonus - Tone or tonicity; the slight, continuous contraction of a muscle, which in skeletal muscles aids in the maintenance of posture and in the return of blood to the heart and many other nuances related to general vitality.

Trabeculations - Anchoring strands of connective tissue that loosely connect the pia mater and the arachnoid membrane. These trabecular anchoring strands allow for independent movement between these two layers of membrane. The term may also be used in many other anatomical situations in order to refer to supporting and/or anchoring structures.

Transillumination - A screening test of brain size and symmetry in which a flashlight is shined through the newborn's head from back to front. The amount of light coming through the orbits of both eyes should be equal. If the brightness of light is greater in one eye than the other, there may be a discrepancy in the size of the two hemispheres of the brain.

Tricuspid Valve - The structure between the right atrium and the right ventricle of the heart through which venous, oxygen-poor blood passes for future oxygenation by circulating through the pulmonary system.

Trigeminal Cranial Nerve (V) - The cranial nerve responsible for sensation from the eye, nose, teeth and gums. It also has motor control over the muscles related to the jaws, and gives you the ability to bite and chew.

Trigeminal Ganglion - The large ganglionic aggregation of nerve-cell bodies related to our masticatory system, as well as to some of the sensation receptors of the eyes and nose.

Triune Brain Model - Developed by Paul D. MacLean, M.D., the triune brain model consists of three separate but functionally and structurally integrated brains that cap the neural chassis. These three "brains" are the reptilian brain, the mammalian brain and the neocortex.

Trochlear Cranial Nerve (IV) - The cranial nerve that innervates the superior oblique muscle of the eyeball. This nerve has to do with eyeball rotation as it attempts to maintain a horizontal position in relation to the horizon as the head is cocked to one side. It also aids in vertical and lateral eyeball movement.

Trophoblast - The peripheral cells of the blastocyst, which attach the fertilized egg to the uterine wall and through which the embryo receives nourishment from the mother. It contributes to the formation of the placenta.

Tunnel Vision - Loss of peripheral vision. It occurs when there is loss of function of the sensory fibers that pass through the optic chiasm, often due to a tumor in this region. It is as though the subject/patient is looking through a tunnel.

Tympanum - The ear drum.

Urethra - The membranous canal through which urine is discharged from the bladder to the exterior of the body.

Vagus Cranial Nerve (X) - A major cranial nerve that offers a wide motor supply to muscles of the larynx and pharynx. It also provides some controlling nerve supply to the heart, blood vessels, trachea, bronchi, the gastrointestinal tract from pharynx to the colon (except for its last two or three feet), and to all the associated glands. In addition, it controls sensations from parts of the meninges, the ear and the eardrum, some taste, the soft palate, and a small amount of motor control to major neck muscles.

Ventricle of the Heart - One of the two lower chambers of the heart. The ventricles perform the stronger pumping tasks. The right ventricle pumps blood through the pulmonary system and the left ventricle pumps blood into the body.

Ventricular System of the Brain - A system of four interconnected cavities in the brain substance within which cerebrospinal fluid is formed from blood and circulated throughout the intradural compartment.

Vernix Caseosa - The fatty substance formed from the sebaceous glands that covers the skin of the fetus. It is a mixture of sebum and dead skin cells that have been sloughed off.

Vertebral Arteries - The left and right vertebral arteries arise from the subclavian arteries in the lower neck/upper thorax. They travel up the neck through the foramina in the transverse processes of cervical vertebra 6 through 1. They then enter the skull and soon join to form the basilar artery, which empties into the circle of Willis.

Vertebral Canal - Also called the spinal canal, it is the canal in which the spinal cord is formed, housed and protected. It extends throughout the length of the vertebral or spinal column in a space formed just behind the vertebral bodies by the pedicles and lamina of these vertebrae.

Vertebral Column - The spinal column. It consists of seven cervical vertebrae atop twelve thoracic vertebrae atop five lumbar vertebrae which rest upon the sacrum. It includes the coccyx, which extends caudad from the lower end of the sacrum. The coccyx is not weight-bearing in the upright position, as are the other vertebrae and the sacrum.

Vesicles - Small membranous sacs containing liquid.

Vestibular Apparatus - One of the inner structures of the ears, it helps with balance and equilibrium.

Vestibulocochlear Cranial Nerve (VIII) - Also known as the acoustic cranial nerve or the auditory nerve, it controls equilibrium, balance and hearing.

Wernicke's Area - An area of the cerebral cortex described by Carl Wernicke, a German neurologist and psychiatrist. This cortical area has to do with speech motor function.

Wolffian Bodies - In an embryo, they represent the beginnings of the urinary system.

Yolk - The stored nutrient of the ovum.

Yolk Sac - The container for a temporary food supply to the embryo.

Zona Pellucida - A clear, non-cellular material encased by a tough, transparent membrane that encloses the human egg, or ovum.

Zygote - The cell resulting from the union of a sperm and an ovum; the fertilized egg.

Index

Page references in italics indicate drawings.